*B*EHÇET

*A C*ontemporary *S*ynopsis

Edited by

Gary R. Plotkin

Chief, Infectious Disease
Department of Medicine
VA Medical Center
Wilkes-Barre, Pennsylvania
Clinical Assistant Professor of Medicine
Hahnemann University School of Medicine
Philadelphia, Pennsylvania

John J. Calabro

Professor of Medicine and Pediatrics
University of Massachusetts Medical School
Director of Rheumatology
Saint Vincent Hospital
Worcester, Massachusetts

J. Desmond O'Duffy

Professor of Medicine
Mayo Medical School
Consultant in Internal Medicine
Mayo Clinic
Rochester, Minnesota

FUTURA PUBLISHING CO., INC.
Mount Kisco, New York
1988

Library of Congress Cataloging-in-Publication Data

Behçet's disease.

Includes bibliographies and index.
1. Behçet's disease.   I. Plotkin, Gary R.
II. Calabro, John J.   III. O'Duffy, J. Desmond.
[DNLM: 1. Behcet's Syndrome.   WW 240 B4188]
RC122.B4B42   1988   616.9   87-19733
ISBN 0-87993-313-5

"Behcet's Disease: A Contemporary Synopsis"
reprinted with permission by Joanne Zeis.
This edition has been reprinted by arrangement
with Futura Publishing Company, Inc.

Copyright © 1988
Futura Publishing Company, Inc.

Published by
Futura Publishing Company, Inc.
295 Main Street, P.O. Box 330
Mount Kisco, New York 10549

L.C. no.: 87-19733
ISBN no.: 0-87993-313-5

All rights reserved.
No part of this book may be translated or reproduced in any form without
the written permission of the publisher.

Printed in the United States of America

Contributors

Raphael J. DeHoratius, M.D., F.A.C.P.
Professor of Medicine
Director, Division of Clinical
  Immunology/Rheumatology
Department of Medicine
Hahnemann University
Philadelphia, Pennsylvania

Scott Dinehart, M.D.
Chief Resident and Assistant
  Clinical Instructor
Department of Dermatology
The University of Texas Medical
  Branch
Galveston, Texas

John J. Gohmann, M.D.
Division of Hematology/Oncology
Department of Internal Medicine
University of Kentucky Medical
  School
Lexington, Kentucky

Marc C. Hochberg, M.D., M.P.H.
Associate Professor of Medicine
  and Epidemiology
Johns Hopkins Medical Institutions
Baltimore Maryland

Joseph L. Jorizzo, M.D.
Professor and Chairman
Department of Dermatology
Wake Forest University
The Bowman Gray School of
  Medicine
Winston-Salem, North Carolina

Scott Korn, M.D.
Fellow in Rheumatology
Hahnemann University
Philadelphia, Pennsylvania

Sharad Lakhanpal, M.B.B.S., M.D., F.A.C.P.
Department of Internal Medicine
Division of Rheumatic Diseases
The University of Texas
Health Science Center at Dallas
Southwestern Medical School
Dallas, Texas

Robert S. Lesser, M.D.
Fellow in Rheumatology
Hahnemann University
Philadelphia, Pennsylvania

J. T. Lie, M.D., M.S., F.A.C.C., F.A.C.A., F.A.R.A.
Professor of Pathology, Mayo
  Medical School and Mayo
  Graduate School of Medicine
Consultant in Pathology and
  Cardiovascular Diseases, Mayo
  Clinic and Mayo Foundation
Rochester, Minnesota

Ewa Marciniak, M.D.
Division of Hematology/Oncology
University of Kentucky Medical
  Center
Lexington, Kentucky

M. Ernest Marshall, M.D.
Division of Hematology/Oncology
University of Kentucky Medical
  Center
Lexington, Kentucky

Mark S. Teter, M.D.
Postdoctoral Fellow, Rheumatology
Johns Hopkins University School
  of Medicine
Baltimore Maryland

PREFACE

ALTHOUGH BEHÇET'S DISEASE (Behçet's syndrome) is of worldwide distribution, certain geographic predilections do exist, and thus, for the physician practicing in North America, this disorder may indeed represent an uncommonly encountered illness. Nevertheless, the number of articles published in recent years has risen significantly, with an increasing proportion being published in the English language. Many of these publications have emphasized the protean multisystemic manifestations of this disease, thus expanding the original description of Behçet's disease as a triple symptom complex into a generalized systemic disorder. In light of these recent developments, a need for a contemporary synopsis of Behçet's disease was envisioned by the editors. It is with this primary objective that the following monograph has been written, with emphasis on the epidemiology, immunology, pathology, clinical features, and treatment of this syndrome.

Although certain controversies related to Behçet's disease have historically abounded in the literature, a multitude of scientific investigators are actively and critically studying this disease, as evidenced by the increasing number of papers presented at each international symposium on Behçet's disease. Indeed, at the last international conference held at the Royal College of Physicians in London, in September 1985, 100 papers representing a multitude of countries were presented reviewing the etiology, pathogenesis, immunology, clinical features, and treatment of Behçet's disease. Where controversy exists, the editors of this monograph have attempted to present the various observations impartially, and, when theoretically feasible, to integrate the scientific data into either coherent hypotheses or a unified theory. Nevertheless, since Behçet's disease is an international illness, the editors acknowledge that there may be geographic variations of many aspects of the disease. With the advancement of modern technology, one has indeed gained much insight into the understanding of Behçet's disease, and consequently, future international meetings should definitely result in even a higher level of comprehension of Hulûsi Behçet's triple symptom complex.

CONTENTS

1

HISTORY AND EVOLUTION

J. Desmond O'Duffy

HULÛSI BEHÇET (Fig. 1) was born in
Istanbul on February 20, 1889, and
graduated in 1910 from Gülhane
Military Medical School. He
worked in military hospitals, first
as a resident and then on the staff,
until the end of World War I. After
a year of training abroad, first in
Budapest and then in Berlin, he
returned to Turkey in 1919. With
the exception of a year in private
practice, it was at the Guraba
Hospital, Istanbul, that he was to
spend the rest of his career. This
hospital was incorporated into the
faculty of Medicine of the University of Istanbul in 1933 with Beh-

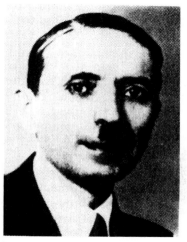

Figure 1.

çet as Director of the Department of Dermatology and Syphilol-
ogy.[1,2]

In 1937 he published his observations, in German, on two patients with the triple symptom complex of recurrent oral and genital ulcerations as well as hypopyon-iritis.[3] The first patient, a man,

From *Behcet's Disease: A Contemporary Synopsis*, edited by Gary R. Plotkin, M.D.,
John J. Calabro, M.D., and J. Desmond O'Duffy, M.B. © 1988, Futura Publishing
Company, Inc., Mount Kisco, NY.

had erythema nodosum and developed blindness from uveitis; while his second patient, a woman, had oral and vulvar ulcers and uveitis. Behçet conducted numerous biopsies and microbiological tests on the lesions of both these patients. Using Herzberg's Victoria blue and Giemsa stains, he reported inclusion bodies in the ulcerations. He therefore proposed a viral etiology; however, this theory has not been validated by rigorous modern virologic technics. In the next three years he described four more cases and claimed that the triple symptom complex was a unique disease.[4]

Acceptance of this entity was difficult initially, especially among dermatologists. There may have been several reasons for the slow recognition of his diagnostic entity. First, there was already a nomenclature for the various components of his new syndrome; for example, ulcus vulvae acutum of Lipschütz was the accepted term for aphthous ulcerations of the vulva.[5] Second, other oculo-muco-cutaneous syndromes had recently been described by other investigators. The syndromes of Reiter and of Stevens and Johnson could be, and were, confused with Behçet's syndrome, since they too could involve the eye and mucous membranes. Third, there had been several recent reports of patients with clinical illnesses resembling Behçet's and these could raise some questions about the originality of Behçet's observations. Behçet, naturally, chose the journal *Dermatologische Wochenscrift* for his presentation, since he had joined its editorial board the previous year. He continued to publish additional articles on the subject in journals written in French and English in order to consolidate his syndrome. He had a difficult personality, divorced his wife, and lived alone in his later years. He smoked incessantly, had tobacco-induced lung disease, and ischemic heart disease, and died in 1948 of these conditions.

Earlier Observations

Did Hippocrates scoop Behçet? In *Epidemics Book III*, Hippocrates is translated from the Greek by the surgeon Francis Adams[6] in 1849: "But, there were also other fevers, as will be described. Many had their mouths affected with aphthous ulcerations. There were also many defluxions about the genital parts, and ulcerations, boils (phymata), externally and internally about the groins." The annotation by Adams here is of interest: "This description apparently can refer to nothing but pestilential buboes."[6] The translation continues: "Watery ophthalmies of a chronic character, with pains; fungous excrescences of the eyelids, externally and internally, called fici, which destroyed the sight of many persons." Adams' explanation of this passage is also trenchant: "It is impossible not to recognize this as a description of purulent ophthalmia." The translation proceeds: "There were fungous growths, in many other instances, on ulcers, especially on those seated on the genital organs."

Feigenbaum, himself a student of Behçet's disease, concluded that Hippocrates was describing a syndrome that was only later to become identifiable as Behçet's.[7] However, Feigenbaum could not explain the growths on the exterior of the lids as being part of Behçet's disease, and it was difficult to accept his explanation that over the centuries the condition had evolved from an epidemic to a sporadic one.

Patients with Behçet's syndrome had been reported prior to 1937. Blüthe, in his inaugural dissertation at Heidelberg,[8] and later Planner and Remenowsky[9] and Adamantiades[10] mentioned the association of iritis with aphthous oral ulcerations and genital ulcerations. However, these and other earlier authors had attributed their patients' illness to well-known infections such as tuberculosis, syphilis, or staphylococcal disease. It is reasonable, therefore, to attribute the seminal description of this disease to Behçet who, while proposing a viral etiology, discarded existing bacterial theories and delineated the specific morbid entity that now bears his name.[3]

Evolution of Behçet's Syndrome

"During the past years I have had the opportunity to follow a patient who furnished a typical picture of this syndrome. The peculiarity of this case was that disturbances of the central nervous system developed almost abruptly and caused the death of the patient."[11] This quotation is from Dr. Berlin of Tel Aviv describing a patient who, along with the usual features, had a catastrophic three-month terminal illness with headaches, convulsions, and coma. The cerebrospinal fluid had 95 cells/dL with 55% lymphocytes. At postmortem examination, perivascular infiltrates were found in the brain, meninges, and scrotum. The central retinal artery, examined through the cranium since an anterior approach was not permitted, was infiltrated by round cells.

Besides emphasizing the importance of vasculitis in the pathogenesis of Behçet's syndrome, Berlin made astute observations on the chronic and relapsing nature of the illness. Moreover, he noticed that injections of saline solution into the conjunctiva led to abscesses at the injection sites; in retrospect, this was an early description of "pathergy." His patient was also colonized with staphylococci on other mucosal lesions.

The credit, however, for noticing a cutaneous hypersensitivity to needle prick (pathergy) is usually given to Blobner,[12] even though Blobner's patient had only ocular and genital disease. This phenomenon of "pathergy" remains controversial and appears to have a geographic bias. Although Japanese and most Turkish observers continue to report it, a well-controlled study of this phenomenon awaits publication. Interestingly, Curth did not observe it in her early reports of North American cases.[13]

Helen Curth, a New York dermatologist, was the first American author to write a comprehensive review of the condition which up to then had mainly been reported from Europe.[13] She described two cases, one with the fully developed triple syndrome, while the other only had oral and vulvar lesions. She was willing to make the diagnosis in the presence of only two clinical features. Her liberal interpretation had some adherents but, in general, as the widening range of target organs was evident, there was continuing demand that an acceptable diagnosis required three or more cardinal features.[14-16] The widening spectrum of the disease was later to embrace synovitis,[17] cutaneous vasculitis,[18,19] thrombophlebitis,[17] major artery inflammation with and without aneurysms,[20] discrete ulcerations of the bowel,[21] as well as meningeal and parenchymal disease of the brain.[11]

The Growing Scope of Behçet's Disease

Since most patients having the disease live in the eastern Mediterranean countries or in Japan, it was logical that the early international congresses were held in Rome in 1966, Istanbul in 1977, and Tokyo in 1981. The published proceedings of these meetings had 9, 57, and 61 papers, respectively, and are referenced under the bibliographic numbers 19, 20, and 21. The title "Behçet's disease," and not "Behçet's syndrome," was used in all these symposia. The disease is now of great interest in the English-speaking world. Table 1 lists the growing number of *Index Medicus* citations on Behçet's disease from 1945 to 1985. It is noteworthy that nowadays, about half of the articles are in journals that are published in English. Thus, no longer is Behçet's disease an exotic "foreign" malady.

Under the auspices of the Royal Society of Medicine, the Fourth International Congress on Behçet's Disease was held in London in 1985. The emphasis of the international meetings, and of the world literature, has been changing from purely clinical and pathological descriptions to investigations on the immunology, epidemiology, and treatment. However, good clinical observations remain crucial to future advances, and these are likely to emanate from regions where patients are plentiful and medical technology is scarce. One is reminded that the fundamental pathology of the retinal vasculitis was observed by the serial fundoscopic observations of Jebejian and Kalfayan[22] in Lebanon. Moreover, it was from the same country that Mamo and Azzam first reported on the beneficial effects of chlorambucil on the uveitis.[23] The most comprehensive review of Behçet's disease is by Mishima and colleagues from Japan,[24] a country where the disease is nationally targeted for investigations since it is one of the leading causes of blindness.

Table 1

Index Medicus Citations on Behçet's Disease		
Year	Total Number	English Language
1945	2	0
1955*	5	2
1966	18	8
1975	48	19
1985	141	74

*Source is current list of medical literature.

References

1. Saylan T. Commemorative lecture for Professor Dr. Hulûsi Behçet. In Dilşen N, Koniçe M, Övül C, eds: *Behçet's Disease. Proceedings of an International Symposium on Behçet's Disease, Istanbul, 29–30 September 1977*. Amsterdam-Oxford: Excerpta Medica, 1979:1–5.
2. Kyle RA, Shampo MA. Hulusi Behçet. *JAMA* 1982; 247:1925.
3. Behçet H. Über rezidivierende, aphthose, durch ein Virus verursachte Geschwüre am Mund, am Auge und an den Genitalien. *Dermatologische Wochenschrift* 1937; 36:1152–1157.
4. Behcet H. Some observations on the clinical picture of the so-called triple symptom complex. *Dermatologica* 1940; 81:73–83.
5. Lipschütz B. Ulcer vulvae acutum (Lipschür). In Jadassohn J: *Handbuch der Haut- und Geschlechtskrankheiten*. Berlin: Julius Springer, 1927; 21:392.
6. Hippocrates. The genuine works of. Translated from Greek. A preliminary discourse and annotations. Francis Adams. Vol 1. *Epidemics III*. p. 403, 1849.
7. Feigenbaum A. Description of Behçet's syndrome in the Hippocratic third book of endemic diseases. *Br J Ophthalmol* 1956; 40:355–357.
8. Blüthe L. Zur Kenntnis des recidiverenden Hypopyons. Inaugural Thesis. Heidelberg, 1908.
9. Planner H, Remenovsky F. Beiträge zur Kenntnis der ulcerationen am aüsseren weiblichen Genitale. *Arch Dermat U Syph* 1922; 140:162–188.
10. Adamantiades B. Sur un cas d'iritis a hypopyon récidivant. *Annales d'oculistique* 1931; 168:271–278.
11. Berlin C. Behçet's syndrome with involvement of the central nervous system. Report of a case with necropsy, of lesions of the mouth, genitalia and eyes; review of the literature. *Arch Dermatol Syphilol* 1944; 49:227–233.
12. Blobner F. Zur recidivierenden hypopyoniritis, *Ztschr f Augenh* 1937; 91:129–139.
13. Curth HO. Recurrent genito-oral aphthosis and uveitis with hypopyon (Behçet's syndrome). Report of two cases. *Arch Dermatol Syphilol* 1946; 54;179–196.
14. Mason RM, Barnes CG. Behçet—Syndrome mit Arthritis. *Schweiz Med Wochenschrift* 1968; 98:665–671.
15. Shimizu T. Behçet's disease. *Jpn J Ophthalmol* 1974; 18:291–294.
16. O'Duffy J, Goldstein NP. Neurologic involvement in seven patients with Behçet's disease. *Am J Med* 1976; 61:170–178.
17. Adamantiades B. Lorando N. Sur le syndrome complexe del' uvéite récidivante ou soi-distant syndrome complexe de Behçet. *Presse Med* 1949; 57:501–503.
18. Touraine A. L'aphthouse. *Bull Soc Franç Derm Syph* 1941; 48:61.
19. Nazzaro P. Cutaneous manifestations of Behçet's disease. Clinical

and histopathological findings. In Monacelli M, Nazzaro P, eds: *Behçet's Disease: International Symposium on Behçet's Disease, Rome 1964.* Basal, S Karger, 1966:15–51.

20. Shimizu T. Clinicopathological studies on Behçet's disease. In Dilşen N, Koniçe M, Övül C, eds: *Behçet's Disease. Proceedings of an International Symposium on Behçet's Disease, Istanbul, 29–30 September 1977.* Amsterdan-Oxford, Excerpta Medica, 1979:9–43.

21. Baba S, Morioka S. Treatment of intestinal Behçet's disease. In Inaba G, ed: *Behçet's Disease. Pathogenetic Mechanism and Clinical Future. Proceedings of the International Conference on Behçet's disease, Tokyo, October 23,24, 1981.* Tokyo, University of Tokyo Press, 1982:559–570.

22. Jebejian R, Kalfayan B. Le syndrome oculo-bucco-génital. *Ann ocul* 1946; 179:481–491.

23. Mamo JG, Azzam SA. Treatment of Behçet's disease with chlorambucil. *Arch Ophthalmol* 1970; 84:446–450.

24. Mishima S, Masuda S, Izawa Y, et al. The eight Frederick H. Verhoeff lecture, presented by Saiichi Mishima, MD. Behçet's disease in Japan: Ophthalmologic aspects. *Trans Am Ophthalmol Soc* 1979; 77:225–279.

2

DIAGNOSTIC CRITERIA AND EPIDEMIOLOGY

Mark S. Teter and Marc C. Hochberg

THE EPIDEMIOLOGY AND CLINICAL ASPECTS of Behçet's disease are closely related. Thoughts on diagnostic criteria and clues to etiology have been influenced by studies describing population trends and immunogenetics. Accordingly, this chapter will review and discuss the evolution of diagnostic criteria, descriptive epidemiology, and theories on etiology, including the role of hereditary factors, allergies, infectious agents, and other environmental factors.

Diagnostic Criteria

It is typical of the difficulty in making the clinical diagnosis of Behçet's disease that an informal criteria committee of the International Symposium on Behçet's Disease held in Istanbul in September, 1977, was unable to reach agreement on standardized diagnostic criteria.[1] Behçet's original description in 1937 of aphthous oral ulcerations, genital ulcerations, and iritis initiated a

From *Behcet's Disease: A Contemporary Synopsis*, edited by Gary R. Plotkin, M.D., John J. Calabro, M.D., and J. Desmond O'Duffy, M.B. © 1988, Futura Publishing Company, Inc., Mount Kisco, NY.

[1]Supported in part by an Arthritis Foundation Clinical Research Center Grant. Dr. Hochberg is the recipient of an Arthritis Investigator Award, The Arthritis Foundation.

debate over clinical, laboratory, epidemiologic, and philosophical classification schema that continues to the present. Behçet himself drew attention to the difficulty of diagnosis due to the lack of simultaneity of oral and genital ulcerations and the absence in some patients of iritis at the time of diagnosis.[2] Since the time of that observation, various investigators have proposed diagnostic criteria that have ranged from challenging the necessity that all components of the triple symptom complex be required for diagnosis,[3-8] to a "spectral" approach in which various combinations of clinical symptoms are grouped and categorized as subtypes of Behçet's disease.[9-11] Furthermore, some authors feel that a distinction should be made between the terms Behçet's disease and Behçet's syndrome, with the former reserved for those patients meeting all criteria for diagnosis without the presence of a concomitant disorder that might account for some manifestations of disease, and the latter term to describe patients in whom classic features of the disease exist, but in whom an associated disease is present that may be responsible for most clinical manifestations.[12]

In 1946 Curth published a series of patients which she felt represented a clinical spectrum of Behçet's disease despite the common absence of iritis.[3] Curth believed that the triple symptom prerequisite for the diagnosis of Behçet's disease led to many cases being overlooked and suggested that two of the three components of the triad were sufficient to establish the diagnosis.

Over the next 20 years several reports of patient series demonstrated a variety of clinical manifestations of disease, often in the presence of only two of the three requisite symptoms.[4-6] Most authors argued for a liberalization of diagnostic criteria. This trend culminated in 1969 with the publication of Mason and Barnes' proposal for multitiered diagnostic criteria.[7] In that report, 25 patients were compared with regard to various symptoms and two groups of criteria were proposed representing "major" and "minor" disease manifestations (Table 1). The major criteria of buccal ulceration, genital ulceration, eye lesions, and skin lesions were separated not on the basis of disease severity, but on their more common prevalence in those patients thought to have definite Behçet's disease. The minor criteria of gastrointestinal lesions, thrombophlebitis, cardiovascular lesions, arthritis, central nervous system lesions, and family history, occurred less commonly but, when present, added significantly to the impression of a valid

Table 1

Diagnostic Criteria for Behçet's Disease: Mason and Barnes

Major:	Buccal ulceration
	Genital ulceration
	Eye lesions
	Skin lesions
Minor:	Gastrointestinal lesions
	Thrombophlebitis
	Cardiovascular lesions
	Arthritis
	Central nervous system lesions
	Family history

NB: Diagnosis based on the presence of a minimum of three major or two major and two minor criteria.

clinical diagnosis. The authors suggested that a diagnosis of Behçet's disease was assured with a minimum of three major or two major and two minor criteria present.

In the United States, O'Duffy[8] reported 10 patients with Behçet's disease and suggested that the disease often passes unrecognized in this country. He agreed with Curth and Mason and Barnes that the prerequisite of the original triple symptom complex for the diagnosis of Behçet's disease would lead to underdiagnosis. O'Duffy[13] found a high frequency of neurological disease in patients seen over the ensuing five years and by 1976, suggested a diagnostic scheme based on equal weighting of the most common clinical manifestations but requiring the presence of recurrent aphthous ulceration and at least two other criteria (Table 2).

Table 2

Diagnostic Criteria for Behçet's Disease: O'Duffy and Goldstein

Suggested criteria:
   Aphthous stomatitis, aphthous genital ulceration, uveitis, cutaneous vasculitis, synovitis and meningoencephalitis
Diagnosis:
   At least three criteria present, one being recurrent aphthous ulceration
Incomplete form:
   Two criteria present, one being recurrent aphthous ulceration
Exclusions:
   Inflammatory bowel disease, systemic lupus erythematosus, Reiter's disease and herpetic infections

As various investigators attempted to identify specific clinical criteria that would ensure a homogeneous and reproducible categorization of patients, attention turned toward identification of various immunological and laboratory findings that were characteristic if not pathognomonic for disease. The most attractive of these was the skin pathergy test. First described by Blobner,[14] the phenomenon of hypersensitivity to subcutaneous needle pricks was subsequently shown in several series to be both sensitive and specific in Behçet's disease patients.[15-17] While some series disputed the sensitivity of this test,[8] others have incorporated the less specific term of skin hyperirritability into proposed diagnostic criteria.[18,19]

The most complex scheme for diagnosis incorporating skin hyperirritability was proposed by the Behçet's Disease Research Committee of Japan[18] (Table 3). Returning to Mason and Barnes' concept of major and minor criteria, this group also formalized the concept of incomplete versus complete Behçet's disease and included the categories of suspect and possible disease. While the authors point out that this design better serves the purpose of classification than discrimination, they propose that complete Behçet's disease is characterized by the appearance of four specific major symptoms in a given patient's clinical course. Incomplete Behçet's disease is diagnosed either by the appearance of three of four major symptoms or by a combination of recurrent hypopyon-iritis or typical chorioretinitis and one other major symptom. Suspect Behçet's disease is defined as symptomatology at two major sites, and possible disease by involvement at one major site.

As recently as September 1985, criteria proposals were presented at an international conference on Behçet's disease without worldwide consensus. A Turkish group proposed a scheme in which major and minor criteria are used to supplement a separate "specific" diagnostic criterion defined as a positive skin pathergy test.[20] This group felt that Behçet's disease could be diagnosed by the presence of skin pathergy plus one major criterion (including thrombophlebitis), or by a combination of major and minor criteria in the absence of skin pathergy.

Concomitant with the development of clinical diagnostic criteria, a spectral approach to the classification of Behçet's disease has been proposed.[9] Touraine proposed in 1941 the concept of "aphthosis," suggesting that oral and genital ulcerations are

Table 3

Diagnostic Criteria for Behçet's Syndrome: Behçet Disease Research Committee of Japan

Major criteria
1. Recurrent aphthous ulceration in the mouth
2. Skin lesions
   a. Erythema nodosum-like eruptions
   b. Subcutaneous thrombophlebitis
   c. Hyperirritability of the skin
3. Eye lesions
   a. Recurrent hypopyon iritis or iridocyclitis
   b. Chorioretinitis
4. Genital ulcerations

Minor criteria
5. Arthritic symptoms and signs (arthralgia, swelling, redness)
6. Gastrointestinal lesions (appendicitis-like pains, melena, etc.)
7. Epididymitis
8. Vascular lesions (occlusion of blood vessels, aneurysms)
9. Central nervous system involvements
   a. Brain stem syndrome
   b. Meningoencephalomyelitic syndrome
   c. Confusional type

Types of Behçet syndrome
1. Complete type: all four major symptoms appear in the clinical course of the patient.
2. Incomplete type:
   a. Three of four major symptoms appear in the clinical course of the patient
   b. Recurrent hypopyon-iritis or typical chorioretinitis and one other major symptom appear in the clinical course of the patient
3. Suspect: involvement at two major sites
4. Possible: involvement at one major site

mucosal manifestations of systemic disease. He classified Behçet's disease into three groups based on other symptoms associated with mucosal ulceration:

a) Mucosal aphthosis, in which oral and genital ulceration alone are present;

b) Mucocutaneous apthosis, in which cutaneous lesions are present in addition to mucosal lesions;

c) General aphthosis, characterized by combinations of mucocutaneous, ocular, neurological, articular, and visceral symptoms.

Lehner[10] elaborated on this concept, arguing that diverse clinical manifestations may have diagnostic and prognostic significance and might be correlated with immunological categorization. He grouped his patients into four categories:

1) Mucocutaneous type: oral and genital ulcers with or without skin manifestations;
2) Arthritic type: with joint involvement and two or more of the mucocutaneous manifestations;
3) Neurological type: with brain involvement and some or all of the lesions found in the mucocutaneous and arthritic types;
4) Ocular type: with uveitis and some or all of the mucocutaneous, arthritic, and neurological manifestations.[11]

It is apparent from this review that nearly 50 years after Behçet's first description of the triple symptom complex that bears his name, the diagnosis of Behçet's disease rests solely on clinical manifestations in the absence of known laboratory, immunological, or pathological diagnostic features. Diagnosis continues to be a process of assigning relative weight to various clinical symptoms and matching these to arbitrarily selected known clinical features of the disease, while carefully avoiding the diagnosis in patients with features of other better-defined illnesses.

Prevalence and Incidence

A number of factors account for the difficulty of estimating the worldwide prevalence of Behçet's disease. The absence of uniform diagnostic criteria has resulted in an inability to confidently compare case reports from divergent geographical sources without specifying the basis for diagnosis in each series. In the 721 cases reviewed by Chajek and Fainaru[21] in 1975, diagnostic criteria varied from one series to another. O'Duffy[8] has suggested that the disease often goes unrecognized and other cases may be mislabeled as Reiter's syndrome, Stevens-Johnson syndrome, or periodic disease.[12] Furthermore, exclusions to diagnosis of inflammatory bowel disease, systemic lupus erythematosis, and herpetic infections have been suggested by some authors and not considered by others.[13] Consequently, while it is apparent that Behçet's disease occurs worldwide, it is useful from an epidemiologic point of view to refer to reports from diverse geographical sources on their own terms and to refrain from extrapolating specific observations into generalized trends.

Most cases of Behçet's disease have been reported from the eastern Mediterranean countries and Japan.[6,21] However, numerous series have been reported from Great Britain, France, Scandinavia, the United States, and Australia, among others.[7,8,22–24] Data on prevalence vary greatly (Table 4). In certain areas of Japan, the estimated prevalence of Behçet's disease is 1 per 10,000 population, but in the Hokkaido district of northern Japan it may be as high as 1 per 7,500.[25] Curiously, there are no reported cases in Okinawa or among Japanese-Americans in Hawaii, although cases of Behçet's disease among other ethnic groups in Hawaii have been reported.[26] The overall incidence patterns in Japan have shown variability with a dramatic upsurge of newly diagnosed cases in the years following World War II but with an apparent decline from 1977 through 1979.[25]

O'Duffy (personal communication) has estimated the prevalence in the United States to be 5 per 100,000 population based on the experience at the Mayo Clinic in residents of Olmsted County, Minnesota. Chamberlain[22] reported 32 cases in northern England with an estimated prevalence of 6.4 per 1,000,000 population.

Effects of Age and Sex

Most reports of Behçet's disease have demonstrated a preponderance of males with a mean age of disease onset in the third decade of life (Table 5). In a Japanese series reported by Oshima

Table 4

Prevalence of Behçet's Disease

Country (Reference)	Prevalence (per 100,000)
Japan[25]	10
Hokkaido District, Japan[25]	13.3
Olmsted County, U.S.A.[66]	4.0
Yorkshire, U.K.[22]	0.64

Table 5

Age and Sex Distribution of Behçet's Disease from Selected Reports

Author	*Origin*	*No. of Patients*	*Male:Female*	*Age of Onset Mean*	*Age of Onset Range*
Oshima[6]	Japan	85	1.7:1	27	6–65
Chajek[21]	Israel	41	4.9:1	27.4	15–54
Chajek[21]	Various	683	2.3:1	25.9	6–72
Chamberlain[22]	U.K.	32	0.6:1	24.7	< 10–61+
O'Duffy[8]	U.S.A.	10	0.4:1	35.2	16–67

and others[6] in 1963, 53 of 85 subjects were male, giving a male:female ratio of 1.7:1. Chajek and Fainaru[21] reported 41 patients seen in an Israeli clinic, of whom 34 were male (male:female ratio 4.9:1), and in reviewing the 683 cases in the world literature up to 1975, found a male:female ratio of 2.3:1. The extensive epidemiologic survey conducted in Japan from 1972 to 1973 confirmed the predominance of males for the complete type of Behçet's disease but suggested that for the incomplete type, sex ratios were essentially unity.[18] However, more recent reports have suggested a reversal with the male-to-female ratio of new cases between 1977 through 1979 being 0.77:1.[25]

Differences exist between these findings and series reported from Great Britain and the United States. Chamberlain[22] described 32 patients seen in Yorkshire County of whom 20 were female (male:female ratio 0.6:1). O'Duffy[8,13] has found a predominance of females in two separate series.

There is more consistency in reported age distribution patterns with the mean age of disease onset in various series ranging from 24.7 to 35.2 years, with extremes ranging from 2 months to 72 years. Oshima and others[6] found a mean age of onset of 27 years with a range of 6 to 65 years in Japan. In the Israeli series, the mean age of onset was 27.4 years with a range of 15 to 54 years.[21] In the English series there was a mean age of 24.7 years with a similar range,[22] and in the American series, the age of onset ranged from 16 to 67 with a mean of 35.2 years.[8] A more recent report from Ammann and others[27] in San Francisco suggested that Behçet's disease may be more common in children than previously reported and listed six cases ranging in age from 2 months to 11 years.

In one of the few longitudinal studies of prognosis in Behçet's disease, Yazici and others[26] reported on 51 patients followed up at 4½ years after initial presentation. At the time of first presentation they found that eye disease, arthritis, folliicuitis, and thrombophlebitis were more common among males and erythema nodosum among females. Regardless of sex, younger patients (age of onset 24 years or less) had a higher incidence of eye disease and total clinical disease activity compared to older patients (age of onset 25 years or more). In follow-up, disease activity became significantly less after 4½ years in all groups, with the best prognosis present in older females.

Genetic Factors

Familial Occurrence

Isolated reports of familial clustering of Behçet's disease led Mason and Barnes[7] to include a positive family history among their minor diagnostic criteria. Aoki[29] subsequently reported a series of 223 Behçet's patients, eight of whom had affected first-degree relatives, and two of whom had affected second-degree relatives. Chamberlain[30] surveyed 32 patients in the United Kingdom and noted an increase in symptoms associated with Behçet's disease among first-degree relatives, although none of these relatives fulfilled Mason and Barnes' diagnostic criteria. Most other reports are limited to accounts of isolated kindred without a consistent inheritence pattern.[31-34] In 1986 Stewart[35] tested an autosomal recessive pattern of Mendelian inheritance on 15 British and 9 Turkish families and found no consistent inheritance pattern of any classic Mendelian type. However, patterns of disease distribution and HLA associations with disease have continued to suggest a genetic influence on disease susceptibility.

Immunogenetic Studies

In 1973 Ohno[36] reported a strong association in Japan between Behçet's disease and HLA-B5. Further reports confirmed this observation, demonstrating this particular antigen in 75% of Japanese patients compared to 30.8% of controls.[37] Similar reports of an association of HLA-B5 with disease were reported in Turkish[38] and Mexican Mestizo Indian populations[39] (Table 6).

In a collaborative study of British and Turkish populations, Yazici, Chamberlain, and others[40] confirmed the striking increase in frequency of HLA-B5 among Turkish patients, with a relative risk of 7.5 which increased to 13.3 if the HLA-Bw51 antigen, a split of HLA-B5, was considered. The distribution of HLA-B5, -Bw51, and -Bw52 was not significantly different in the British patient and control groups. A modest increase in HLA-B27 in British patients was suggested but not analyzed owing to a small sample size.

This observation was consistent with Chamberlain's previous report of the lack of association between Behçet's disease and HLA-B5 in northern England.[41] This in turn supported other British reports in which no excess of HLA-B5 could be demonstrated.[42] Because of clinical similarities between Behçet's disease and the seronegative spondyloarthropathies, attention focused on

Table 6

Selected Immunogenetic Studies in Behçet's Disease

Author	Country	HLA Phenotype	Frequency (%)*	
			Patients	Controls
Ohno[36]	Japan	B5	75	30.8
Lavalle[38]	Mexico	B5	70	31
Yazici[40]	Turkey	B5	86.3	42.3
		Bw51	82	23
	Britain	B5	28.6	17.8
		Bw51	21	12
O'Duffy[44]	United States	B5+	12	10
Lehner[47]	Britain	B12/DR2	64.7	37.7
		DR7	39	17
		B5/Bw51	25	12
		MT2(DRw52)	64.7	36.7
		MT3(DRw53)	66.7	46.7
Okuyama[48]	Japan	Bw51	56.8	12.2
		DRw52	86.1	52.1
	Italy	Bw51	80	10.8
		DRw6	30	19.1
		DRw8	20	4.4

*Comparisons between patients and controls showed significant differences ($p < 0.05$) in all cases except where indicated by "+" next to HLA phenotype.

potential associations with HLA-B27. An early British report suggested such an association,[30] but a subsequent report in 1983 showed no association of HLA-B27 and Behçet's disease in a series of 14 British patients, despite the presence in seven patients of mild erosive sacroiliitis.[43]

O'Duffy[44] has found no association between any HLA antigen and Behçet's disease among his patients in the United States, although the Bw51 antigen was not tested at the time this study was completed. This observation is particularly noteworthy when linked to the lower prevalence, later age of disease onset, and reversed male-to-female ratio of the U.S. patients compared to eastern Mediterranean and Japanese series.

Lehner's[11] spectral classification of Behçet's disease allowed for more specific associations between HLA type and clinical manifestations of disease.[11] Lehner and Batchelor[45] found the mucocutaneous type to be associated with HLA-B12, the arthritic type with HLA-B27, and the ocular type with HLA-B5. A Turkish study attempted to confirm these findings but failed to find a correlation.[46] While confirming the strong association in Turkey between HLA-B5 and disease, the authors found no difference in mean age of onset or frequency of ocular disease, arthritis, or vascular involvement between HLA-B5 positive and negative patients. However, further studies by Lehner and others[47] continued to demonstrate associations between HLA type and disease classification. Their subsequent report suggested an association of HLA-B12 and/or DR2 with the mucocutaneous and arthritic types and DR7 with the ocular and neurological types. HLA-B5 and especially the -Bw51 split continued to be strongly associated with the ocular type of Behçet's disease. Furthermore, this study found an increase in MT2 (DRw52) with neurological disease and MT3 (DRw53) with ocular disease.

Collaborative studies between investigators in Japan and Italy in 1984 confirmed a strong association between HLA-Bw51 and Behçet's disease in both populations.[48] Also implicated were Class II antigens with HLA-DRw52 increased in Japanese patients and HLA-DRw6 and DRw8 slightly increased in Italian patients. Interestingly, while HLA-Bw51 and -DRw52 appeared to segregate independently in the Japanese patients, HLA-Bw51 and -DRw52 tended to exist on the same haplotype in Italian patients. Both groups showed an association between HLA-Bw51 and positive skin pathergy. Later studies confirmed the double association of HLA-Bw51 and -DRw52 in Japan and suggested a negative association between HLA-DR1 and HLA-DQw1 and disease.[49]

As immunogenetic studies on Behcet's disease continue, investigations are now directed toward clarifying discrepancies between HLA associations in various populations with particular attention toward correlations of clinical manifestations with HLA phenotype.

Environmental Factors

The etiology of Behçet's disease is unknown. Behçet[2] himself described what may have represented viral inclusion bodies in hypopyon fluid and oral exudates of his patients, and other investigators have found evidence suggesting an infectious etiology.[26, 50–57] Some studies have supported environmental or allergic associations.[1,18,25,58,59]

Infectious Agents

Sezer[50] conducted extensive studies of body fluids from Behçet's patients in 1953 and claimed to have isolated a specific causative virus. In these experiments vitreous fluid from one Behçet's patient and subretinal serous fluid from two others were inoculated into the chorioallantoic membranes of fertile eggs. Inoculations of ground membrane into the brains of 10 mice resulted in various manifestations of encephalitis, and ground brain tissue was then reinoculated into fertile eggs and maintained for more than 30 passages. Intraperitoneal inoculations of ground membrane into guinea pigs resulted in fatal hemorrhagic lobar pneumonia and direct inoculation into the anterior chamber of rabbits resulted in hypopyon formation. Sezer then identified by electron microscopy what he felt was the causative virus. In further clinical studies on Behçet's patients, Sezer provided evidence of documented viremia in patients with active disease and demonstrated renal excretion of this same virus.[51] These studies have not been confirmed.

Evans, Pallis, and Spillane[52] described three cases of Behçet's disease in 1957, all with central nervous system involvement. Inoculations of anterior chamber fluid and brain tissue from one deceased patient onto chick embryo chorioallantoic membrane resulted in virus outgrowth. Furthermore, increased levels of viral neutralizing antibody were found in serum of patients with active disease. Later studies by Noyan and others[53] produced a meningoencephalitic syndrome in mice by intracerebral inoculation of cerebral spinal fluid from a Behçet's patient.

Other investigators have failed to demonstrate a virus in patients with active disease. Katzenellenbogen[54] failed to produce a reaction in a rabbit cornea after inoculation of material from oral and genital ulcers. France and others[55] showed no pathological changes in a guinea pig inoculated with fluid from an articular effusion and no growth on chick embryos injected with joint fluid and scrapings from a mouth ulcer. Braley[56] found no evidence of virus or bacteria in purulent fluid aspirated from an affected eye, and Breslin[57] cultured blood, urine, and anterior chamber fluid with negative results.

In a 1961 review on virologic aspects of Behçet's disease, Dudgeon[60] found the studies to date to be unconvincing. He argued that the most compelling evidence for a viral etiology was the lack of another etiology. The lack of epidemics or focal outbreaks of disease and the rarity of familial disease were incongruent with the natural history of other known viruses. Sezer's[51] claim of prolonged viremia in the presence of antibody was likewise contrary to known viral infections, as was the absence of acquired immunity in a recurrent illness.

However, recent studies have continued to implicate, via indirect measures, a viral etiology for Behçet's disease. Denman and others[61] evaluated the lymphocytes of 86 Behçet's patients for two parameters consistent with a persistent viral infection. They found lymphocyte chromosomal abnormalities in 16 of 38 patients compared to only 1 of 17 healthy controls, and found the lymphocytes of 37% of Behçet's patients imparied the ability of Herpes-Simplex I virus to replicate in lymphocyte cultures stimulated by phytohemagglutinin compared to no impairment by all healthy controls. In 1982, Eglin, Lehner and Subak-Sharpe[62] demonstrated that part of the Herpes-Simplex virus genome was transcribed in peripheral blood mononuclear cells of patients with ocular and arthritic types of Behçet's disease and in patients with recurrent aphthous ulcers. As recently as 1981, conflicting evidence regarding a viral etiology was presented at the Third International Conference on Behçet's Disease.[26]

Nonviral infectious agents have also been implicated. Feigenbaum and others characterized Behçet's disease as "sepsis lenta" caused by staphylococci, dependent upon resistance lowered by past exposure to tuberculosis.[63] In 1985, Namba[64] presented evidence of a persistent streptococcal antigen in the plasma of patients with ocular disease, both active and in remission. Electron microscopy was suggestive of the presence of streptococcal L-forms in patient plasma and leukocytes.[64]

Other Factors

Environmental factors in etiology have been investigated with increasing interest in Japan where the incidence of Behçet's disease increased dramatically with post-World War II industrialization.[18] Behçet's patients have been reported to have increased tissue levels of such environmental pollutants as organochloride, organophosphate, inorganic copper, benzene hexachloride, chlorophenothane, polychlorinated biphenyls, bromide, chromium, zinc, and cyclic guanosine 5'-monophosphate.[1,26] Relative concentrations of trace elements may also be significant; one study reported increased tissue copper levels and decreased zinc levels in patients compared to controls.[58]

Allergic factors have also been suggested in the etiology of Behçet's disease. McMenemey and Lawrence[59] described the histopathology of brain tissue from two cases which they felt were consistent with allergic changes. Suggestions for antigenic stimuli have included environmental pollutants, bacterial infections and food allergies including English walnuts, gingko nuts, casein, α-lactalbumin, β-lactoglobulin, and gluten.[10,18]

The search for the etiology of Behçet's disease continues. Recent trends have shifted back toward a viral etiology in conjunction with genetic factors.[26] Viruses, particularly slow-viruses, in a genetically receptive host offer a chance of reconciling conflicting opinions regarding the classification of Behçet's disease as an infectious or autoimmune disorder.

Summary and Conclusions

Behçet's disease is a heterogeneous clinical entity. In the absence of pathognomonic diagnostic indicators, it is apparent that differences in diagnostic standards account for some, if not all, discrepancies in epidemiologic, genetic, and etiologic studies.

The most compelling correlations demonstrating a single disease process between divergent populations occur between Japanese and eastern Mediterranean patients. Prevalence data, clinical homogeneity, and genetic factors as indicated by HLA tissue typing suggest that in these two areas which account for the bulk of worldwide disease, a common pathogenetic mechanism may be at work. Ohno[65] provides data which suggest a common population bond, where HLA-Bw51 and Behçet's disease are seen to be coincident along the historical Silk Route bridging the Mediterranean and the Far East.

British and American studies suggest divergent patient populations which, although they share clinical characteristics with Mediterranean and Japanese studies, differ in prevalence of specific disease manifestations, demographics, and HLA associations. Lehner's[11] subclassification of Behçet's disease with the specific HLA associations may account for part of this discrepancy, in which some types of Behçet's disease in British populations are more closely reminiscent than others of Mediterranean and Japanese disease.

If the various reports of Behçet's disease indicate a heterogeneous spectrum of disease as opposed to a single specific illness, then genetic and other etiologic hypotheses may be seen as multifactorial but with a common theme. Genetic predisposition combined with a triggering exogenous factor, be it environmental, infectious, or allergic, may set in motion a cascade of immunological responses resulting in clinical manifestations of disease. As such, variations in any one of these factors may determine characteristics of the host which vary with geography and genetic composition.

Acknowledgement: The authors wish to thank Ms Angie Rutkowski for her expert clerical and editorial assistance.

References

1. O'Duffy JD. Summary of international symposium on Behçet's disease, Istanbul, September 29–30, 1977. *J. Rheumatol* 1978; 5:229–233.
2. Behçet H. Über rezidivierende, aphthose, durch ein Virus verursachte Geschwüre am Mund, am Auge und an den Genitalien. *Derm Wscmr* 1937; 105:1152–1157.
3. Curth HO. Behcet's syndrome, abortive form (?) (recurrent genital ulcerations). *Arch Dermatol Syphilol* 1946; 54:481–484.
4. Phillips DL, Scott JS. Recurrent genital and oral ulceration with associated eye lesions; Behçet's syndrome. *Lancet* 1955; 1:366–371.
5. Strachan RW, Wigzell FW. Polyarthritis in Behçet's multiple symptom complex. *Ann Rheum Dis* 1963; 22:26–35.
6. Oshima Y, Shimizu T, Yokohari R, et al. Clinical studies on Behçet's syndrome. *Ann Rheum Dis* 1963; 22:36–45.
7. Mason RM, Barnes CG. Behçet's syndrome with arthritis. *Ann Rheum Dis* 1969; 28:95–103.
8. O'Duffy JD, Carney JA, Deodhar S. Behcet's disease. Report of 10 cases, 3 with new manifestations. *Ann Intern Med* 1971; 75:561–570.
9. Touraine A. L'aphthose. *Bull Soc Franç Derm Syph* 1941; 48:61–68.
10. Lehner T. Oral ulceration and Behçet's syndrome. *Gut* 1977; 18:491–511.
11. Lehner T, Barnes CG. Criteria for diagnosis and classification of Behçet's syndrome. In Lehner T, Barnes CG, eds: *Behçet's Syndrome. Clinical and Immunological Features. Proceedings of a Conference Sponsored by Royal Society of Medicine, February 1979.* London, Academic Press, 1979:1–9.
12. Ehrlich GE. Intermittent and periodic arthritic syndromes. In McCarty DJ, ed: *Arthritis and Allied Conditions. A Textbook of Rheumatology.* Philadelphia, Lea and Febiger, 1985:891–896.
13. O'Duffy JD, Goldstein NP. Neurologic involvement in seven patients with Behçet's disease. *Am J Med* 1976; 61:170–178.
14. Blobner F. Zur rezidivieren hypopion-iritis. *Zeitschrift Augenheilk* 1937; 91:129.
15. Jensen T. Sur les ulcérations aphtheuses la mugueuse de la bouche et de la peau génitale combinées avec les symptômes oculaires (syndrome de Behçet). *Acta Derm Venereol* 1941; 22:64–79.
16. Katzenellenbogen I. Survey of 22 cases of Behcet's disease: The significance of specific skin hyperreactivity. *XIII Congressus Internationalis Dermatologiae, Munchen.* Berlin, Springer, 1967:321.
17. Tüzün Y, Yazici H, Pazarli H, et al. The usefulness of nonspecific skin hyperreactivity (the pathergy test) in Behçet's disease in Turkey. *Acta Derm Venereol* (Stockh) 1979; 59:77–79.
18. Shimizu T, Ehrlich GE, Inaba G, Hayashi K. Behçet disease (Behçet syndrome). *Semin Arthritis Rheum* 1979; 8:223–260.
19. Wong RC, Ellis CN, Diaz LA. Behçet's disease. *Int J Dermatol* 1984; 23:25–32.

20. Dilşen N, Koniçe M, Aral O. Our diagnostic criteria in Behçet's disease (BD) (abstract 44). Royal Society of Medicine international conference on Behçet's disease, September 5 and 6, 1985, London, England.
21. Chajek T, Fainaru M. Behçet's disease. Report of 41 cases and a review of the literature. *Medicine* 1975; 54:179–196.
22. Chamberlain MA. Behçet's syndrome in 32 patients in Yorkshire. *Ann Rheum Dis* 1977; 36:491–499.
23. Sulheim O, Dalgaard JB, Anderson SR. Behçet's syndrome. Report of case with complete autopsy performed. *Acta Path Microbiol Scand* 1959; 45:145–158.
24. Cooper DA, Penny R. Behçet's syndrome: clinical, immunological, and therapeutic evaluation of 17 patients. *Med J Aust* 1974; 4:585–592.
25. Aoki K, Fujioka K, Katsumata H, et al. Epidemiological studies on Behcet's disease in the Hokkaido district. *Jpn J Clin Ophthal* 1971; 25:2239–2248.
26. O'Duffy JD, Lehner T, Barnes CG. Summary of the third international conference on Behçet's disease, Tokyo, Japan, October 23–24, 1981. *J Rheumatol* 1983: 10:154–158.
27. Ammann AJ, Johnson A, Fyfe GA, et al. Behçet syndrome. *J Pediatr* 1985; 107:41–43.
28. Yazici H, Tüzün Y, Pazarli H, et al. Influence of age of onset and patient's sex on the prevalence and severity of manifestations of Behçet's syndrome. *Ann Rheum Dis* 1984; 43:783–789.
29. Aoki K, Ohno S, Ohguchi M, Sugiura S. Familial Behçet's disease. *Jpn J Clin Ophthal* 1978; 22:72–75.
30. Chamberlain MA. A family study of Behçet's syndrome. *Ann Rheum Dis* 1978; 37:459–465.
31. Goolamali SK, Comaish JS, Hassanyeh F, Stephens A. Familial Behçet's syndrome. *Br J Dermatol* 1976; 95:637–641.
32. Berlin C. Behçet's disease as a multiple symptom complex. Report of ten cases. *Arch Dermatol* 1960; 82:73–79.
33. Forbes IJ, Robson HN. Familial recurrent orogenital ulceration. *Br Med J* 1960; 1:599–601.
34. Fowler TJ, Humpston DJ, Nussey AM, Small M. Behçet's syndrome with neurological manifestations in two sisters. *Br Med J* 1968; 2:473–474.
35. Stewart JAB. Genetic analysis of families of patients with Behçet's syndrome: Data incompatible with autosomal recessive inheritance. *Ann Rheum Dis* 1986; 45:265–268.
36. Ohno S, Aoki K, Sugiura S, et al. Immunohematological studies on Behçet's disease. *Acta Soc Ophthalmol Jpn* 1973; 77:1452–1458.
37. Ohno S, Nakayama E, Sugiura S, et al. Specific histocompatibility antigens associated with Behçet's disease. *Am J Ophthalmol* 1975; 80:636–641.
38. Yazici H, Akokan G, Yalcin B, Muftuoglu A. The high prevalence of HLA-B5 in Behçet's disease. *Clin Exp Immunol* 1977; 30:259–261.

39. Lavalle C, Alarcon-Segovia D, Del Guidice-Knipping JA, Fraga A. Association of Behçet's syndrome with HLA-B5 in the Mexican mestizo population. *J Rheumatol* 1981; 8:325–327.
40. Yazici H, Chamberlain MA, Schreuder I, et al. HLA antigens in Behçet's disease: A reappraisal by a comparative study of Turkish and British patients. *Ann Rheum Dis* 1980; 39:344–348.
41. Chamberlain MA. Behçet's disease (letter). *Br Med J* 1978; 2:1369–1370.
42. Jung RT, Chalmers TM, Joysey VC. HLA in Behçet's disease (letter). *Lancet* 1976; 1:694.
43. Caporn N, Higgs ER, Dieppe PA, Watt I. Arthritis in Behçet's syndrome. *Br J Radiol* 1983; 56:87–91.
44. O'Duffy JD, Taswell HF, Elveback LR. HL-A antigens in Behçet's disease. *J Rheumatol* 1976; 3:1–3.
45. Lehner T, Batchelor JR. Classification and an immunogenetic basis of Behçet's syndrome. In Lehner T, Barnes CG, eds: *Behçet's Syndrome. Clinical and Immunological Features. Proceedings of a Conference Sponsored by the Royal Society of Medicine, February 1979*. London, Academic Press, 1979:13–32.
46. Müftüoğlu AU, Yazici H, Yurdakul S, et al. Behçet's disease: Lack of correlation of clinical manifestations with HLA antigens. *Tissue Antigens* 1981; 17:226–230.
47. Lehner T, Welsh KI, Batchelor JR. The relationship of HLA-B and DR phenotypes to Behçet's syndrome, recurrent oral ulceration and the class of immune complexes. *Immunology* 1982; 47:581–587.
48. Okuyama T, Kunikane H, Kasahara, et al. Behçet's disease. In Albert ED, et al, eds: *Histocompatibility Testing 1984*. Berlin, Springer-Verlag, 1984:397–402.
49. Ohno S, Matsuda H. Studies of HLA antigens and Behçet's disease (abstract 1). Royal Society of Medicine international conference on Behçet's disease, September 5 and 6, 1985, London, England.
50. Sezer FN. The isolation of a virus as the cause of Behçet's disease. *Am J Ophthalmol* 1953; 36:301–315.
51. Sezer FN. Further investigations on the virus of Behçet's disease. *Am J Ophthalmol* 1956; 41:41–55.
52. Evans AD, Pallis CA, Spillane JD. Involvement of the nervous system in Behçet's syndrome. Report of three cases and isolation of virus. *Lancet* 1957; 2:349–353.
53. Noyan B, Gursoy G, Akin E. Inoculationsversuche bei Mausen mit dem Liquor eines Falles von Neuro-Behcetscher Krankheit. *Acta Neuropath* 1969; 12:195–199.
54. Katzenellenbogen I. Recurrent aphthous ulceration of oral mucous membrane and genitals associated with recurrent hypopyoniritis (Behçet's syndrome). Report of three cases. *Br J Dermatol* 1946; 58:161–172.
55. France R, Buchanan RN, Wilson MW, Sheldon MB. Relapsing iritis with recurrent ulcers of the mouth and genitalia (Behçet's syn-

drome). Review: With report of additional case. *Medicine* 1951; 30:335–355.

56. Braley AE. A case of Behçet's disease. *Trans Am Acad Ophthalmol Otolaryngol* 1958; 62:712–715.

57. Breslin HJ. Behçet's disease. Report of a case history of seventeen years' duration. *Am J Ophthalmol* 1962; 53:132–136.

58. Cengiz K. Serum zinc, copper, and magnesium in Behçet's disease (abstract 22). Royal Society of Medicine international conference on Behçet's disease, September 5 and 6, 1985, London, England.

59. McMenemy WH, Lawrence BJ. Encephalomyelopathy in Behçet's disease: Report of necropsy findings in two cases. *Lancet* 1957; 2:353–358.

60. Dudgeon JA. Virological aspects of Behçet's disease. *Proc R Soc Med* 1961; 54:104–106.

61. Denman AM, Fialkow PJ, Pelton BK, et al. Lymphocyte abnormalities in Behçet's syndrome. *Clin Exp Immunol* 1980; 42:175–185.

62. Eglin RP, Lehner T, Subak-Sharpe JH. Detection of RNA complementary to Herpes-simplex virus in mononuclear cells from patients with Behçet's syndrome and recurrent oral ulcers. *Lancet* 1982; 2:1356–1361.

63. Feigenbaum A, Kornblueth W. Behçet's disease as manifestation of a chronic septic condition connected with a constitutional disorder, with a report of 4 cases. *Acta Med Orient* 1946; 5:139–151.

64. Namba K. Behçet's disease and streptococcal infection (abstract 20). Royal Society of Medicine international conference on Behçet's disease, September 5 and 6, 1985, London, England.

65. Ohno S, Ohguchi M, Hirose S, et al. Close association of HLA-Bw51 with Behcet's disease. *Arch Ophthalmol* 1982; 100:1455–1458.

66. O'Duffy JD. Behçet's disease. In Kelly WN, Harris Ed Jr, Ruddy S, Sledge CB, eds: *Textbook of Rheumatology*. Philadelphia, WB Saunders, 1985:1174–1178.

3

IMMUNOLOGY: HUMORAL IMMUNITY

Scott Korn and Raphael J. DeHoratius

MULTIPLE STUDIES HAVE EXAMINED the humoral immune response in Behçet's disease (BD), and this chapter will review those alterations in B lymphocyte function and immunoglobulin production that have been reported in the literature and will summarize the scientific data supporting the role of circulating immune complexes and autoantibodies in the pathogenesis of Behçet's syndrome. Correlations between the humoral immunological phenomena and the clinical activity of BD will be emphasized; and where relevant data are available, comparisons between the immunological alterations in idiopathic recurrent oral ulceration (ROU) and BD will be reviewed in their proper perspective.

B Lymphocytes

The B lymphocyte, which is the principle cell type involved in humoral immunity, normally comprises 5 to 15% of peripheral blood lymphocytes and is characterized by the presence of IgG or IgM immunoglobulin on its surface, as well as C3, Fc, and immunoglobulin receptors, and an antigen determined by the Class II MHC gene.[1] Both B and T lymphocytes can be enumerated by

From *Behcet's Disease: A Contemporary Synopsis*, edited by Gary R. Plotkin, M.D., John J. Calabro, M.D., and J. Desmond O'Duffy, M.B. © 1988, Futura Publishing Company, Inc., Mount Kisco, NY.

applying monoclonal antibodies directed against surface antigens, and studies of peripheral blood from patients with BD have re-

As a result of being exposed to the proper antigenic stimulus, B cells respond by differentiating, proliferating, and producing immunoglobulin. Normally the circulating B lymphocytes are in variable states of activation, ranging from resting to fully differentiated plasma lymphocytes which are actively secreting immunoglobulin. When resting B lymphocytes are exposed to the T-cell-independent B-cell mitrogen, *Staphylococcus aureus* Cowen 1 (SAC), in the presence of T-cell-derived soluble factors, the B lymphocytes are normally activated and produce immunoglobulin. Suzuki and colleagues[3] recently studies B-lymphocyte function in 23 BD patients with varying degrees of clinical activity. When B lymphocytes from normal controls and patients with inactive BD were stimulated by SAC in the presence of T-cell-derived soluble factors, similar amounts of immunoglobulin were produced. However, when B lymphocytes from patients with active BD were exposed to the same stimuli, a decreased amount of immunoglobulin was produced as compared to the control and inactive cases. These data suggested that the percentage of circulating B lymphocytes in the resting state was reduced in active BD. The second phase of Suzuki's study involved exposing B lymphocytes to pokeweed mitogen (PWM), a T-cell-dependent polyclonal activator, in the presence of autologous T lymphocytes and their soluble factors. Normally, B lymphocytes that were partially activated will proliferate and produce immunoglobulin in response to these stimuli; however, the B lymphocytes from both active and inactive BD failed to produce increased immunoglobulin in response to PWM. When T lymphocytes from controls were substituted for the autologous T lymphocytes, the B lymphocytes from patients with BD still failed to respond, suggesting an intrinsic defect in the partially activated lymphocytes. The clinical significance of this proposed defect was unknown. The final phase of the study involved estimating the proportion of fully activated B lymphocytes in BD by measuring the spontaneous production of immunoglobulin. The investigators concluded that there was a fivefold increase in the number of fully differentiated, immunoglobulin-secreting B lymphocytes in patients with active BD. Since IgA, IgM, and IgG production were all increased, Suzuki and colleagues[3] suggested a state of polyclonal activation. In contrast, the cells from inactive BD patients spontaneously produced normal amounts of immunoglobulins. Cell cycle analysis and cell size profile studies confirmed that in active BD there was an increased and decreased percentage, respectively, of activated and resting circulating B lymphocytes.[3]

Behçet's disease is not the only disorder characterized by polyclonal B-cell activation; certain viral infections and several autoimmune disorders, including systemic lupus erythematosus (SLE), are associated with polyclonal immunoglobulin production. Normally, marcophages and T lymphocytes, both helper and suppressor, regulate the immune response and modulate B-cell immunoglobulin production. Macrophages synthesize interleukin-1 (IL-1), and among its other functions, IL-1 appears to be involved in stimulating B-lymphocyte proliferation and differentiation. T lymphocytes produce B-cell growth factor and T-cell replacing factor, which are both involved in the differentiation of B lymphocytes into plasma cells. T lymphocytes also produce interleukin-2 (formerly called T-cell growth factor) which is involved in activating T lymphocytes; however, the direct effects of this lymphokine on the proliferation or differentiation of B cells remains controversial.[4] The various hypotheses concerning etiologic agents in BD are discussed elsewhere in this book, and the exact nature of the immunoregulatory disturbances resulting in polyclonal B cell activation have not yet been established. Nevertheless, the stimulation of humoral immunity in BD which is marked by B-lymphocyte activation and immunoglobulin production, is not completely the result of an intrinsic B-lymphocyte abnormality but must also be dependent upon "a complex imbalance of T lymphocyte subsets,"[5] as discussed in the next chapter.

Serum Immunoglobulins

Several studies have commented on the increased immunoglobulin production observed in BD. In 1963, Oshima and colleagues[6] reported elevated levels of alpha 1, alpha 2, and gamma globulins in many of their 85 Japanese patients with definite or probable BD. Kalbian and Challis[7] reported 12 cases from Israel all of whom had a decreased serum albumin and increased serum globulin, most notably the alpha 2 fraction. O'Duffy[8] and his colleagues studied 9 patients with BD, 8 of whom had an elevated alpha 2 globulin level. They further characterized the immunoglobulin isotypes and noted four of nine had a polyclonal increase in IgA, four of nine had an increase in IgM, and only one of nine had an increase in IgG, with some patients having elevations of two of the immunoglobulin classes.

One of the most comprehensive studies of serum immunoglobulins in BD was reported by Scully, Lehner and Harfitt.[9] They evaluated 64 patients with BD (classified into neurological, ocular, arthritic, and mucocutaneus subgroups), 75 patients with ROU (classified as minor aphthous lesions, major aphthous lesions, or herpetiform ulcerations) and 27 healthy controls. The most striking observation was a statistically significant increase in serum IgA in patients with the neurological, ocular, and arthritic subgroups of BD ($p < 0.05$). Patients with the mucocutaneous form of BD as well as those with ROU also had an increased serum IgA level, but the difference was not statistically significant. When serum IgG was examined, elevations were noted in the arthritic and neurological subgroups of BD as well as the major form of ROU, but none of the increases was statistically significant. Increased serum IgM levels were noted in the mucocutaneous form of BD and the major and herpetiform types of ROU, but again, these increases were not statistically significant. In the 20 patients with ocular BD, the mean IgM was slightly lower than that of the healthy controls. In contrast, three of the four patients with an elevated IgM in O'Duffy's series[8] had ocular involvement. Two other studies[10,11] agreed with the British group's observations that serum IgA levels were frequently increased in BD, but serum IgM was also increased in 18 of 32 patients.[11] While Scully et al.[9] noted a trend of increased levels of IgA in all types of ROU with IgG or IgM elevations in some of the subsets of ROU, another study which did not examine subsets of patients noted normal levels of IgG and IgA in Israeli patients with ROU.[12]

While the results from the various studies of serum immunoglobulins may appear contradictory (Table 1), several conclusions can be supported by the published data. First, many patients with BD have a disorder of the IgA system, although some will have

Table 1

Serum and Secretory Immunoglobulins in Behçet's Disease

	Mucocutaneous	Ocular	Arthritic	Neurological
Serum immunoglobulins				
IgG			↑	↑
IgA	↑		↑↑	↑↑	↑↑
IgM		↓		
Salivary IgA levels				
unstimulated mixed saliva	↑	↑	↑	
stimulated parotid saliva	↓↓	↓↓	↓↓	
Lacrimal immunoglobulins				
IgG		↑	↑	
IgA	↑	↑↑	↑↑	
IgM	↑	↑	↑↑	

↑ represents an increase that is not statistically significant.
↑↑ represents a statistically significant increase.
Data are from Scully et al.[9] Conflicting data are discussed in the text of this article.

other immunoglobulin disturbances. These immunoglobulin variations may relate to the different patient groups studied with their heterogeneity of disease manifestations as well as their genetic composition. In studies of aphthous ulcerations, conflicting results have been obtained when the incidence of HLA types has been examined in patients with ROU.[13] HLA-B12 is associated with the mucocutaneous form of BD which was the one type not noted to have increased IgA levels in the large British study.[9] HLA-B5 has been linked with the ocular form of BD in which Scully et al.[9] noted IgA elevations. Second, ROU (also known as recurrent aphthous stomatitis) and BD may represent opposite ends of a continuous spectrum of disease which develops in response to an as yet undetermined stimulus. Subgroups of patients with either BD or ROU may have abnormalities of immunoglobulin concentrations, and perhaps the immunogenetic factors controlling immunoglobulin production also determine those variable genital and nonmucosal manifestations of BD which are absent in ROU. If this is correct, then the question that must be raised is whether the various immunoglobulin alterations are directly responsible for the clinical manifestations or are they merely a result of nonspecifically activated B lymphocytes?

Secretory Immunoglobulins

In attempts to understand the possible role of immunoglobulin alterations in producing the mucosal lesions, investigators have studied immunoglobulin concentrations in saliva (Table 1). The IgA levels in mixed saliva of patients with BD[9] and ROU[12] do not differ significantly from those of normal controls. However, when parotid saliva was separately collected and examined, a decrease in the secretion rate with resultant decrease in the total IgA produced by the parotid gland was noted in patients with the arthritic and ocular forms of BD and less so in the mucocutaneous type.[9] Furthermore, while the total IgA level in saliva may be normal despite the diminished parotid contribution, the IgA may be qualitatively abnormal. Saliva examined from 4 patients with BD, 4 with ROU, and 12 controls revealed a markedly decreased level of secretory component, in both its free and bound forms, in the saliva of the BD patients.[14] Secretory IgA, which is responsible for mucous membrane host defense, is composed of a dimer of serum IgA, a J-chain, and a polypeptide known as the secretory component. Abdou and colleagues[14] hypothesized that a deficiency of secretory component may lead to impaired mucous membrane defense and allow the entrance of antigens into the tissues to trigger the immune response with resultant oral ulceration.

Determinations of immunoglobulin levels in lacrimal fluid have also been performed (Table 1). Sculley and coworkers[9] noted significantly increased amounts of IgA in the lacrimal fluid of patients with BD, specifically those with the ocular and arthritic forms of the disease. These authors noted a positive correlation between the lacrimal and serum IgA levels in their patients, and a negative correlation between the salivary and lacrimal IgA levels. Lacrimal IgA levels in patients with ROU were normal. Lacrimal fluid IgG was increased in both the patients with BD and those with ROU, but the increase did not reach statistical significance for either group. Lacrimal fluid IgM was significantly increased in both groups, especially the ocular BD cases. Although the ocular pathology in BD rarely involves the conjuctiva,[15] the lacrimal fluid immunoglobulin elevations may reflect intraocular pathology.[9] In addition, the elevated immunoglobulins in the lacrimal fluid may protect the ocular conjuctiva while the oral mucosal lesions may develop secondary to a deficiency of IgA in the parotid fluid.

Cerebrospinal Fluid Immunoglobulins

Behçet's disease often involves the central nervous system and measurements of cerebrospinal fluid (CSF) immunoglobulins have been performed by various investigators. Elevated CSF IgA and to a lesser extent IgG in patients with neuro-Behçet's have been noted,[16] while elevations of serum IgA are also common in patients with the neurological complications. One must, however, distinguish between elevated CSF immunoglobulins due to leakage through an impaired blood-brain barrier and that due to increased intrathecal synthesis.[17] Simultaneous serum and CSF IgM, IgA, and IgG were measured in 12 patients with neurological involvement secondary to BD during periods in which the neuropsychiatric manifestations were either active or quiescent. CSF IgM levels were increased in 10 patients, IgA levels were increased in 11, and IgG levels were increased in 6. When an index of CSF immunoglobulin production was derived using the simultaneous serum values, an increased CSF IgM index was noted in the patients with active neurological Behçet's disease. Since the IgG and IgA indices were normal in the neuro-Behçet's patients despite elevations of CSF IgG or IgA, only isolated increased intrathecal IgM production occurred in active neuro-Behçet's.[17] An elevated IgM index was not observed in either the patients without BD or those with BD without neurological involvement. In addition, the IgM index has been shown to decrease in BD with successful treatment of the central nervous system manifestations. However, this index was not specific for neuro-Behçet's, since it has been reported elevated in infectious meningoencephalitis.[18]

Circulating Immune Complexes

Cryoglobulins are immunoglobulins that have the unusual physicochemical characteristic of reversibly precipitating at low temperatures,[19] and their detection reflects the presence of circulating immune complexes (CIC). Cryoglobulins can consist of a monoclonal protein or two or more types of immunoglobulins (mixed); and they have been associated with various infectious, autoimmune, and lymphoproliferative disorders. Investigators have searched for cryoglobulins in BD patients with variable results. In one series of six patients, cryoglobulins were not detected,[20] but in an isolated case report, a mixed (IgA and IgG) cryoglobulinemia was noted in a patient with BD and a pericardial effusion. The cryoglobulin titer correlated directly with the disease activity.[21] Lehner,[22] however, found that 64% of his patients with ROU and 75% of the BD patients had cold precipitating immunoglobulins when serum was allowed to clot at 37°C for four hours followed by storage at 4°C for seven days.[22] Cryoglobulins were found in all four forms of BD (mucocutaneous, arthritic, neurological, ocular), and serial studies demonstrated a positive correlation between remissions or exacerbations and decreases or increases of IgM or IgG type cryoglobulins. In contrast, a negative correlation was seen between disease activity and cold precipitable IgA.[22] While cryoglobulins in patients without BD often demonstrate rheumatoid factor activity (IgM directed against IgG), rheumatoid factor is unusual in the sera of patients with BD.

There are various other techniques that may be more sensitive measures of CIC than testing for cold insoluble proteins. The Raji cell assay as well as the Clq binding assay measure different size CIC; in one study,[23] 44% of BD cases had a positive Raji cell assay, while 50% had a positive Clq assay. The presence of CIC did not correlate either with the duration of disease or specific organ involvement, but did correlate with an index of disease activity.[23] In another investigation,[22] measurement of the inhibition of agglutination of IgG or IgM-coated latex particles demonstrated IgG type complexes in 52% of the 42 patients with ROU and 59% of the 64 patients with BD. In the ROU group, there was a trend to increased levels of IgG CIC with increasing severity of the ulcerations. In BD, the arthritic, neurological, and ocular forms had a slightly greater prevalence of IgG CIC than the mucocutaneous form. IgA-type CIC were found in 40% of the ROU and 47% of the BD cases. In the ROU patients, the herpetiform ulceration group had the lowest prevalence of IgA CIC. In BD, the neurological group had the highest prevalence, while the other three groups had basically normal mean levels although there was marked overlap of the individual values. With the application of the Clq assay, only 5% of the ROU and 20% of the BD patients had detectable CIC with the highest prevalence being in the neurological and ocular groups. As in the studies of cryoglobulins, a direct correlation of IgM or IgG CIC and a negative correlation of IgA CIC with clinical activity were noted in patients with BD. The investigators did not attempt to correlate the size of the CIC with the particular organ manifestations.[22] It is not surprising that more patients did not demonstrate CIC, since there are well-recognized limitations in the sensitivity of the various quantitative assays. Also, the different prevalence rates of CIC in the various forms of ROU and BD may reflect the underlying genetic control of immunoregulation and the different HLA types of the study samples.

Whenever CIC are demonstrated, the question arises whether they have an integral function in the pathogenesis of the disease or merely represent epiphenomena of the pathological process. Several of the above studies have correlated levels of CIC with disease activity, and although these data are suggestive, there is no conclusive proof that the immune complexes produce the disease manifestations. However, the differential prevalence rates of the various immune complexes among the subgroups of BD also suggest a role for the CIC in the production of specific organ dysfunction. Uveitis has been associated with other classical immune complex diseases; and one study[24] noted an increase in the CIC in a patient with ocular BD immediately before and during the early phase of disease exacerbation; but this, too, is only circumstantial evidence for the pathogenetic role of immune complexes. In one case report[25] an infant developed transient mucocutaneous lesions resembling Behçet's, presumably secondary to transplacental transfer of a factor (? IgG) from his mother who had BD; however, immunoglobulins and CIC were not measured in the infant.

Immune Complex Deposition

In order to further understand the role of CIC, tissue studies have also been performed in BD. In an unusual case of both lung and renal involvement in BD, glomerulonephritis and pulmonary vasculitis were histologically demonstrated in tissue sections.[26] IgG, C3, and fibrinogen deposits were noted in renal and pulmonary specimens, and CIC were detected by Raji cell assay. Thus, the histologic hallmark of BD is a vasculitis, probably immune-complex-mediated, principally involving veins, venules, and capillaries. Another study,[27] which examined oral ulcerations and erythema nodosum-like lesions in a patient with BD, demonstrated the presence of inflammatory infiltrates as well as IgM deposition and positive immunofluorescence to antistreptococcal group D sera in the vessel walls. Additionally, IgM and IgG deposits have been detected in vascular walls, especially venules, in the cutaneous lesions of a patient with BD.[28] Williams and Lehner[29] performed immunofluorescent studies on oral lesions in ROU and BD and noted similar findings with C3± IgM in vessel walls; patients with nonaphthous oral lesions did not demonstrate these deposits. However, complement and immunoglobulin deposition have been documented in apparently normal mucosa by at least one investigator.[13]

Pathergy

Pathergy, also called the needle-stick reaction, is a common, but nonspecific clinical finding in BD which is characterized by the development of pustular vasculitic lesions 24 hours after trauma to the skin.[30] The importance of immune complexes in the development of these lesions has been suggested by the histamine trap test in which a baseline skin biopsy was performed followed by a repeat biopsy four hours after the intradermal injection of histamine. In one study, Jorizzo et al.[2] studied five patients with BD and detected CIC in one of five by Raji cell and zero of five by the Clq assay. Baseline skin biopsies were performed in five patients and five controls after which histamine was injected into two sites. Biopsy of one site four hours after injection revealed deposition of immunoglobulin and/or C3 in all five patients and in none of the controls. Examination of the other site at 24 hours revealed trace purpura in the BD patients. Light microscopy of these experimentally induced lesions revealed a true leukocytoclastic vasculitis (endothelial swelling of dermal blood vessels, polymorphonuclear [PMN] cells within vessel walls, fibrinoid necrosis, and leukocytoclasis or disruption of PMN) in one patient and a "pathergy-like" picture in the other four (endothelial swelling and PMN accumulation without leukocytoclasis or fibrinoid necrosis). These histologic findings were similar to the spontaneously formed classic pustular lesions of BD.[2] The same group of investigators later reported similar findings of variable deposits of Clq, fibrin, IgM, and C3 in biopsies performed after histamine injection in patients with BD prior to initiating thalidomide therapy.[31] In this later study, Jorizzo et al.[31] commented on the histologic similarity of the lesions to those seen in Sweet's vasculitis (neutrophilic vascular reaction) which resembled leukocytoclastic vasculitis except for the absence of fibrinoid necrosis. A pathergy-like phenomenon has also been described in the synovium of patients with BD.[32] In essence, the above histologic studies have implicated the role of immune complexes in the pathogenesis of at least the cutaneous manifestations of BD. In addition, since synovitis, uveitis, and meningoencephalitis occur in various disorders marked by immune complex deposition, CIC may contribute to these clinical manifestations in BD.

Chemotaxis and Immunoglobulin

In addition to the deposition of immune complexes, an increase in PMN chemotaxis which characterizes BD has been postulated to contribute to the pathergy phenomenon. In various experiments, sera from patients with BD produced increased chemotaxis of normal PMN while the Behçet's PMN failed to demonstrate increased chemotaxis when exposed to control sera.[2] Enhanced granulocyte chemotaxis was noted in Behçet's, while in contrast, normal chemotaxis was observed in patients with ROU.[33] However, polymorphonuclear cells (PMN) from Behçet's patients demonstrated increased chemotaxis when exposed to either pooled AB serum or autologous serum,[33] while inulin stimulation of PMN from Behçet's failed to produce increased chemotaxis compared to controls.[34] Other studies have demonstrated a cytoplasmic factor in the Behçet's PMN which increased chemotaxis of normal PMN although this factor may have been an absorbed serum factor.[35] While the majority of the studies have noted increased chemotaxis in BD secondary to a serum factor, experiments of the phagocytic capabilities of the PMN have shown variable results.[36] A strong negative correlation was observed between PMN chemotaxis in BD and the level of IgA cryoglobulins during inulin activation studies, while a positive correlation was noted between chemotaxis and IgG cryoglobulin levels. Additionally, when normal PMN were exposed to IgA complexes, a concentration-dependent depression of chemotaxis was noted; and thus investigators have postulated that IgA immune complexes blocked the PMN chemotaxis receptors and impaired the clearance of other immune complexes responsible for tissue damage.[34] An additional study[37] of the effects of various immune complexes on normal neutrophil chemotaxis also concluded that IgA immune complexes did indeed have a suppressive effect.

Complement Activity and Immunoglobulin

One possible mechanism by which immune complexes can affect chemotaxis is by activating the complement cascade. Immune complexes containing IgM or IgG can activate the cascade through the classic pathway, producing C3a and C5a, both chemotactic factors. In contrast, IgA complexes cannot activate the classic pathway. In light of the previous discussion of the effects of immune complexes on chemotaxis in BD, IgM and IgG immune complexes may promote PMN migration by activating complement while IgA complexes may have a suppressant chemotactic effect by their inability to activate complement.[34] Moreover, the C3b receptors are under genetic control and variability in the number of these receptors in BD may be one other factor responsible for altered chemotaxis.

The previously discussed histologic studies have documented C3 deposition in various tissues in BD, suggesting that complement activation may contribute to the pathogenesis of the lesions. Additionally, electron microscopic examination of CIC and membrane fragments in the sera of patients with BD has disclosed 10 nm holes in these fragments.[38] These holes appeared identical to those produced by complement activation in other diseases, again suggesting complement activation in BD. Studies of various complement components in the sera of patients with BD, however, have failed to conclusively document consumption of these components. Normal CH50 levels may occur in patients with BD,[8] and in one study[39] of 15 patients with BD and 17 patients with rheumatoid arthritis (RA); serum C3, C4, and CH50 were normal or elevated in the two patient groups compared to control specimens. The level of disease activity in these patients, however, was not mentioned. Synovial fluid C3, C4, and CH50 were also determined in the two groups of patients and the values were higher in BD than in RA. The normal serum to synovial fluid complement ratio was 3:1. In the BD patients, the ratio of serum to synovial fluid CH50, C3, or C4 averaged 2, while in RA the average ratio was 4, suggesting less complement consumption in the inflamed synovium of BD than in RA.[39] Complement activation may still be occurring when the serum C3 and C4 levels are normal if the changes in concentrations are not significant enough to fall outside the "normal range." The complement proteins behave as acute-phase reactants with increased production occurring in inflammatory conditions, and elevated levels of C9 in the serum have, in fact, been documented in active BD and ROU.[40] In one study, the elevation of C9 plasma levels correlated with disease activity, whereas normalization of C9 concentration occurred during periods of disease quiescence.[41] Similarly, Factor B, which is involved in the alternate pathway of complement activation, has also been found to be increased in active BD, especially the neurological type. Increased Factor B was rarely observed in ROU.[40] Therefore, complement activation may be occurring in BD, but the increased rate of production of the components due to inflammation may equal or exceed the increased rate of consumption, thereby maintaining normal or elevated serum levels. Since a low transitional value of CH50 may be observed immediately prior to an ocular flare of BD, complement activation may indeed have an important role in the pathogenesis of the acute attack.[42]

Antigen Characterization

In order to further characterize the immunological phenomena occurring in BD, investigators[43] have attempted to identify the antigens present in the CIC. The CIC of 18 patients with BD and 7 with ROU were isolated, and the immune complexes after being disassociated were permitted to cross-react. The

CIC of one patient with BD cross-reacted with the CIC of the other 17 patients with Behçet's, but only with one of the non-Behçet's patients, thus suggesting a common antigen contained within the immune complexes in BD. Moreover, the immune complexes of two other patients with BD cross-reacted with two different subgroups of Behçet's patients, suggesting that different antigens in addition to a common antigen were present in the sera of subgroups of BD patients.[43] In a recent abstract, Mowbray[44] updated his original work and confirmed the presence of IgG complexes of two major antigenic types associated with different clinical presentations as well as having detected an antigen common to all patients tested with BD. To date, studies to identify the common and group-specific antigens precisely have been unsuccessful.[44]

Autoantibodies

In addition to directly identifying the antigens in the immune complexes, investigators have searched for the presence of antibodies to self antigens. Generally, antinuclear antibodies (ANA) were not found in BD,[8] although 6% of the Behçet's patients in one study had a low ANA titer.[45] None of the 50 patients had antibodies to native DNA, histones, and Sm, RNP, SSB or Scl-70 antigens.[45] In 1963, using the tanned red cell hemagglutination technique, autoantibodies against oral mucous membrane were detected in 17 of 40 (42%) Behçet's patients, 4 of 25 patients with other diseases, and 0 of 18 healthy controls.[6] The titer of the antibody increased before disease flares and was often negative during remission. In 1965, the low titer (1:2 to 1:8) antibody to guinea pig lip cytoplasmic antigen was found in 8 of 8 definite Behçet's patients, but only 3 of 60 other patients[46]; however, the significance of this antibody was unknown.

In 1967, tests for antibodies to fetal oral mucosa in patients with BD and ROU used the three techniques of hemagglutination, complement fixation, and Ouchterlony's precipitation.[47] The results were stratified according to the type of ulceration present (aphthous or herpetiform). The hemagglutination test detected antibody at a titer of 1:80 to 1:640 in 18 of 21 (85%) Behçet's patients regardless of the type of ulceration. Of the patients with

ROU, 30% of the herpetiform and 70% of the focal aphthous types had positive titers. In comparison to the hemmagglutination assay, the complement fixation and precipitation tests detected a lower number of positive results in each group. Of note, 100% of the Behçet's patients with ocular involvement had a positive antibody titer by hemagglutination. Lehner[47] postulated that it was unlikely for the antibodies to develop in response to nonspecific muscosal damage since he could not detect significant antibody levels in patients with other diseases and ulcerating mouth lesions. In contrast, O'Duffy[8] detected anticytoplasmic antibodies in five of five Behçet's patients using an indirect immunofluorescent technique with human cadaver esophageal cells as substrate but doubted that these antibodies had a causative role despite the absence of a positive test in 20 controls.

In support of a possible infectious etiology for Behçet's disease, antibodies to various bacteria have been examined.[48] Serum antibodies to *Streptococcus salivarius* have been found in elevated titers in Behçet's and recurrent aphthous stomatitis patients, and immunofluorescent studies have implicated group D streptococcal antigen in the oral ulcerations of BD.[36,48]

Since ocular and neurological involvement may occur in BD, investigators have researched for antibodies directed at ocular or neural tissue. One study[49] noted antiretinal antibodies in low titer in ocular Behçet's and two other forms of posterior uveitis believed to be autoimmune in origin. Two Japanese studies[50,51] have examined antibodies to various glycolipids which may function as receptors on cell surfaces or recognition sites for cell-to-cell interaction. Antibodies against glycolipids have been described in autoimmune diseases (such as SLE), neoplastic diseases, and multiple sclerosis. Investigators, using an assay based on complement-mediated lysis of liposomes containing various glycolipids, evaluated sera from patients with Behçet's and healthy controls.[51] Among both groups they found low titer antibodies to several glycosphingolipids present on human red blood cell membranes, but the patients had a higher incidence and titer of antibodies to GA-2, GA-1, GM-1, and GM-3. GA-2 is normally found on guinea pig erythroctyes, GM-3 on equine erythrocytes, GA-1 on mouse NK cells, and GM-1 is present in human brain tissue. There was no apparent correlation of the antibody titer with either the organ system involved or the disease activity.[51] Inaba and Aoyama[50] examined antibodies against various gangliosides (glycolipids containing sialic acid often found on cell surface membranes of neural tissue), including GM-1, GM-2, and GM-4. Serum antibodies against these three glycolipids have been found in multiple sclerosis, while antibodies directed against GA-1 (asialo GM-1) have been detected in SLE with cerebral involvement. This group used ELISA tests to assay for antibodies to gangliosides in Behçet's patients with neurological involvement, Behçet's without neurological signs, other neurological or collagen diseases, and healthy controls. They noted a significantly greater incidence of IgM antibodies to GM-1 and GA-1 in the neuro-Behçet's cases compared to the other diseases. Employing a complement fixation assay, they studied the anti-GA1 antibodies and found high titers in the neuro-Behçet's patients as well as one patient with multiple sclerosis and one with SLE. Only 7 of 36 (19%) nonneurological Behçet's patients had elevated titers compared to 91% of the neuro-Behçet group. A temporary fall in antibody titer was noted prior to exacerbations in some patients.[50] Both groups of investigators[50,51] commented on the variety of technical difficulties in their assays, but both studies demonstrated the presence of antibodies against antigens on neural membranes although a cause and effect relationship was not confirmed.

Several other antibody systems have been examined in Behçet's disease. In one study, antibodies to lipopolysaccharide (endotoxin) were elevated in Behçet's compared to healthy controls, but the antibodies were also present in patients with SLE and rheumatoid arthritis. Additionally, antibodies have been isolated from synovial fluid in Behçet's cases, but the clinical significance of this finding was not known.[52] Antibodies to 10 nm intermediate filaments of the cytoskeleton have also been detected in 47% of Behçet's patients. However, these antibodies were found in 35% of RA patients, 16% of SLE patients, and 9% of the controls. While the antibody titer correlated with the C-reactive protein level and disease activity, it was nonetheless a nonspecific finding.[53]

Recently an association has been recognized between anticardiolipin antibodies and vascular thrombosis in SLE. In view of the high incidence of thrombophlebitis in Behçet's, two British studies[54,55] examined antibodies to cardiolipin, a phospholipid related to sphingomyelin, in a series of Behçet's cases. In one study of

25 Behçet's patients with superficial thrombophlebitis, 60% of the patients had a major vessel thrombosis.[54] Only two of the 25 cases (8%) had antibodies to cardiolipin and neither of these patients had documented cerebral, pulmonary, or retinal vascular disease or deep vein thrombosis. Of note, 22 of the 25 were on corticosteroids or immunosuppressives known to suppress antibodies to cardiolipin. The other study,[55] using the same technique and criteria for diagnosis of Behçet's, examined 70 patients from three centers. Thirteen of the 70 had cardiolipin antibodies, either IgG (7), IgM (3), or both (3). Seven of the 13 had retinal vascular disease, two of 13 had thrombophlebitis (superficial or deep), and one had a cerebral infarction. Using fluorescein angiography, 54% of the antibody-positive patients had retinal vascular disease compared to 23% of the antibody negative; and thus, there was a significant statistical difference. While the second study[55] did demonstrate a correlation of anticardiolipin antibodies with retinal vascular disease, neither study demonstrated a significant correlation with pulmonary, cerebral, or deep vein thrombosis. In contrast to the SLE patients who had cardiolipin antibodies, none of the Behçet's patients was noted to have a positive VDRL test.[55]

Acute-Phase Reactants

Many of the immunological phenomena (circulating immune complexes, cryoglobulin, antibodies to oral mucosa) already mentioned have been found to correlate generally with Behçet's disease activity. These tests were not routinely performed by all investigators and were often studied only on a research basis. Two commonly available laboratory tests, the erythrocyte sedimentation rate (ESR) and C-reactive protein (CRP) level, also correlated with disease activity in at least some patients with Behçet's. Most review articles on Behçet's have commented on the elevated ESR. Oshima[6] noted an increased ESR in 60% of his patients, and O'Duffy[8] noted an elevated ESR in 8 of his 9 patients not on corticosteroids. In a review of 41 cases, an elevated ESR was noted during many exacerbations of disease activity, and the ESR became normal during remissions.[20] Adinolfi and colleagues[40] were often able to correlate ESR levels with disease activity in the mucocutaneous, arthritic, and ocular forms of Behçet's, as well a: the major type of ROU; however, neuro-Behçet's disease activit' did not correlate with the ESR. In contrast, in a recent prospectiv(study of 150 patients with Behçet's, an elevated ESR was as sociated with erythema nodosum, thrombophlebitis, and acut(arthritis; but this association was absent in those with th(mucocutaneous, ocular, and neurological manifestations.[56]

Although C-reactive protein is normally present in the plasm; in trace amounts, CRP commonly acts as an acute-phase reactant In Oshima's series, 45% had an elevated C-reactive protein.' Adinolfi et al.[40] noted that 30% of the herpetiform type of ROU anc 50% of the Behçet's cases, especially those with the mucocutane ous, arthritic, and ocular types, had elevated CRP levels, wherea: the neuro-Behçet's patients rarely had elevated values. Müf tüoğlu[56] recently reported the results of his prospective study not ing an association between qualitatively elevated CRP levels anc erythema nodosum or acute thrombophlebitis in BD. When quan titative CRP levels were performed in 50 patients, increases ir clinical disease activity were accompanied by slight to moderat(rises in CRP and ESR in many, but not all, of the patients. None o the patients in "complete remission" was noted to have an ele vated CRP level.[56]

Conclusion

Several aberrations in the humoral immune system have beer described in patients with Behçet's disease. While some of the im munological alterations appear to correlate with clinical diseas(activity, the precise role of the humoral immune system in produc ing the clinical manifestations remains to be established. Studie: of the cellular immune functions may contribute further insigh into the role of humoral immunity in the pathogenesis of Behçet': disease.

References

1. Katz P. Clinical and laboratory evaluation of the immune system
   Med Clin North Am 1985; 69:453–464.

2. Jorizzo JL, Hudson RD, Schmalstieg FC, et al. Behçet's syndrome: Immune regulation, circulating immune complexes, neutrophil migration, and colchicine therapy. *J Am Acad Dermatol* 1984; 10:205–214.
3. Suzuki N, Sakane T, Ueda Y, Tsunematsu T. Abnormal B cell function in patients with Behçet's disease. *Arthritis Rheum* 1986; 29:212–219.
4. Stobo JD. Lymphocytes: Structure and function. In McCarty DJ, ed: *Arthritis and Allied Conditions. A Textbook of Rheumatology.* Philadelphia, Lea & Febiger, 1985:309–323.
5. Valesini G, Pivetti-Pezzi P, Mastrandrea F, Moncada A. Evaluation of T cell subsets in Behçet's syndrome using anti-T cell monoclonal antibodies. *Clin Exp Immunol* 1985; 60:55–60.
6. Oshima Y, Shimizu T, Yokohari R, et al. Clinical studies on Behçet's syndrome. *Ann Rheum Dis* 1963; 22:36–45.
7. Kalbian VV, Challis MT. Behçet's disease. Report of twelve cases with three manifesting as papilledema. *Am J Med* 1970; 49:823–829.
8. O'Duffy JD, Carney JA, Deodhar S. Behçet's disease. Report of 10 cases, 3 with new manifestations. *Ann Intern Med* 1971; 75:561–570.
9. Scully CM, Lehner T, Harfitt R. Serum, salivary and lacrimal immunoglobulins in Behçet's syndrome and recurrent oral ulcers. In Lehner T, Barnes CG, eds: *Behçet's Syndrome. Clinical and Immunological Features. Proceedings of a Conference Sponsored by the Royal Society of Medicine, February 1979.* London, Academic Press, 1979:77–89.
10. Aoki K. Studies on plasma protein in Behçet's disease. *Jpn J Ophthal* 1972; 16:93–98.
11. Chamberlain MA. Behçet's syndrome in 32 patients in Yorkshire. *Ann Rheum Dis* 1977; 36:491–499.
12. Ben-Aryeh H, Malberger E, Gutman D, et al: Salivary IgA and serum IgG and IgA in recurrent aphthous stomatitis. *Oral Surg Oral Med Oral Pathol* 1976; 42:746–752.
13. Editorial. Aphthous immunology. *Lancet* 1978; 2:412–413.
14. Abdou NI, Schumacher HR, Colman RW, et al. Behçet's disease: Possible role of secretory component deficiency, synovial inclusions, and fibrinolytic abnormality in the various manifestations of the disease. *J Lab Clin Med* 1978; 91:409–422.
15. Colvard DM, Robertson DM, O'Duffy JD. The ocular manifestations of Behçet's disease. *Arch Ophthalmol* 1977; 95:1813–1817.
16. Aoyama J, Inaba G, Shimizu T. Third complement component in cerebrospinal fluid in neuro-Behçet's syndrome. Conversion patterns by crossed immunoelectropheresis. *J Neurol Sci* 1979; 41:183–190.
17. Hirohata S, Takeuchi A, Miyamato T. Association of cerebrospinal fluid IgM index with central nervous system involvement in Behçet's disease. *Arthritis Rheum* 1986; 29:793–796.
18. Sindic CJM, Cambiaso CL, Depré A, et al. The concentration of IgM in the cerebrospinal fluid of neurological patients. *J Neurol Sci* 1982; 55:339–350.

19. Rodman GP, Schumacher HR, Zvaifler AJ, eds. Cryoglobulinemia. In *Primer on the Rheumatic Diseases*. Atlanta, Arthritis Foundation, 1983:82–83.
20. Chajek T, Fainaru M. Behçet's disease. Report of 41 cases and a review of the literature. *Medicine* 1975; 54:179–196.
21. Scarlett JA, Kistner MI, Yang LC. Behçet's syndrome. Report of a case associated with pericardinal effusion and cryoglobulinemia treated with indomethacin. *Am J Med* 1979; 66:146–148.
22. Levinsky RJ, Paganelli R, Lehner T. Immune complexes and their characterization in Behçet's syndrome and recurrent oral ulcers. In Lehner T, Barnes CG, eds: *Behçet's Syndrome. Clinical and Immunological Features. Proceedings of a Conference Sponsored by the Royal Society of Medicine, February 1979*. London, Academic Press, 1979:33–43.
23. Gupta RC, O'Duffy JD, McDuffe FC, et al. Circulating immune complexes in active Behçet's disease. *Clin Exp Immunol* 1978; 34:213–218.
24. Inoue T, Oniki S. Kajiyama K, Jimi S. Circulating immune complexes in Behçet's disease. *Jpn J Ophthalmol* 1983; 27:35–39.
25. Fam AG, Siminovitch KA, Carette S, From L. Neonatal Behçet's syndrome in an infant of a mother with the disease. *Ann Rheum Dis* 1981; 40:509–512.
26. Gamble CN, Wiesner KB, Shapiro RF, Boyer WJ. The immune complex pathogenesis of glomerulonephritis and pulmonary vasculitis in Behçet's disease. *Am J Med* 1979; 66:1031–1039.
27. Kaneko F, Takahashi Y, Muramatsu Y, Miura Y. Immunological studies on aphthous ulcer and erythema nodosum-like eruptions in Behcet's disease. *Br J Dermatol* 1985; 113:303–312.
28. Reimer G, Luckner L, Hornstein OP. Direct immunofluorescence in recurrent aphthous ulcers and Behçet's disease. *Dermatologica* 1983; 167:293–298.
29. Williams BD, Lehner T. Immune complexes in Behçet's syndrome and recurrent oral ulceration. *Br Med J* 1977; 1:1387–1389.
30. Haim S. Pathogenesis of lesions in Behçet's disease. *Dermatologica* 1979; 158:31–37.
31. Jorizzo JL, Schmalstieg FC, Solomon AR, et al. Thalidomide effects in Behçet's syndrome and pustular vasculitis. *Arch Intern Med* 1986; 146:878–881.
32. Giacomello A, Taccari E, Zoppini A. Marked synovial sensitivity to pricking in Behçet's syndrome. *Arthritis Rheum* 1980; 23:259–260.
33. Djawari D, Hornstein OP, Schötz J. Enhancement of granulocyte chemotaxis in Behçet's disease. *Arch Dermatol Res* 1981; 270:81–88.
34. Abdulla YH, Lehner T. The effect of immune complexes on chemotaxis in Behçet's syndrome and recurrent oral ulcers. In Lehner T, Barnes CG, eds: *Behçet's Syndrome. Clinical and Immunological Features. Proceedings of a Conference Sponsored by the Royal Society of Medicine, February 1979*. London, Academic Press, 1979:55–66.

35. Takeuchi A, Kobayashi K, Mori M, Mizushima Y. Mechanism of hyperchemotaxis in Behçet's disease. *J Rheumatol* 1981; 8:40-44.
36. O'Duffy JD, Lehner T, Barnes CG. Summary of third international conference in Behçet's disease. Tokyo, Japan, October 23-24, 1981. *J Rheumatol* 1983; 10:154-158.
37. Ito S, Mikawa H, Shinomiya K, Yoshida T. Suppressive effect of IgA soluble immune complexes on neutrophil chemotaxis. *Clin Exp Immunol* 1979; 37:436-440.
38. Lehner T, Almeida JD, Levinsky RJ. Damaged membrane fragments and immune complexes in the blood of patients with Behçet's syndrome. *Clin Exp Immunol* 1978; 34:206-212.
39. Hamza M'H, Ayed K, el Euch M, et al. Synovial fluid complement levels in Behçet's disease (letter). *Ann Rheum Dis* 1984; 43:767.
40. Adinolfi M, Beck SE, Lehner T. Serum levels of acute phase proteins, C9, factor B and lysozyme in Behçet's syndrome and recurrent oral ulcers. In Lehner T, Barnes, CG, eds: *Behçet's Syndrome. Clinical and Immunological Features. Proceedings of a Conference Sponsored by the Royal Society of Medicine, February 1979.* London, Academic Press, 1979:107-125.
41. Rumfeld WR, Morgan BD, Campbell AK. The ninth complement component in rheumatoid arthritis, Behçet's disease and other rheumatic diseases. *Br J Rheumatol* 1986; 25:266-270.
42. Kogure M, Shimada K, Hara H. Complement titer in patient with Behçet's disease. *Acta Soc Ophthalmol Jpn* 1971; 75:1260-1268.
43. Burton-Kee EJ, Lehner T, Mowbray JF. Antigens in circulating immune complexes of Behçet's syndrome. In Lehner T, Barnes CG, eds: *Behçet's Syndrome. Clinical and Immunological Features. Proceedings of a Conference Sponsored by the Royal Society of Medicine, February 1979.* London, Academic Press, 1979:45-54.
44. Mowbray JF. Immune complexes and complement in Behçet's disease (abstract 17). Royal Society of Medicine international conference on Behçet's disease, September 5 and 6 1985, London, England.
45. Moroi Y, Takeuchi A, Mori M, et al. Antinuclear antibody in Behçet's disease (letter). *J Rheumatol* 1982; 9:809-810.
46. Shimizu T, Katsuta Y, Oshima Y. Immunological studies on Behçet's syndrome. *Ann Rheum Dis* 1965; 24:494-499.
47. Lehner T. Behçet's syndrome and autoimmunity. *Br Med J* 1967; 1:465-467.
48. Nagumo M, Sakurada S, Hayashi Y, Kakuta S. The interaction of leukocytes and oral bacteria in the pathogenesis of recurrent aphthous ulcerations. In Inaba G, ed: *Behçet's disease. Pathogenetic Mechanism and Clinical Future. Proceedings of the International Conference on Behçet's Disease, October 23-24, 1981, Tokyo.* Tokyo, University of Tokyo Press, 1982:291-300.
49. Chan C-C, Palestine AG, Nussenblatt RB, et al: Anti-retinal autoantibodies in Vogt-Koyanagi-Harada syndrome, Behçet's disease, and sympathetic ophthalmia. *Ophthalmology* 1985; 92:1025-1028.
50. Inaba G, Aoyama J. Anti-glycolipid antibodies in neuro-Behçet's

syndrome. In Inaba G, ed: *Behçet's Disease. Pathogenetic Mechanism and Clinical Future. Proceedings of the International Conference on Behçet's Disease, October 23–24, 1981, Tokyo.* Tokyo, University of Tokyo Press, 1982:145–152.

51. Yasuda T, Ueno J, Matuhasi T. Antiglycolipid antibodies in Behçet's disease. In Inaba G, ed: *Behçet's Disease. Pathogenetic Mechanism and Clinical Future. Proceedings of the International Conference on Behçet's Disease, October 23–24, 1981, Tokyo.* Tokyo, University of Tokyo Press, 1982:413–420.

52. Noguchi Y, Furusawa S. Study of anti-LPS antibodies in Behçet's disease. In Inaba G, ed: *Behçet's disease. Pathogenetic Mechanism and Clinical Future. Proceedings of the International Conference on Behçet's Disease, October 23–24, 1981, Tokyo.* Tokyo, University of Tokyo Press, 1982:369–375.

53. Akoğlu T, Kozokoğlu H, Akoğlu E, Erken E. Antibody to intermediate filaments of the cytoskeleton in patients with Behçet's disease (abstract 21). Royal Society of Medicine international conference on Behçet's disease, September 5 and 6, 1985, London, England.

54. Efthimiou J, Harris EN, Hughes GRV. Negative anticardiolipin antibodies and vascular complications in Behçet's syndrome (letter). *Ann Rheum Dis* 1985; 44:725–726.

55. Hull RG, Harris EN, Gharavi AE, et al. Anticardiolipin antibodies: Occurrence in Behçet's syndrome. *Ann Rheum Dis* 1984; 43:746–748.

56. Müftüoğlu AÜ, Yazici H, Yurdahul S, et al. Behçet's disease. Relation of serum C-reactive protein and erythrocyte sedimentation rates to disease activity. *Int J Dermatol* 1986; 25:235–239.

4

IMMUNOLOGY: CELL-MEDIATED IMMUNE SYSTEM

Scott Dinehart and Joseph L. Jorizzo

ACTIVE RESEARCH HAS REVEALED NUMEROUS aberrations and dysfunctions of cell-mediated immunity in patients with Behçet's syndrome. Considerable dispute exists as to whether these are primary or secondary events. Intricate and complex interactions between cell-mediated immunity, effector cells, and humoral immunity make this determination even more difficult. It is the purpose of this chapter to summarize, and when possible, to explain those changes in cell-mediated immunity that characterize Behçet's syndrome.

Skin Tests and Mitogenic Response of Lymphocytes

There is no in-vivo impairment of cell-mediated immunity in Behçet's syndrome as tested by intradermal delayed skin hypersensitivity with PPD, Candida, and streptokinase-streptodornase antigens.[1-5] Moreover, there have not been any reported increases in the incidence or severity of viral or fungal infections in patients with Behçet's syndrome who have not received immunosuppres-

From *Behcet's Disease: A Contemporary Synopsis*, edited by Gary R. Plotkin, M.D., John J. Calabro, M.D., and J. Desmond O'Duffy, M.B. © 1988, Futura Publishing Company, Inc., Mount Kisco, NY.

sive therapy. Enhanced delayed hypersensitivity skin reactions can also be observed when streptococcal vaccines are injected intradermally,[6,7] and an intact delayed hypersensitivity type of skin reaction to skin homogenates has been described by Haim et al.[8] However, diminished percentages of positive responses to the dinitrochlorobenzene (DNCB) patch test, an in-vivo measure of type IV hypersensitivity independent of intradermal injection, occurs in the order of decreasing frequency in patients with possible, suspected, incomplete, and complete types of Behçet's syndrome.[9] With respect to the enhanced cutaneous responses noted after the intradermal injection of certain antigens, these reactions may be related to the pathergy phenomenon which is proposed to occur by a nondelayed hypersensitivity mechanism.

In-vitro lymphocyte cultures have shown both decreased and normal transformation responses to standard mitogens, such as phytohemagglutinin or concavalin A.[3-5,8,10-13] Mixed lymphocyte response, using autologous B cells to stimulate T cells, has been found to be markedly diminished at the onset of disease exacerbations.[12] In addition, standard mixed lymphocyte culture response has also been shown to be depressed in patients with Behçet's syndrome.[2]

Searches for the role of specific antigens that may trigger the symptoms of Behçet's syndrome are critical to the understanding of the immunopathology of this disease. In an effort to incriminate specific provoking antigens, homogenates of oral mucosa have been shown to induce a significant transformation in lymphocytes from patients with Behçet's disease, but not in controls.[1,14] This evidence is not definitive proof of a causal relationship but may merely represent lymphocyte sensitization following nonspecific tissue injury. A reduced in-vitro T-cell reactivity to both walnut extract and candidal antigens in both Behçet's patients and controls is seen after ingestion of walnuts. Despite these findings, oral mucosal trauma, and not walnut hypersensitivity, is the probable precipitating event for the well-documented post-walnut flares characteristic of Behçet's syndrome.[15,16]

Peripheral Blood T Cells

T cells are intricately involved in Type IV hypersensitivity reactions and are considered to be the principal effectors of the cellular-mediated immune system. Numerous reports concerning quantitation and characterization of peripheral T lymphocytes by E rosettes and monoclonal antibodies have been published in patients with Behçet's syndrome, and the results of these studies are summarized in Table 1. The divergent findings may be related to differences in populations, techniques, or activity of the disease. The most consistent characteristics appear to be a decreased number of total peripheral T lymphocytes and a decreased T-cell helper to suppressor ratio. This decreased ratio is consistent with other in-vitro evidence for diminished cell-mediated immunity.[17] However, one disadvantage to these types of immunological studies is that relative cell numbers may not accurately reflect functional capability. One investigator has furthermore described diminished numbers of T cells but indicated that these cells may function at increased levels of activity.

Cytotoxicity, NK Cells, Interferon, Interleukin-2

Circulating lymphocytes that are cytotoxic for oral mucosa have been demonstrated in patients with Behçet's syndrome using a trypan blue dye exclusion macroassay.[18] Using a radiolabeled chromium release macroassay, others have confirmed the presence of antibody-independent lymphocytotoxicity.[19,20] It is possible that the positive lymphocytotoxicity is generated by sensitized lym-

Table 1

Abnormalities of T-Cell Subsets in the Peripheral Blood of Patients with Behçet's Syndrome

- Elevated or normal values for total T cells[3,5,8,10,40]
- Decreased helper T cells, increased suppressor T cells, decreased helper/suppressor ratio[12,41]
- Decreased helper T cells[42]
- Decreased total T cells, decreased helper T cells, decreased suppressor T cells, unchanged helper/suppressor ratio[43,44]
- Decreased helper T cells, increased suppressor T cells, decreased helper/suppressor ratio, increased natural killer cells[45]
- Decreased helper/suppressor ratio[4]
- Decreased total T cells[8,13]
- Decreased mature T cells, increased suppressor T cells, decreased helper/suppressor ratio, presence of immature T cells[46]

phocytes via specific recognition of antigenic structures on oral target cells.

Natural killer (NK) cells were originally discovered as naturally occurring cells that were cytotoxic to various tumor cell lines, and they have been shown to be responsible, in close collaboration with interferon and macrophages, for a variety of immunological phenomena. During ocular exacerbations of Behçet's syndrome, peripheral blood NK activity is decreased, and explanations for this immunological observation include the trapping of peripheral NK cells in the tissues and inhibition of NK activity by circulating immune complexes.[21]

Decreased peripheral blood NK activity during exacerbation of Behçet's syndrome as compared to normals and patients with inactive disease has been confirmed by Kaneko et al.[22] In this latter study, however, actual numbers of NK cells were increased in the peripheral blood of patients with active disease. Since the addition of gamma-interferon to these cells produced increased NK activity,[22] patients with active Behçet's syndrome may have adequate numbers of NK cells but lack a factor that activates them.

Interferons, which are proteins produced by lymphocytes as well as by other cells including lymphoblasts and fibroblasts, are potent stimulators of NK cells and have been implicated in the control of early viral infections. In patients with Behçet's syndrome, gamma-interferon is produced spontaneously by cultures of T lymphocytes and is detected in the peripheral circulation.[23–25] However, these findings are also observed in patients with Vogt-Koyanagi-Harada disease, but not in normal controls.[26] T lymphocytes from patients with Behçet's disease appear spontaneously to produce elevated levels of gamma-interferon independent of accessory cells, such as macrophages, or of serum factors. In addition, levels of gamma-interferon are dependent on disease activity, with higher values being seen during the convalescent stage.[24] The lower levels of gamma-interferon occurring during active disease may represent a failed attempt to increase NK cell activity.

Elevated levels of gamma-interferon are present in cultured cells of patients with viral infections and in the serum of patients with autoimmune diseases such as systemic lupus erythematosus.[26] Besides its well-defined role in control of viral infection, gamma-interferon also has many nonviral activities including immune regulation. The interaction of interferon with humoral immunity is now under intense investigation. There also is evidence that changes in circulating immune complexes (known to occur in Behçet's syndrome) may affect interferon activity. As a result of the abnormalities of interferon activity present in Behçet's syndrome, a viral or a viral-associated autoimmune pathogenesis of the disease has been postulated by various investigators. The definitive cause of the enhanced interferon production in Behçet's syndrome, however, remains unidentified.

Interleukin-2 (IL-2) or T-cell growth factor (TCGF) is synthesized by T cells activated by antigen or mitogen in the presence of interleukin-1. As a consequence of stimulation by IL-2, subpopulations of T cells possessing surface receptors for this lymphokine subsequently proliferate, resulting in the expansion of T cells with helper, suppressor, or cytotoxic functions.[27] T cells from patients with Behçet's disease have been shown to produce normal amounts of IL-2 in response to phytohemagglutinin stimulation; however, regardless of disease activity, the responsiveness to IL-2 was deficient in the concanavalin A-activated lymphoblasts. There also was a decreased number of T cells with IL-2 receptors in patients with early active Behçet's disease, while in those with either chronic active or inactive disease, there was diminution in the density of IL-2 receptors on the T cells. The inadequate response of T cells to IL-2 in Behçet's disease may contribute to the immunological abnormalities present in this disease.[28]

Leukocyte Inhibitory Factor and Macrophage Inhibitory Factor

Immobilization of phagocytes once they are present in an area of tissue inflammation occurs by various tissue mediators, including leukocyte migration inhibitory factor (LIF) and macrophage migration inhibitory factor (MIF). Produced by activated T lymphocytes, LIF and MIF are used as in-vitro parameters of cell-mediated immunity, and their functions may be related to delayed hypersensitivity in vivo. Anterior chamber fluid from Behçet's syndrome patients with ocular involvement contains higher levels of MIF than the anterior chamber fluid from control patients, and synovial fluid from Behçet's disease patients with articular involvement also inhibits macrophage migration. In addition, macrophage migration in serum has been shown to be abnormal in patients with Behçet's syndrome.[10,29,30]

When compared to normal controls, levels of LIF were reported diminished in 20 patients with active Behçet's disease.[31] Certain tissue specimens from normal individuals failed to inhibit leukocyte migration in patients with Behçet's syndrome, whereas in the latter patients, autologous antigens such as vitreous, aqueous humor, and spinal fluid produced inhibition of leukocytes.[32] In another study, LIF was reduced in Behçet's disease patients in clinical remission as compared to controls. During relapse the LIF levels were significantly higher than during remission and slightly higher than in controls.[33]

Histopathology and Cell-Mediated Immunity

The histopathological findings in established lesions of Behçet's syndrome are often reported as supporting a cell-mediated immune mechanism for the disease. Similarity of the histologic changes in lesions of Behçet's disease to those of known delayed hypersensitivity (tuberculin skin test intradermal reaction) suggests a disordered cellular immunity. Routine light microscopy of early oral ulcers reveals a chronic inflammatory reaction with aggregations of lymphocytes and monocytes infiltrating the dermis and epidermis as well as occurring around the dermal blood vessels.[16] Additionally, electron microscopic studies have confirmed the prominence of lymphocytes and monocytes in the oral ulcers of Behçet's syndrome. Atypical lymphocytes, probably representing transformed T cells, have been seen even in the preulcerative specimens taken from the buccal and gingival mucosa,[34] and macrophages have been observed in association with these cells. By cytological analyses of the inflammatory infiltrates of oral ulcers and erythema nodosum-like lesions of Behçet's syndrome, the infiltrating cells have been mainly composed of helper T lymphocytes and macrophages in association with natural killer cells.[35] These data have suggested participation of both humoral and cellular immunity in the production of the pathological lesions of Behçet's syndrome. NK cells, however, have been reported to be absent in the gastrointestinal lesions[36]; while the Langerhans cell, an integral component of cutaneous Type IV hypersensitivity, may contribute to the production of cutaneous lesions in Behçet's disease, as suggested by the histologic findings of an increased number of these cells in pathergy lesions.[37] Although not increased in number, Langerhans cells were larger, had more granules, and were believed to be in a more active metabolic state in the erythema nodosum-like lesions.[38]

Nevertheless, there are indications that the lymphocyte-predominant histology present in biopsy specimens from patients with Behçet's disease represents late findings and that the neutrophilic infiltrates reflect early histologic changes. Many investigators do not dispute the presence of neutrophils but contend, and have documented, that early lesions are predominantly composed of lymphocytes and macrophages. Perhaps as a response to infiltrating T helper cells, plasma cells and neutrophils increase in number and in association with circulating immune complexes precipitate a Type III reaction.[39]

Summary

Evidence has been received which highlights involvement of the cell-mediated immune system in the pathogenesis of Behçet's syndrome. Abnormalities of in-vitro measures of cell-mediated immunity include altered transformation of lymphocytes to standard mitogens, decreased peripheral blood T lymphocytes with a depressed T-cell helper-to-suppressor ratio, altered peripheral blood NK activity, and increased production of lymphokines important to the development of a cell-mediated immune response. Interpretation of these immunological and histological observations is difficult owing to the complex interactions between cell-mediated and humoral immunity. Identification of causal agents or antigens will help in synthesizing a coherent etiologic theory which explains the clinical, immunological, and histopathological findings. It is evident by the preceding discussion that certain defects in the regulation of cell-mediated immunity exist in patients with Behçet's disease. However, it is unknown whether these abnormalities are a direct cause or a result of Behçet's syndrome.

References

1. Lehner T. Immuno-pathology of Behçet's syndrome. In Lehner T, Barnes CG, eds: *Behçet's Syndrome. Clinical and Immunological Features. Proceedings of a Conference Sponsored by the Royal Society of Medicine, February 1979.* London, Academic Press, 1979:127–139.
2. Berkel Aİ, Ersoy F, Firat T, Kazokğlu H. Immunologic studies in Behçet's disease. In Dilşen N, Koniçe M, Övül C, eds: *Behçet's Disease. Proceedings of an International Symposium on Behçet's Disease, Istanbul, 29–30 September 1977.* Amsterdam-Oxford, Exerpta Medica, 1979:254–257.
3. Abdou NI, Schumacher HR, Colman RW. Behçet's disease: Possible role of secretory component deficiency, synovial inclusions, and fibrinolytic abnormality in the various manifestations of the disease. *J Lab Clin Med* 1978; 91:409–422.
4. Lee S, Kim DH, Bang DS, et al. Immunologic aspects in each type of Behçet's disease (abstract 11). Royal Society of Medicine international conference on Behçet's disease, September 5 and 6, 1985, London, England.
5. Yazici H, Yalçin B, Akokan G, et al. Immunological and rheumatological studies in Behçet's disease. In Dilşen N, Koniçe M, Övül C, eds: *Behçet's Disease. Proceedings of an International Symposium on Behçet's Disease, Istanbul, 29–30 September 1977.* Amsterdam-Oxford, Exerpta Medica, 1979:258–260.
6. Graykowski EA, Barile MF, Lee WB, Stanley HR Jr. Recurrent aphthous stomatitis. Clinical, therapeutic, histopathologic, and hypersensitivity aspects. *JAMA* 1966; 196:637–644.
7. Kaneko F, Kaneda T, Ohnishi O, et al. Behçet's syndrome and infection allergy. 1. Defection of chronic infectious foci and immune responses to bacterial vaccines *in vivo* and *in vitro. Jpn J Allergology* 1978; 27:440–447.
8. Haim S. Mekori T, Sobel JD, Robinson E. Aspects of lymphocyte function in Behçet's disease. *Dermatologica* 1976; 153:34–37.
9. Bang DS, Lee S, Kim DH, Nam IW. DNCB responsiveness in patients with Behçet's syndrome (abstract 12). Royal Society of Medicine international conference on Behçet's disease, September 5 and 6, 1985, London, England.
10. Djawari D, Hornstein OP. Cellular immune status and macrophage function in Behçet's disease. *Z Hautkr* 1980; 55:271–292.
11. Victorino RMM, Ryan P, Hughes GRV, Hodgson HJF. Cell-mediated

immune functions and immunoregulatory cells in Behçet's syndrome. *Clin Exp Immunol* 1982; 48:121–128.

12. Sakane T, Kotani H, Takada S, Tsunematsu T. Functional aberration of T cell subsets in patients with Behçet's disease. *Arthritis Rheum* 1982; 25:1343–1351.

13. Ahmed AR. Lymphocyte studies in Behçet's syndrome. *Dermatologica* 1982; 164:175–180.

14. Lehner T. Stimulation of lymphocyte transformation by tissue homogenates in recurrent oral ulceration. *Immunology* 1967; 13:159–166.

15. Marquardt JL, Synderman R, Oppenheim JJ. Depression of lymphocyte transformation and exacerbation of Behçet's syndrome by ingestion of English walnuts. *Cell Immunol* 1973; 9:263–272.

16. O'Duffy JD. Behçet's disease. In Kelley WN, Harris ED Jr, Ruddy S, Sledge CB, eds: *Textbook of Rheumatology*. Philadelphia, WB Saunders, 1981:1174–1178.

17. Morimoto C, Reinherz EL, Nadler LM, et al: Comparison in T- and B-cell markers in patients with Sjögren's syndrome and systemic lupus erythematosus. *Clin Immunol Immunopathol* 1982; 22:270–278.

18. Rogers RS III, Sams WM Jr, Shorter RG. Lymphocytotoxicity in recurrent apthous stomatitis. Lymphocytotoxicity for oral epithelial cells in recurrent aphthous stomatitis and Behçet syndrome. *Arch Dermatol* 1974; 109:361–363.

19. Reimer G, Steinkohl S, Djawari D, Hornstein OP. Lytic effect of cytotoxic lymphocytes on oral epithelial cells in Behçet's disease. *Br J Dermatol* 1982; 107:529–536.

20. Reimer G, Djawari D. Lymphocytotoxicity for oral epithelial cells in Behçet's disease. A case report. *Dermatologica* 1982; 164:82–89.

21. Watanabe K, Ohashi Y. Natural killer cell activity in patients with Behçet's disease (letter). *Am J Ophthalmol* 1984; 98:813–814.

22. Kaneko F, Takahashi Y, Muramatsu R, et al. Natural killer cell numbers and function in peripheral lymphoid cells in Behçet's disease. *Br J Dermatol* 1985; 113:313–318.

23. Fujii N, Minagawa T, Nakane A, et al. Spontaneous production of γ-interferon in cultures of T lymphocytes obtained from patients with Behçet's disease. *J Immunol* 1983; 130:1683–1686.

24. Ohno S, Kato F, Matsuda H, et al. Detection of gamma interferon in the sera of patients with Behçet's disease. *Infect Immun* 1982; 36:202–208.

25. Ohno S, Kato F, Matsuda H, et al. Studies on spontaneous production of gamma-interferon in Behçet's disease. *Ophthalmologica* 1982; 185:187–192.

26. Ohno S. Immunological aspects of Behçet's and Vogt-Koyanagi-Harada's diseases. *Trans Opthal Soc UK* 1981; 101:335–341.

27. Smith KA. Interleukin-2. *Ann Rev Immunol* 1984; 2:319–333.

28. Sakane T, Suzuki N, Ueda Y, et al. Analysis of interleukin-2 activity in patients with Behçet's disease. Ability of T cells to produce and respond to interleukin-2. *Arthritis Rheum* 1986; 29:371–378.

29. Shimizu T. Clinicopathological studies on Behçet's disease. In Dilşen N, Koniçe M, Övül C, eds: *Behçet's Disease. Proceedings of an International Symposium on Behçet's Disease, Istanbul, 29–30 September 1977.* Amsterdam-Oxford, Excerpta Medica, 1979:9–43.
30. Shimizu T, Ehrlich GE, Inaba G, Hayashi K. Behçet disease (Behçet syndrome). *Semin Arthritis Rheum* 1979; 8:223–260.
31. Ünal S, Dündar S, Özerkan K. LIF in Behçet's disease (abstract 28). Royal Society of Medicine international conference on Behçet's disease, September 5 and 6, 1985, London, England.
32. Sanefuji J. Cell mediated immunity in uveitis 3. Leukocyte inhibition test in Behçet disease. *Acta Soc Ophthalmol Jpn* 1974; 78:408–412.
33. Haim S, Gilhar A. Mekori T, Segal R. Leukocyte migration inhibition in Behçet's disease. *Dermatologica* 1979; 159:302–306.
34. Honma T, Saito T, Fujioka Y. Intraepithelial atypical lymphocytes in oral lesions of Behçet's syndrome. *Arch Dermatol* 1981; 117:83–85.
35. Kaneko F, Takahashi Y, Muramatsu Y, Miura Y. Immunological studies on aphthous ulcer and erythema nodosum-like eruptions in Behçet's disease. *Br J Dermatol* 1985; 113:303–312.
36. Yamana S, Jones SL, Shimamoto T, et al. Immunohistological analysis of lymphocytes infiltrating the terminal ileum in a patient with intestinal Behçet's disease (abstract 32). Royal Society of Medicine international conference on Behçet's disease, September 5 and 6, 1985, London, England.
37. Saito T, Honma T, Saigo K. Epidermal Langerhans' cells after the prick test for Behçet's disease. *Dermatologica* 1980; 161:152–160.
38. Kohn S, Haim S, Gilhar A, et al. Epidermal Langerhans' cells in Behçet's disease. *J Clin Pathol* 1984; 37:616–619.
39. Müller W, Lehner T. Quantitative electron microscopical analysis of leukocyte infiltration in oral ulcers of Behçet's syndrome. *Br J Dermatol* 1982; 106:535–544.
40. Matsumura Y, Mizushima Y, Morito T, et al. Disorders of inflammatory and immunological responses in Behçet's disease. In Dilşen N, Koniçe M, Övül C, eds: *Behçet's disease. Proceedings of an International Symposium on Behçet's Disease, Istanbul, 29–30 September 1977.* Amsterdam-Oxford, Exerpta Medica, 1979:215–218.
41. Lim SD, Haw CR, Kim NI, Fusaro RM. Abnormalities of T-cell subsets in Behçet's syndrome. *Arch Dermatol* 1983; 119:307–310.
42. Kaneko F, Takahashi Y, Muramatsu R, Minagawa T. Natural killer (NK) cell activity and subpopulation of peripheral blood lymphoid cells (PBLC) in Behçet's disease (abstract 16). Royal Society of Medicine international conference on Behçet's disease, September 5 and 6, 1985, London, England.
43. Kansu E, Kayserili B, Aktan S, et al. Immunological features of neuro-Behçet's syndrome (abstract 14). Royal Society of Medicine international conference on Behçet's disease, September 5 and 6, 1985, London, England.
44. Kansu E, Unal S, Karacadağ S, et al. T-lymphocyte subsets in Behçet's

disease (abstract 13). Royal Society of Medicine conference on Behçet's disease, September 5 and 6, 1985, London, England.

45. Ayed K, Hamza M, Hamzaoui K. Evaluation of lymphocytes subpopulations by monoclonal antibodies (OKT_3, OKT_4, OKT_8, Leu-7) in Behçet's disease (abstract 15). Royal Society of Medicine international conference on Behçet's disease, September 5 and 6, 1985, London, England.

46. Valesini G, Pivetti-Pezzi P, Mastrandrea F, et al. Evaluation of T cell subsets in Behçet's syndrome using anti-T cell monoclonal antibodies. *Clin Exp Immunol* 1985; 60:55–60.

5

IMMUNOLOGY: NEUTROPHIL, CIRCULATING IMMUNE COMPLEXES, COMPLEMENT

Scott Dinehart and Joseph L. Jorizzo

IMMUNOLOGICAL MECHANISMS HAVE LONG BEEN suspected to play a role in the development of the lesions of Behçet's syndrome. Early studies, influenced by lesional histology that showed lymphocytes, led investigators to postulate dysfunction of delayed hypersensitivity in the pathogenesis of Behçet's disease. Recently, reexamination of the histology of mucocutaneous lesions and accumulation of additional information concerning neutrophils, circulating immune complexes, and complement have suggested that a Type III hypersensitivity phenomenon may be responsible for many of the clinical, histologic, and laboratory findings of Behçet's syndrome. A hypothesis involving the interaction between immune complex-mediated vessel damage and enhancement of neutrophil chemotaxis will be presented which may indeed explain the cutaneous, mucosal, and perhaps visceral lesions of Behçet's disease. However, in order to understand this pathogenetic mechanism, one must review certain immunological events characteristic of Behçet's disease. Since certain aspects of this immunology have already been discussed in this monograph, they will only be briefly reviewed in this chapter for clarification.

From *Behcet's Disease: A Contemporary Synopsis*, edited by Gary R. Plotkin, M.D., John J. Calabro, M.D., and J. Desmond O'Duffy, M.B. ©1983 , Futura Publishing Company, Inc., Mount Kisco, NY.

Neutrophil

Early studies in Japan, followed by confirmation from investigators in the Middle East and Europe, showed that neutrophils from patients with Behçet's syndrome demonstrated increased migration to standard chemoattractants (as assessed by either Boyden chamber or subagarose methods) when compared to neutrophils from a normal control population.[1-4] This early work questioned whether the mechanism of increased neutrophil migration was serum-induced or related to the inherent properties of the neutrophil itself.[2,5] Based upon electron microscopic studies, Saga and Matsuda[6] have reported an increase in the number of microtubules in the neutrophils of six patients with active Behçet's disease as compared to three control subjects. Since colchicine was known to affect neutrophil adherence,[7] locomotion,[8,9] and phagocytosis,[10] possibly via an effect on microtubules; various investigators have advocated systemic colchicine therapy in Behçet's syndrome as a means of modifying this enhanced chemotaxis.

However, data generated from studies of six patients with Behçet's syndrome by Dr. Jorizzo et al.[11] have shown that the enhancement of neutrophil migration resulted from a heat stable serum factor. Interestingly, pretreating patients with oral colchicine (0.6 mg, by mouth, three times daily for 4 weeks, followed by 4 weeks of "off" treatment, followed by 4 weeks of "on" treatment) did not appreciably affect the inherent migration of the neutrophil. Moreover, the ability of serum from patients with Behçet's syndrome to enhance the migration of neutrophils from either patients or controls was completely eliminated when one compared serum obtained from colchicine treated with untreated patients. Additional preliminary results from studies in this area suggested that the enhancement of neutrophil migration, observed when sera from Behçet patients were mixed with agar using the subagarose method, may not be detected when using a more adherence-independent system such as collagen.[11]

Thalidomide therapy has been demonstrated to be beneficial for the mucocutaneous and arthritic manifestations of Behçet's syndrome.[12] Despite in-vitro evidence from France which revealed a potentially inhibitory effect of thalidomide on neutrophil migration, chemotaxis was not affected in patients with Behçet's disease treated with this experimental medication.[12,13] Therefore, thalidomide's mechanism of action may be dependent upon its inhibitory effects on circulating immune complex–induced vasculitis which is characteristic of Behçet's syndrome. In one experiment, the LFA/Mac-1/p150,95 family of glycoproteins, which has been associated with neutrophil adherence, was studied qualitatively by tritium labeling of neutrophil cell surfaces. As a result, recent evidence has suggested that the LFA-1/Mac-1/p150,95 family of cell surface glycoproteins was necessary for optimal neutrophil adherence, chemotaxis, and phagocytosis. Also, in patients with Behçet's disease, there weren't any quantitative abnormalities in this group of glycoproteins either prior to or during treatment with thalidomide.[12]

In addition to increased neutrophil chemotaxis and random motility, there has been documentation of increased enzymatic (methyltransferase, phospholipase A2) activities in the neutrophil cell membranes[14] and enhanced production of oxygen intermediates by the neutrophil.[15] Enhanced neutrophil phagocytic activity[16,17] and uptake of immunoglobulins[18] and other phagocytes[19] by neutrophils are further support of the potentiated functions of the polymorphonuclear leukocyte in Behçet's syndrome.

Circulating Immune Complexes

Circulating immune complexes may be detected in serum from more than half of patients with Behçet's syndrome[11,20-25]; and the clinical manifestations of uveitis, erythema nodosum, and arthritis have been variably ascribed to the presence of these immune complexes. A significant correlation has been shown between the presence of circulating immune complexes, as detected by an agglutination inhibition test and by Clq binding and Raji cell assays, and disease activity.[21,26] Both IgG- and IgA-containing circulating immune complexes have been found in the sera of patients with Behçet's disease. The nature of the antigens contained in these complexes is unknown, however, investigations using an immunoblot technique are in progress to identify any common antigen.[13] Identification of specific antigens both in circulating immune complexes and tissue will of course be required to establish the functions of circulating immune complexes in disease pathogenesis.

Complement

The complement system in Behçet's syndrome has been evaluated by several investigators, and elevations in total serum complement and complement components, particularly C5, C8, C9, and factor B, have been noted in various studies.[27,28] These elevations may be helpful in identifying subsets of patients with characteristic features of Behçet's syndrome and in predicting response to therapy with corticosteroids and other immunosuppressive agents.[27] Of the various complement components, levels of C9 seem to correlate most favorably with disease activity since normalization of raised valves occurs during disease quiescence. Elevated levels of complement components may either contribute to cellular damage or may function as acute-phase proteins modulating the immune response to damaged tissue.

Although many studies have reported normal serum concentrations of C3 and C4 in Behçet's disease, low levels of C2, C3, and C4 present before an attack of uveitis may implicate complement consumption by the classic pathway in the pathogenesis of certain complications of this disorder.[29] Biopsy of oral ulcers has revealed deposition of C3 and C9 in blood vessel walls and C9 in the basement membrane zone.[30] However, the specificity and significance of these findings are not known. In light of the occurrence of IgA-containing circulating immune complexes, elevated serum IgA levels, and the mucosal nature of the clinical symptoms in Behçet's syndrome, the alternative pathway of complement may also participate in the pathogenesis of the basic disease process. Unfortunately, study of specific complement components has provided minimal evidence for activation of the alternative pathway. Since membrane fragments with complement holes have been found by electron microscopy in the sera of some patients with Behçet's syndrome, complement components may be responsible for lysis of the affected cells.[22]

Correlation with Histopathology

Many reports of the histopathologic features of Behçet's syndrome have been published based on autopsy registry data.[31] The study of late lesions with their almost exclusively mononuclear cell infiltrations, has led to theories of pathogenesis that ignore the neutrophils that are present in the early lesions. Since the histologic features vary with time, the evaluation of neutrophilic to lymphohistiocytic histopathology may represent leukocytoclastic vasculitis in which the early diagnostic neutrophil-dominated histopathological changes are replaced rapidly by nondiagnostic lymphocytic changes after 24 to 36 hours.[32] Thus, one must not dismiss the finite life span of lesions when attempting to draw mechanistic conclusions from morphological data.

Recent interpretations of light, electron, and immunofluorescent microscopic data from the earliest mucosal or cutaneous lesions in Behçet's syndrome are compatible with an underlying neutrophilic vascular reaction.[11,12,24,33,34] Cutaneous pathergy lesions produced by needle prick, which are particularly suitable for study of the early histologic changes, have shown a vascular reaction composed mainly of neutrophils at six hours. At 24 hours there is a dense neutrophilic infiltrate along with a large number of mast cells.[35] In addition, the histopathological findings of the pathergy lesions are similar to those of the erythema nodosum-like lesions of Behçet's disease.

Immunohistologic evaluation using a modification of Braverman's histamine trap test has supported the concept of a predominance of neutrophils in the early cutaneous lesions of Behçet's syndrome.[11,12,33] This test is particularly relevant in the assessment of patients with Behçet's syndrome since pathergy lesions (the development of cutaneous pustular vasculitic lesions after trauma to the skin) may be induced by intradermal injection of this mediator of inflammation. In one study, test sites have been assessed by immunofluorescent microscopy (4 hours) and by routine light microscopy (24 hours), using suitable controls, for the presence of immunoreactant and fibrin deposition (4 hours) and neutrophilic vascular reaction (24 hours), after intradermal injection of histamine. Ten patients with Behçet's syndrome tested during active disease had evidence of neutrophilic vascular reactions detected by routine microscopic assessment of histamine-induced lesions. Histologically, these lesions showed endothelial cell swelling, a perivascular neutrophilic infiltrate with lysis of these cells (leukocytoclasis), invasion of neutrophils into blood vessel walls, and extravasation of erythrocytes. These neutrophilic vascular reactions differed histologically from leukocytoclastic vasculitis only by the absence of fibrinoid necrosis. Eight of these ten patients also had immunoreactants (usually Clq, C2, or IgG) or fibrin detected in dermal blood vessels by immunofluorescent microscopy from biopsies taken four hours after histamine injection. Six patients were retested during disease remission, and the skin biopsies of all patients showed changes on routine histology similar to those seen in normal controls. During disease remission, immunofluorescent microscopic analysis of biopsied skin was negative in five of the six patients.

Concept of Pustular Vasculitis

The concept that pustular vasculitis may explain the cutaneous pathergy and mucocutaneous lesions characteristic of Behçet's syndrome is supported by the presence of circulating immune complexes, enhanced migration of neutrophils, complement and immunoglobulin deposition, and an early neutrophilic vascular histology. Although this pathogenetic mechanism is most evident in the mucocutaneous lesions, it may also explain the visceral and ophthalmologic lesions in Behçet's syndrome. This postulated theory of pathogenesis of Behçet's disease may begin with exposure to an unknown antigen which stimulates production of antibodies, and thus circulating immune complexes. The antigen(s) may be either endogenous or exogenous stimuli to which the individual reacts in an abnormal manner immunologically because of genetic predisposition. As a result, cutaneous or synovial trauma could result in endogenous release of histamine from mast cells which promotes circulating immune complex deposition and subsequent vasculitis at the trauma site. Neutrophils may then converge at the site with resultant enhancement of subsequent neutrophil migration. This polymorphonuclear leukocyte infiltration produces pustular instead of simple purpuric lesions. Signs and symptoms of serum sickness including arthralgias, arthritis, and fever, develop as the Type III hypersensitivity reaction progresses immunologically. Other syndromes, whose lesions may occur by a similar pustular vasculitic mechanism, include the bowel bypass syndrome, bowel-associated dermatosis-arthritis syndrome, and the disseminated gonococcal dermatitis-arthritis syndrome.[36,37] This discussion has thus attempted to integrate the observed immunopathology of Behçet's syndrome into a hypothesis that may explain the pathogenesis of this disease. Additional studies are of course necessary for confirmation of this theory.

References

1. Djawari D, Hornstein OP, Schötz J. Enhancement of granulocyte chemotaxis in Behçet's disease. *Arch Dermatol Res* 1981; 270:81–88.
2. Mizushima Y, Matsumura N, Mori M. Chemotaxis of leukocytes and colchicine treatment in Behçet's disease. *J Rheumatol* 1979; 6:108–110.
3. Sobel JD, Haim S, Obendeanu N, et al. Polymorphonuclear leukocyte function in Behçet's disease. *J Clin Pathol* 1977; 30:250–253.
4. Takeuchi A, Kobayashi K, Mori M, Mizushima Y. The mechanism of hyperchemotaxis in Behçet's disease. *J Rheumatol* 1981; 8:40–44.
5. Miyachi Y, Taniguchi S, Ozaki M, Horio T. Colchicine in the treatment of the cutaneous manifestations of Behçet's disease. *Br J Dermatol* 1981; 104:67–69.
6. Saga T, Matsuda H. Microtubules in neutrophils of patients with Behçet's disease. *Jpn J Ophthalmol* 1985; 29:31–36.
7. MacGregor RR. The effect of anti-inflammatory agents and inflammation on granulocyte adherence. Evidence for regulation by plasma factors. *Am J Med* 1976; 61:597–607.
8. Borel JF. Effect of some drugs on the chemotaxis of rabbit neutrophils in vitro *Experimentia* 1973; 27:676–678.
9. Valerius NH. In vitro effects of colchicine on neutrophil granulocyte locomotion. Assessment of the effect of colchicine on chemotaxis, chemokinesis and spontaneous motility, using a modified reversible Boyden chamber. *Acta Pathol Microbiol Scand (B)* 1978; 86B:149–154.
10. Lehrer RI. Effects of colchicine and chloramphenicol on the oxidative metabolism and phagocytic activity of human neutrophils. *J Infect Dis* 1973; 127:40–48.
11. Jorizzo JL, Hudson RD, Schmalstieg FC, et al. Behçet's syndrome:

Immune regulation, circulating immune complexes, neutrophil migration, and colchicine therapy. *J Am Acad Dermatol* 1984; 10:205–214.

12. Jorizzo JL, Schmalstieg FC, Solomon AR Jr, et al. Thalidomide effects in Behçet's syndrome and pustular vasculitis. *Arch Intern Med* 1986; 146:878–881.

13. Jorizzo JL. Behçet's disease. An update based on the 1985 international conference in London. *Arch Dermatol* 1986; 122:556–558.

14. Niwa Y. Methlytransferase and phospholipase A2 activity in the membrane of neutrophils and lymphocytes from patients with Behçet's disease (abstract 24). Royal Society of Medicine international conference on Behçet's disease, September 5 and 6, 1985, London, England.

15. Niwa Y, Miyake S, Sakane T, et al. Auto-oxidative damage in Behçet's disease-endothelial cell damage following the elevated oxygen radicals generated by stimulated neutrophils. *Clin Exp Immunol* 1982; 49:247–255.

16. Takabatake M. Cytologic studies of the aqueous humor II. Electron microscopic observations of floating cells in the anterior chamber in various ocular diseases. *Folia Ophthal Jpn* 1975; 26:138–145.

17. Takeda N. Studies on phagocytic function in patients with collagen diseases and Behçet's disease. *Fukush Med J* 1979; 29:37–51.

18. Shimizu T, Katsuta Y, Oshima Y. Immunologic studies on Behçet's syndrome. *Ann Rheum Dis* 1965; 24:494–500.

19. Noguchi Y, Hashimoto T, Yanagida T, et al. Mononuclear cell with phagocytized leukocyte(s) in synovial fluid taken from patients with Behçet's disease. In Inaba G, ed: *Annual Report 1978, Studies on Etiology, Treatment and Prevention of Behçet's Disease.* Behçet Disease Research Committee of Japan, Ministry of Welfare, 1978:1–7.

20. Gamble CN, Wiesner KB, Shapiro EF, Boyer WJ. The immune complex pathogenesis of glomerulonephritis and pulmonary vasculitis in Behçet's disease. *Am J Med* 1979; 66:1031–1039.

21. Gupta RC, O'Duffy JD, McDuffie FC, et al. Circulatory immune complexes in active Behçet's disease. *Clin Exp Immunol* 1973; 34:213–218.

22. Lehner T. Almeida JD, Levinsky RJ. Damaged membrane fragments and immune complexes in the blood of patients with Behçet's syndrome. *Clin Exp Immunol* 1978; 34:206–212.

23. Lehner T, Welsh KL, Batchelor JR. Relationship of HLA phenotype to immunoglobulin class present in immune complexes from patients with Behçet's syndrome. *Tissue Antigens* 1981; 17:357–361.

24. Valesini G, Picardo M, Pastore R, et al. Circulating immune complexes in Behçet's syndrome: Purification, characterization and cross-reactivity studies. *Clin Exp Immunol* 1981; 44:522–527.

25. Williams BD, Lehner T. Immune complexes in Behçet's syndrome and recurrent oral ulceration. *Br Med J* 1977; 1:1387–1389.

26. Levinsky RJ, Lehner T. Circulating soluble immune complexes in recurrent oral ulceration and Behçet's syndrome. *Clin Exp Immunol* 1978; 32:193–198.

27. Lehner T, Adinolfi M. Acute phase proteins, C9, factor B, and lysozyme

in recurrent oral ulceration and Behçet's syndrome. *J Clin Pathol* 1980; 33:269–275.

28. Yamamoto M. Immunologic abnormalities in patients with Behçet's disease I. Complement system in patients with Behçet's disease. *Okayama Igakkai Zasshi* 1983; 95:17–24.
29. Shimada K, Kogure M, Kawashima T, Nishioka K. Reduction of complement in Behçet's disease and drug allergy. *Med Biol* 1974; 52:234–239.
30. James DG. Behçet's syndrome. *N Engl J Med* 1979; 301:431–432.
31. Lakhanpal S, Tani K, Lie JT, et al. Pathologic features of Behçet's syndrome: A review of Japanese autopsy registry data. *Hum Pathol* 1985; 16:790–795.
32. Sams WM Jr, Thorne EG, Small P, et al. Leukocytoclastic vasculitis. *Arch Dermatol* 1976; 112:219–226.
33. Jorizzo JL, Solomon AR, Cavallo T. Behçet's syndrome. Immunopathologic and histopathologic assessment of pathergy lesions is useful in diagnosis and follow up. *Arch Pathol Lab Med* 1985; 109:747–751.
34. Müller W, Lehner T. Quantitative electron microscopical analysis of leukocyte infiltration in oral ulcers of Behçet's syndrome. *Br J Dermatol* 1982; 106:535–544.
35. Tüzün Y, Altaç M, Yazici H, et al. Nonspecific skin hyperactivity in Behcet's disease. Iperrealtivita' cutanea asepcifica nel morbo di Behçet. *Haematologica* 1980; 65:395–398.
36. Jorizzo JL. Pustular vasculitis: An emerging disease concept. *J Am Acad Dermatol* 1983; 9:160–162.
37. Jorizzo JL, Schmalstieg FC, Dinehart SM, et al. Bowel-associated dermatosis-arthritis syndrome. Immune complex-mediated vessel damage and increased neutrophil migration. *Arch Intern Med* 1984; 144:738–740.

6

HEMATOLOGIC ASPECTS

*M. Ernest Marshall, John J. Gohmann, and
Ewa Marciniak*

Behçet's disease has been characterized clinically and pathologically as a systemic inflammatory disorder for which the etiology remains unknown. While a number of hematologic abnormalities have been described in patients with this illness, detailed studies of the underlying pathophysiological mechanisms of these abnormalities have been hindered by the relatively uncommon occurrence of this disease. In the present review emphasis is focused on those aspects of the hematologic system that have been characterized in greatest detail in patients with Behçet's disease. Therefore, this chapter includes discussions of coagulation, fibrinolysis, polymorphonuclear leukocytes, platelets, and endothelial cell damage as they relate to the pathogenesis of Behçet's disease.

Anemia

Anemia, defined as a hemoglobin of ≤ 10 g/dL, is an inconstant feature of Behçet's disease, and in one review, anemia occurred in less than 20% of patients.[1] A satisfactory description of the mechanism(s) of anemia in this disease is lacking. Furthermore,

From *Behcet's Disease: A Contemporary Synopsis*, edited by Gary R. Plotkin, M.D., John J. Calabro, M.D., and J. Desmond O'Duffy, M.B. © 1988, Futura Publishing Company, Inc., Mount Kisco, NY.

there have been no clear correlations between the severity of anemia and disease activity.

Coagulation and Fibrinolysis

Venous thrombosis is a characteristic manifestation of Behçet's disease. Kluft et al.[2] reviewed 266 patients with Behçet's disease within the literature and reported that 77 (30%) had venous thrombosis. Their review indicated that 20% of patients had superficial thrombophlebitis, 12% had deep vein thrombosis, and 6% had vena caval obstruction. A number of authors have attempted to explain this striking incidence of venous thrombosis by examining peripheral blood coagulation parameters in patients with Behçet's disease during periods of disease exacerbation and remission. While definite trends have emerged from a review of this literature, there have been contradictory findings within and among various series.

In a series of 36 patients with Behçet's disease, Haim et al.[3] reported marked elevations in fibrinogen levels in five patients, three of whom had thrombophlebitis. Two patients with venous involvement, however, had normal fibrinogen levels. Chajek et al.[4] recorded marked elevations in fibrinogen levels in nine patients with Behçet's disease, six of whom had thrombophlebitis. In a separate study, Chajek and Fainaru[5] monitored coagulation parameters in 17 patients and found fibrinogen levels to be within normal limits during the remission phase of the disease. Fibrinogen levels were markedly elevated (490–660 mg/dL) in seven patients with active thrombophlebitis and slightly elevated (390–500 mg/dL) in patients without thrombophlebitis during relapses of the mucocutaneous or ocular manifestations of the disease. Toki and Yamura[6] found the fibrinogen levels in the euglobulin fraction of plasma to be within normal physiological ranges in seven patients with Behçet's disease. They speculated that the discrepancy between their findings and the results of others might be due to differences between measurements made on plasma versus the euglobulin fraction. Fibrinogen degradation products were reportedly elevated in one patient[3]; while in a larger series of patients, they were within normal physiological ranges.[5]

Chajek et al.[4,5] have reported that the clotting time, bleeding time, prothrombin time, and partial thromboplastin time were all normal in patients with Behçet's disease. In addition, coagulation Factors V, VII, IX, and X were present in normal levels, while there was a marked elevation of Factor VIII levels that tended to parallel fibrinogen levels, that is, waxing and waning respectively, with relapse and remission of disease activity.[4,5] However, both fibrinogen and Factor VIII are acute-phase reactants, and a causative correlation of their increased levels with thrombosis has not been established.

The most striking, and pathophysiologically most interesting, peripheral blood abnormalities in Behçet's disease have included aberrations in fibrinolysis. Such studies have generally indicated diminished fibrinolytic activity in peripheral blood as quantitated by in-vitro assays.[3-10] In essence, Figure 1 is a simplified schema of the normal mechanism of peripheral blood fibrinolysis. (For a more detailed review of fibrinolysis, consult Francis and Marder.[11]) The proenzyme, plasminogen, is a β-globulin, and in the presence of activators, it is converted to plasmin. Activators are proteolytic enzymes that are derived from plasma (proactivator) or tissue sources. The endopeptidase enzyme plasmin is capable of digesting fibrin, as well as fibrinogen, and is under the control of normally occurring plasma proteinase inhibitors (antiplasmins) which consist of the fast-acting (α_2-antiplasmin) and slow-acting (α_2-macroglobulin) types. Effective thrombus dissolution requires binding of both plasminogen and plasminogen activators to the fibrin surface where rapidly generated plasmin is also partially protected from inactivation by α_2-antiplasmin.

In most of the published reports, fibrinolysis has been evaluated in the laboratory by the euglobulin lysis time (ELT), but this test is not specific and is believed primarily to reflect activator activity in plasma. Confirmatory observations from a number of investigators have indicated that there was a prolonged ELT in patients with Behçet's disease.[3-10] These observations must be tempered by the realization that the ELT is not a specific test and, indeed, may not be very informative. "Hypofibrinolysis" is an ill-defined condition, and the results of laboratory procedures used to evaluate this condition must be viewed with caution.[12] A prolonged ELT is not, however, a universal finding in Behçet's disease since some patients, even during exacerbations of disease activity,

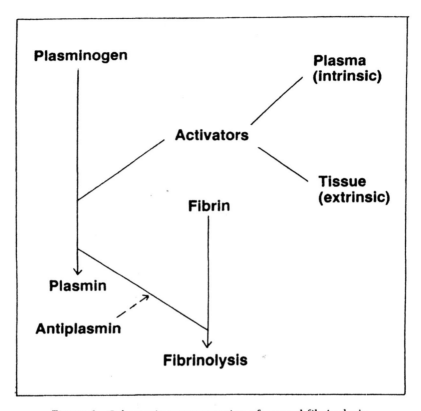

Figure 1—Schematic representation of normal fibrinolysis.

will display a normal ELT[3,5,6,9,10]; and diminished fibrinolytic activity is not a phenomenon unique to this illness. Cunliffe and Menon[9] examined the fibrinolytic activity of 52 patients with cutaneous vasculitis (none of whom had Behçet's disease) and found that 32 had abnormally low activity. They also observed that there was a relationship between the activity of the vasculitis and the lower fibrinolytic activity.[9]

Chajek and Fainaru[5] found the ELT to be normal in 12 of 13 patients during remission of their Behçet's disease. The ELT was markedly elevated in 5 of 7 patients with active thrombophlebitis and in 3 of 4 patients without thrombophlebitis but in exacerbation of other symptoms of the disease. They determined that the decrease in fibrinolytic activity was due to plasma inhibitors of both plasmin and plasminogen activators.[5]

Mishima et al.[10] monitored fibrinolytic activity in 37 patients with Behçet's disease. For purposes of analysis, they identified three subgroups of patients: group 1 consisted of four patients with mucocutaneous symptoms and group 2 consisted of four patients with genital ulcerations and mucocutaneous symptoms. Both groups 1 and 2 were studied during periods of exacerbation of disease activity. Group 3 consisted of 29 patients manifesting ocular and mucocutaneous symptoms, and this group was further separated into 17 patients with exacerbation of symptoms while 12 patients were in the remission phase. The ELT was prolonged in the patients in group 2 and the patients in group 3 who were experiencing active symptoms. Meanwhile, the ELT was within normal ranges in patients in group 1 and in those patients in group 3 who were in a period of symptomatic remission. The authors suggested that the phenomena of genital ulcers and ocular symptoms may be related to decreased levels of activator activity. They suggested, further, that measurement of plasminogen activator activity levels may be useful in monitoring or predicting disease activity.[10] More recently, two patients with Behçet's disease were reported with suppressed release of vascular tissue plasminogen activator stores; however, neither patient had clinically apparent thromboembolic disease.[13]

Toki and Yamura[6] found the ELT to be markedly prolonged in five of seven patients with Behçet's disease; and they reported that the five patients with prolonged ELT had two antiactivators in the plasma, one of which appeared to be an α_2-plasmin inhibitor, that accounted for the impaired fibrinolysis. They suggested that the decrease in activator content in the euglobulin fraction was followed by an increase of antiactivator content in the plasma which might result in the significant prolongation of the ELT.[6]

Venous thromboembolism is a final expression of multiple physiological pathways and complex events. Clotting tests and assays of the concentration of coagulation factors generally have provided minimal insight into the understanding of the thrombotic phenomenon. In addition, there have been no studies regarding the existence of natural coagulation inhibitors such as antithrombin III, protein C, and protein S in patients with Behçet's syndrome.

Because the treatment of Behçet's disease historically has been unsatisfactory, investigators have sought new therapeutic strategies. One such development in the treatment of this disease resulted from the frequent observations of decreased fibrinolytic activity in these patients. Several investigators have used anabolic steroids alone or in combination with phenformin since these agents have been shown to stimulate fibrinolytic activity most likely by increasing the activator content of the vascular wall.[14] Other authorities have used oral therapy with streptokinase which functions as an exogenous plasminogen activator.[5,7-9,15-17]

Most of the reports of the use of fibrinolytic agents have been anecdotal, dealing with single cases or small series of patients. Collum et al.[7] treated four patients with Behçet's disease with oral streptokinase and two of these patients were able to discontinue the use of corticosteroids. All four patients experienced improvement in symptoms with fewer exacerbations of disease activity and remained on therapy for two to eight years with continued clinical benefit and no apparent toxicity from therapy.[7] Chajek and Fainaru[5] treated seven patients with oral streptokinase. Treatment improved acute phlebitis and prevented symptomatic relapses in three patients; however, the treatment was not effective in preventing mucocutaneous recurrences in several patients. It apparently arrested choroiditis in one patient. Cunliffe[8] treated two patients with cutaneous vasculitis with phenformin hydrochloride and ethyloestrenol and noted an improvement in clinical status of the disease and an increase in fibrinolytic activity. One patient described in detail experienced clinical improvement and increased fibrinolytic activity within three weeks on therapy and remained free of clinical disease with normal fibrinolytic activity for 10 months. Amenorrhea, thought to be due to ethyloestrenol, developed after 5 months, and this drug was therefore discontinued after 10 months. Menstruation returned three weeks thereafter but was accompanied by a decrease in fibrinolytic activity and recurrence of cutaneous lesions. The skin manifestations and conjunctival ulcerations improved upon reinstitution of the drug.[8] Menon et al.[15] reported their experience with the use of phenformin hydrochloride and ethyloestrenol in a single patient. Their patient with Behçet's disease experienced multiple recurrences of deep vein thrombophlebitis and pulmonary embolism; however, the ELT was repeatedly within normal ranges. Upon institution of therapy, the clinical condition improved and by eight months the leg ulcerations healed and there was no recurrence of deep vein thrombosis.[15]

Cunliffe and Menon[9] treated 10 patients with cutaneous vasculitis (none of whom had Behçet's disease) with either phenformin hydrochloride 50 mg orally twice daily and ethyloestrenol 2 mg orally four times daily or phenformin hydrochloride and stanozolol 5 mg orally twice daily. Stanozolol had the theoretical advantage of producing weaker androgenic effects. The combination of phenformin hydrochloride plus stanozolol was equally effective as the combination containing ethyloestrenol in this small series. Cunliffe et al.[17] subsequently reported successful therapy of another patient with Behçet's disease using phenformin and stanozolol. While individual reports suggest that a patient with Behçet's syndrome may benefit from therapy with fibrinolytic agents, it is difficult to establish general conclusions because of the great clinical variability inherent in this disease, with its spontaneous remissions and relapses and the small number of patients reported in any series.

Anticardiolipin Antibodies

On the basis of earlier reports describing an association between anticardiolipin antibodies and arterial and venous thrombosis in connective-tissue diseases, Hull et al.[18] measured levels of these antibodies in 70 patients with Behçet's disease. Significant levels of these antibodies comprised from both IgG and IgM classes, were found in 13 of the 70 patients. In seven and three patients, respectively, only the IgG or IgM type was detected, while three had both IgG and IgM antibodies. When the group of patients possessing anticardiolipin antibodies was compared to the group without these immunoglobulins, there was no significant difference with respect to the occurrence of major symptoms, defined as orogenital ulcerations, uveitis, and arthritis. Of 20 patients with retinal vascular disease, 7 had anticardiolipin antibodies, and the difference was statistically significant. Two patients, displaying the highest levels of the antibody, had evidence of either retinal vasculitis, retinal vein occlusion, and cerebral infarction or retinal vasculitis alone. The authors concluded that anticardiolipin antibodies may play a pathogenetic role in a subgroup of patients with Behçet's disease.[18] Efthimiou et al.[19] subsequently reported results of anticardiolipin antibodies in 25 patients with Behçet's disease. Their findings were somewhat contradictory to those of Hull et al.[18]; that is, they found anticardiolipin antibodies in only 2 of the 25 patients. Also, only the IgM species was present in both cases. These authors thus disputed the earlier suggestion that anticardiolipin antibodies may play a major pathogenetic role in the vascular complications of Behçet's disease.[19]

Platelets

Platelet abnormalities in Behçet's disease have been reported by several authors, and one such abnormality involved the phenomenon of platelet rosetting. In a study of one patient with Behçet's disease, Prchal et al.[20] observed platelet rosetting around polymorphonuclear leukocytes (PMN) but not around monocytes, lymphocytes, or other granulocytes. The degree of platelet rosetting paralleled the patient's clinical course, i.e., during clinical remission, platelet rosetting was absent, while in the active phase of the disease, greater than 80% of the granulocytes were surrounded by 5 to 20 platelets. This rosetting phenomenon occurred only in EDTA-anticoagulated blood.[20] Ehrlich et al.[21] observed platelet rosetting in another patient with Behçet's disease. However, when calcium ions were added to heparinized, EDT-treated, and oxalate-treated blood, the platelets migrated away from the granulocytes. Moreover, the addition of serum from a patient with Behçet's disease to granulocytes from a normal donor resulted in platelet rosetting. These results indicated a relationship between calcium ions and the phenomenon of platelet rosetting, and the authors inferred that the presence of a plasma factor accounted for the rosetting phenomenon.

Matsuda et al.[22] confirmed the phenomenon of increased platelet activity in Behçet's disease. They also observed elevated plasma concentrations of platelet Factor 4 in Behçet's disease compared to controls, whereas there was no difference in the levels of β-thromboglobulin. Kirch et al.[23] reported that platelet aggregation was not significantly different in Behçet's disease, compared to controls, during periods of disease quiescence; however, there was increased ADP- and collagen-induced platelet aggregation during periods of active disease.

To further investigate the phenomenon of increased platelet aggregation, Hizli et al.[24] measured peripheral blood levels of prostacyclin (a potent antiplatelet-aggregating substance produced by the vessel wall) in 15 patients with Behçet's disease and 8 normal control subjects. The levels of 6-keto-prostaglandin F$_1\alpha$, a PGI$_2$ (prostacyclin) metabolite, were measured by radioimmunoassay. Patients with Behçet's disease had significantly lower levels of 6-keto-prostaglandin Fα (14.73 ± 3.25 pg/ml) than the normal control subjects (196.11 ± 60.81 pg/ml). Five patients with Behçet's disease had active thrombophlebitis at the time of study, but their prostacyclin levels were not significantly different from the patients without thrombophlebitis. The authors speculated that the low levels of prostacyclin could contribute to the pathogenesis of the venous thrombosis observed in Behçet's disease.[24] The published results of Hizli et al.,[24] however, prompted a contradictory report by Ritter et al.[25] The latter group of investigators claimed that the results of Hizli et al.[24] suffered from a methodological error. Ritter et al.[25] maintained that the radioimmunoassay of Hizli et al.[24] was less sensitive and less accurate than the quantitation of 6-oxoprostaglandin F$_1\alpha$ levels using the technique of gas chromatography/negative ion chemical ionization mass spectrometry. Using this latter technique, Ritter et al.[25] measured plasma 6-oxoprostaglandin F$_1\alpha$, the stable hydrolysis product of prostacyclin, in a patient with Behçet's disease who was experiencing venous and arterial vasculitis. By this method the prostacyclin level was equal to that of normal controls. Studying a sample of surgically obtained vessel wall from the abdominal aortic aneurysm of the Behçet's disease patient, they further demonstrated that the diseased vessel retained the capacity to synthesize prostacyclin in vitro. They concluded that the association between abnormal levels of prostacyclin and Behçet's disease remains unproven.[25] Kansu et al.,[26] however, have studied by radioimmunoassay the production of 6-keto-prostaglandin F$_1\alpha$ by resected segments of the antecubital fossa vein from eight patients with active Behçet's disease, including three with thrombophlebitis and one with neuro-Behçet's disease. Compared to controls, prostacyclin generation as measured by 6-keto-PGF$_1\alpha$ levels was impaired in seven patients with Behçet's disease, and thus, the authors[26] postulated that the abnormality of in-vitro prostacyclin production resulted either from impaired biosynthesis by vascular endothelial cells or by rapid degradation of prostacyclin. Since the endothelial cell is a major site for activation of coagulation inhibitors and neutralization of clotting enzymes, there has been an accumulation of data supporting a new and important role of this cell in the prevention of thrombosis.[27] Evidence for endothelial cell dysfunction in association with Behçet's disease has been reported[28] and currently one can only hypothesize that a dysfunction of the endothelial integrity in any disease entity may affect the balance between anticoagulant and procoagulant tendencies with resultant thrombus formation.

Neutrophil-Mediated Endothelial Injury

Since the polymorphonuclear leukocyte (PMN) normally may contribute to vascular injury, with resultant thrombus formation,[29] the following discussion reviews the interactions of white cells with endothelium in Behçet's disease. Patients with Behçet's disease may have normal peripheral blood leukocyte counts,[1,5,7,9] neutrophilia,[1,5,7] or rarely, neutropenia.[30] Yalçin et al.[1] observed neutrophilia (WBC $> 10,000/mm^3$) in 10 of 74 patients, all with mucocutaneous disease. The remaining patients all displayed normal leukocyte counts even during periods of active disease. Monocytosis (defined as $>500/mm^3$) occurred in 17 of 38 patients but there was no correlation between monocyte count and disease activity.[1] Chajek and Fainaru[5] observed the leukocyte count to be normal in 34 patients during disease remission while exacerbations of disease activity, especially in the presence of fever, were associated with a tendency to leukocytosis with a left shift.[5]

The most striking observations surrounding polymorphonuclear leukocytes in Behçet's disease have been qualitative rather than quantitative. Early reports have indicated that PMN from patients with Behçet's disease displayed increased chemotactic activity, and thus, this cell might be important in the pathogenesis of pathergy or mucocutaneous hyperirritability. Electron microscopic studies of naturally occurring skin lesions in Behçet's disease have revealed perivascular infiltration by large numbers of PMN and mast cells with resultant increased amounts of tissue histamine.[31,32] Jorizzo et al.[33] examined PMN migratory activity in six patients with Behçet's disease and six control subjects. Their study was designed not only to confirm the increased migratory activity of PMN from patients with Behçet's disease, but also to obtain preliminary information as to whether this increased activity was due to a serum factor or to some intrinsic property of the white cell. PMN migration was quantified using an agarose plate method, and the plates contained heat-inactivated serum from either Behçet's disease patients or normal controls. As a result of preincubating the PMN in nutrient medium, patient serum or normal serum, these investigators observed that heat-inactivated serum from patients with Behçet's disease increased the migration of PMN from both patients and the control subjects. Heat-inactivated serum from the control subjects, however, did not produce this effect. PMN migration studies were repeated on four patients with Behçet's disease after taking colchicine for four weeks. Colchicine was known to affect microtubules in the normal PMN, and there were preliminary reports that colchicine could produce clinical improvement in patients with Behçet's disease. In summary, PMN migration studies after colchicine treatment showed decreased cell migration in patients compared to control subjects but the difference was not statistically significant. Colchicine also inhibited the ability of serum from Behçet's patients to enhance the migration of patients' cells as well as the ability of patient serum to enhance the migration of cells from normal subjects. However, the authors[33] did not characterize the nature of the factor in the sera of Behçet's patients that accounted for the increased PMN migratory activity. On the basis of the evidence for a circulating immune complex–mediated vasculitis and increased PMN migration in Behçet's patients, the authors[33] proposed a theory to explain the pustular vasculitis (pathergy) seen in this disease. They speculated that cutaneous or synovial trauma resulted in the release of endogenous histamine and other mediators of inflammation that promoted immune complex deposition. Subsequently, PMN with enhanced migration would converge, followed by additional immunological and hematologic events that were ultimately responsible for the pustular vasculitic lesions of Behçet's disease.

The studies of Jorizzo et al.[33] were somewhat in conflict with previous reports by other investigators. James et al.[34] had reported that when measured in vitro, PMN from patients with Behçet's disease displayed increased migratory activity, but when assessed in vivo by a standard skin chamber technique, there were fewer PMN migrating in the skin chambers in Behçet's patients compared to control subjects. The reasons for this discrepancy were unknown. While Fordham et al.[35] confirmed the findings of increased PMN motility in Behçet's disease, their assays were performed in serum-free medium, which suggests that the observed hypermotility was due to intrinsic properties of the cells. Sobel et al.[32] measured spontaneous and stimulated nitroblue tetrazolium (NBT) reduction, PMN oxygen consumption, and PMN migration in 19 patients with Behçet's disease. Spontaneous NBT reduction was normal in most patients, while NBT reduction after stimulation with endotoxin was decreased in Behçet's patients compared to normal controls. PMN from Behçet's patients displayed lower resting oxygen consumption and less migration than normal controls. However, they also examined the PMN migratory response to *E. coli* lipopolysaccharide, which is known to activate complement-medicated chemotaxis. In response to this antigen, PMN from patients with Behçet's disease displayed increased migratory activity compared to normal controls. PMN from control subjects also demonstrated enhanced migratory activity in the presence of serum from patients with Behçet's disease. Thus, the findings of Sobel et al.[32] suggested that the enhanced chemotactic activity of PMN in Behçet's disease was due to a serum chemotactic factor as well as an intrinsic PMN factor. The results of the NBT studies suggested a minor functional metabolic abnormality in PMN in Behçet's disease, but since patients with Behçet's disease did not have an increased susceptibility to infection, this abnormality did not impair the inflammatory response to extrinsic antigens.[32]

Niwa et al.[36] measured neutrophil-derived oxygen intermediates and lysozomal enzymes in 17 patients with Behçet's disease who were receiving glucocorticosteroids and colchicine. The production of oxygen intermediates by neutrophils was markedly increased during active disease, and the authors postulated that tissue injury in Behçet's disease may be related to excessive generation of oxygen intermediates by stimulated neutrophils. Endothelial cell damage was assessed in a ^{51}Cr-release cytotoxicity assay in which cultured ^{51}Cr-labeled endothelial cells were incubated with PMN from Behçet's patients. ^{51}Cr release from endothelial cells incubated with activated PMN from Behçet's patients was markedly elevated compared to control subjects. Electron microscopic studies revealed destruction of desmosomes and cellular deformation. Their studies suggested that PMN from Behçet's patients generated high levels of oxygen intermediates which, by oxidative damage, resulted in endothelial cell injury. Since their results indicated that oxygen intermediate production was increased more than lysozomal enzyme production, they concluded that oxygen intermediates contributed to tissue damage more than lysozomol enzymes. This hypothesis was supported further by the finding that co-incubation with superoxide dismutase and catalase reduced ^{51}Cr release to control levels. The increased production of oxygen intermediates could not be ascribed to circulating immune complexes.[36] In addition, the production of platelet-activating factor as measured by acetyltransferase activity by both stimulated and nonstimulated neutrophils from patients with either active or inactive Behçet's disease has been reported to be similar to that of a control group.[37]

Summary

Since the etiology of Behçet's disease remains an enigma, there has been no unifying hypothesis to explain the underlying pathogenetic abnormalities observed in this syndrome. Because patients with this disorder constitute a heterogeneous clinical group, it is not surprising that the hematologic and laboratory investigations in this syndrome have yielded varied and frankly contradictory findings. From the present review, one can conclude the following:

1. Anemia is not a constant finding in Behçet's syndrome. The nature of the anemia has been inadequately described, and there is no association between the degree of anemia and disease activity.
2. Fibrinogen levels are markedly elevated in many, but not all, patients with Behçet's syndrome, and in some, fibrinogen

levels parallel disease activity being elevated in exacerbation and normal in quiescent periods. However, these observations have not been universal.

3. Clotting time, bleeding time, prothrombin time, and partial thromboplastin time are normal in Behçet's syndrome.

4. Coagulation Factors V, VII, IX, and X are normal in Behçet's syndrome; however, Factor VIII levels may be elevated and may parallel disease activity. This is probably a nonspecific finding since Factor VIII is an acute-phase reactant.

5. Fibrinolysis might be impaired in many, but not all, patients with Behçet's syndrome. However, impaired fibrinolysis is not a specific finding since it has been observed in a number of other vasculitides. Increased fibrinolytic activity may parallel disease activity in some patients with Behçet's disease.

6. In some patients, decreased fibrinolytic activity might be due to an increased activity of inhibitors of both plasmin and plasminogen activators. Also, decreased levels of plasminogen activators have been variably reported in Behçet's syndrome.

7. Fibrinolytic agents appear to ameliorate clinical phenomena in some patients with Behçet's syndrome.

8. Platelet rosetting around PMN and increased platelet aggregation may occur in Behçet's disease.

9. There is significant evidence suggesting that endothelial cell injury modulated by enhanced PMN activity, increased release of neutrophil-derived oxygen intermediates, and production of anticardiolipin antibodies, plays a pathogenetic role in the development of the vascular complications of Behçet's syndrome.

References

1. Yalçin B, Gürsoy A, Ezer G, et al. Haematological and immunological features of Behçet's disease. *Haematologica* 1980; 65:390–394.
2. Kluft C, Michiels JJ, Wijngaards G. Factual or artificial inhibition of fibrinolysis and the occurrence of venous thrombosis in 3 cases of Behçet's disease. *Scand J Haematol* 1980; 25:423–430.

3. Haim S, Sobel JD, Friedman-Birnbaum R. Thrombophlebitis. A cardinal symptom of Behçet's syndrome. *Acta Derm Venereol* (Stockh) 1974; 54:299–301.
4. Chajek T, Aronowski E, Izak G. Decreased fibrinolysis in Behçet's disease. *Thromb Diath Haemorrh* 1973; 29:610–618.
5. Chajek T. Fainaru M. Behçet's disease. Report of 41 cases and a review of the literature. *Medicine* 1975; 54:179–196.
6. Toki N, Yamura T. Studies on the blood fibrinolytic enzyme system of patients with cutaneous vasculitis. *Br J Dermatol* 1980; 103:41–50.
7. Collum, LMT, Mullaney J, Bowell R. Current concepts of Behçet's disease. *Trans Ophthalmol Soc UK* 1981; 101:422–428.
8. Cunliffe WJ. An association between cutaneous vasculitis and decreased blood-fibrinolytic activity. *Lancet* 1968; 1:1226–1228.
9. Cunliffe WJ, Menon IS. The association between cutaneous vasculitis and decreased blood fibrinolytic activity. *Br J Dermatol* 1971; 84:99–105.
10. Mishima H, Masuda K, Shjimada S, et al. Plasminogen activator activity levels in patients with Behçet's syndrome. *Arch Ophthalmol* 1985; 103:935–936.
11. Francis CW, Marder VJ. Mechanisms of fibrinolysis. In Williams WJ, Beutler E, Erslev AJ, Lichtman MA, eds: *Hematology*. New York, McGraw-Hill, 1983:1266–1276.
12. Davidson JF, Walker ID. Assessment of the fibrinolytic system. In Bloom A, Thomas DP, eds: *Haemostasis and Thrombosis*. New York, Churchill Livingstone, 1981:796–808.
13. Jordan JM, Allen NB, Pizzo SV. Defective release of tissue plasminogen activator in systemic and cutaneous vasculitis. *Am J Med* 1987; 82:397–400.
14. Isaacson S. Nilsson IM. Antithrombotic effect of a combined phenformin ethyloestrenol therapy. In Von Kaulla KN, Davidson JF, eds: Synthetic fibrinolytic thrombolytic agents. Springfield, IL, Charles C Thomas, 1975:171–180.
15. Menon IS, Cunliffe WJ, Dewar HA. Preliminary report of beneficial effect of phenformin in combination with ethyloestrenol in treatment of cutaneous vasculitis and Behçet's syndrome. *Postgrad Med J* 1969 *(May Suppl)*; 45:62–63.
16. Cunliffe WJ, Menon IS. Treatment of Behçet's syndrome with phenformin and ethyloestrenol. *Lancet* 1969; 1:1239–1240.
17. Cunliffe WJ, Roberts BE, Dodman B. Behçet's syndrome and oral fibrinolytic therapy (letter). *Br Med J* 1973; 2:486–487.
18. Hull RG, Harris EN, Gharavi AE, et al. Anticardiolipin antibodies: Occurrence in Behçet's syndrome. *Ann Rheum Dis* 1984; 43:746–748.
19. Efthimiou J, Harris EN, Hughes GRV. Negative anticardiolipin antibodies and vascular complications in Behçet's syndrome (letter). *Ann Rheum Dis* 1985; 44:725–726.
20. Prchal JT, Blakely J. Granulocyte platelet rosettes (letter). *N Engl J Med* 1973; 289:1146.
21. Ehrlich GE, Kajani M, Schwartz IR, McAlack RF. Further studies of

platelet rosettes around granulocytes in Behçet's syndrome. *Inflammation* 1975–76; 1:223–229.

22. Matsuda T, Kaneko K, Hoshi K, Mizushima Y. Platelet function in Behçet's disease (abstract 34). Royal Society of Medicine International conference of Behçet's disease, September 5 and 6, 1985, London, England.

23. Kirch W, Hutt HJ, Dührsen U, Ohnhaus EE. Platelet function in patients with Behçet's syndrome and in healthy subjects (abstract 35). Royal Society of Medicine international conference on Behçet's disease, September 5 and 6, 1985, London, England.

24. Hizli N, Sahin G, Sahin F, et al. Plasma prostacyclin levels in Behçet's disease (letter). *Lancet* 1985; 1:1454.

25. Ritter JM, Barrow SE, Quigley C. Plasma prostacyclin levels in Behçet's disease (letter). *Lancet* 1985; 2:497.

26. Kansu E, Sahin G, Sahin F, et al. Impaired prostacyclin synthesis by vessel walls in Behçet's disease (letter). *Lancet* 1986; 2:1154.

27. Rosenberg RD, Rosenberg JS. Natural anticoagulant mechanisms. *J Clin Invest* 1984; 74:1–6.

28. Schmitz-Huebner U, Knop J. Evidence for an endothelial cell dysfunction in association with Behçet's disease. *Thromb Res* 1984; 34:277–285.

29. Harlan JM. Leukocyte-endothelial interactions. *Blood* 1985; 65:513–525.

30. Leonard RCF, Thompson RB. Behçet's syndrome and neutropenia. *Postgrad Med J* 1981; 54:448–449.

31. Mizushima Y, Matsumura N, Mori M. Chemotaxis of leukocytes and colchicine treatment in Behçet's disease. *J Rheumatol* 1979; 6:108–110.

32. Sobel JD, Haim S, Obedenau N, et al. Polymorphonuclear leukocyte function in Behçet's disease. *J Clin Pathol* 1977; 30:250–253.

33. Jorizzo JL, Hudson RD, Schmalstieg FC, et al. Behçet's syndrome: Immune regulation, circulating immune complexes, neutrophil migration, and colchicine therapy. *J Am Acad Dermatol* 1984; 10:205–214.

34. James DW, Walker JR, Smith MJH. Abnormal polymorphonuclear leucocyte chemotaxis in Behçet's syndrome. *Ann Rheum Dis* 1979; 38:219–221.

35. Fordham JN, Davies PG, Kirk A, Currey HLF. Polymorphonuclear function in Behçet's syndrome. *Ann Rheum Dis* 1982; 41:421–425.

36. Niwa Y, Miyake S, Sakane T, et al. Autooxidative damage in Behçet's disease—Endothelial cell damage following the elevated oxygen radicals generated by stimulated neutrophils. *Clin Exp Immunol* 1982; 49:247–255.

37. Ozaki Y, Ôhashi T, Niwa Y. Evaluation of neutrophil acetyltransferase activity in patients with inflammatory disorders. *Life Sci* 1986; 39:2343–2350.

7

PATHOGENESIS:
MISCELLANEOUS FACTORS

Gary R. Plotkin

THE PRECEDING CHAPTERS HAVE EXTENSIVELY reviewed those functions of inflammation, autoimmunity, coagulation, and fibrinolysis as they relate to the pathogenesis of Behçet's syndrome. Since the etiology of this disease remains an enigma, investigators have studied a multitude of various infectious agents and metabolic, physiological, and biochemical factors in attempts to better understand this disorder. Although these factors have at times been studied as independent variables, their influence may indeed be interrelated, thus emphasizing the potential complexity of the pathogenesis of Behçet's disease. This chapter attempts to review those factors not previously discussed which have received the most attention in the recent literature.

Organic Compounds and Trace Minerals

Since Behçet's disease may have predilections for certain geographic localities (i.e., Japan and the eastern Mediterranean countries), investigators have concentrated on environmental factors to

From *Behcet's Disease: A Contemporary Synopsis*, edited by Gary R. Plotkin, M.D., John J. Calabro, M.D., and J. Desmond O'Duffy, M.B. © 1988, Futura Publishing Company, Inc., Mount Kisco, NY.

explain the pathogenesis of this disorder. According to Ishikawa et al.,[1] chemicals such as organophosphate, organochloride, and inorganic copper compounds are commonly used in Japan and, therefore, an animal model of pedigreed Pitman Moor strain miniature swine was fed these compounds. After 4 to 10 months of administration of these chemicals, the animals developed intestinal and genital ulcers, cutaneous lesions, and oral aphthae which mimicked the human manifestations of Behçet's syndrome. The copper content was highest in the skin and liver.[1] In addition, Hori et al.[2] and Nishiyama et al.[3] reported elevated levels of polychlorinated biphenyls in the sera, and chloride, copper, and phosphorus content in neutrophils, macrophages, vascular endothelial cells, inflammatory cells of skin lesions, and epithelial cells of hair follicles from patients with Behçet's disease. In several studies of patients with Behçet's syndrome, blood and sural nerve levels of organophosphate, organochloride, and inorganic copper were elevated; levels of benzene hexachloride and dichloro-diphenyl trichlorethane were increased in sural nerve specimens; and polychlorinated biphenyls were elevated in the sera, peripheral sural nerve, skin, and blood vessels.[2-4] Shimizu et al.[5] have reported a significant correlation between increased levels of serum copper and the ocular attacks in patients with Behçet's disease and observed that an increase in the serum copper concentration preceded the ocular attacks. Also, the higher the level of this trace element, the more severe the ocular manifestations. Enucleated globes from patients with Behçet's disease contained higher concentrations of copper in the hypopyon, aqueous humor, and vitreous body as compared to controls.[5]

Serum zinc levels have tended to be decreased in patients with Behçet's syndrome, and the absolute levels have been lower in those with the ocular and arthritic manifestations.[6] Zinc concentrations in enucleated eyes from patients with Behçet's disease have not differed from those levels found in the ocular structures obtained from controls.[5] At least in patients with rheumatoid arthritis, plasma zinc and copper levels may be decreased and increased, respectively, and therefore changes in these trace elements are not specific for Behçet's disease. In addition, since the majority of serum copper is complexed to the acute-phase reactant protein ceruloplasmin, elevations of this trace element may be secondary to systemic or tissue inflammation and thus not reflect environmental or nutritional aberrations.[7] Serum magnesium levels have been normal in patients with Behçet's syndrome.[6]

Lipoproteins

Ohguchi et al.[8] have analyzed serum lipid levels in patients with Behçet's disease. They observed normal levels of serum triglyceride and phospholipid; however, high-density lipoprotein cholesterol was decreased while beta-lipoprotein was elevated in a statistically significant proportion of the study sample. Nevertheless, the ranges of the absolute values of the serum lipids overlapped with the normal controls.[8] Since many variables may influence serum lipid concentrations (e.g., diet, medications, exercise, renal disease), additional studies that control for these many variables are necessary to enable one to correlate lipid abnormalities with the pathophysiology and disease activity of Behçet's syndrome. Since the precipitation of immunoglobulin-lipoprotein complexes within tissue may occur in certain disorders characterized by abnormal immunoglobulins such as multiple myeloma, macroglobulinemia, lymphocytic leukemia, and lymphoma,[9] determination of these complexes in patients with Behçet's syndrome may reveal additional insight into the pathogenesis of this disease.

Alpha-1-Proteinase Inhibitor (Antitrypsin)

This glycoprotein, which is an acute-phase reactant, is the major alpha-1-globulin in human serum, and its main function is to inhibit various serine proteases including plasmin, thrombin, Factor XI, Factor XIII, neutrophil proteases elastase and cathepsin G, and pancreatic elastase, trypsin, and chymotrypsin.[10] This serum protease inhibitor, which is primarily of hepatic origin and to a lesser extent mononuclear phagocytes, is the major inhibitor of neutrophil elastase, an enzyme capable of degrading the major connective-tissue components of the extracellular matrix of various tissues.[10,11] Its deficiency in human sera has been reported in patients with idiopathic anterior uveitis.[12-14] The ocular manifestations of Behçet's disease include anterior uveitis and retinal vasculitis[15]; however, Wakefield et al.[14] have reported eight patients with Behçet's syndrome and retinal vasculitis, all of whom possessed normal to elevated serum levels of alpha-1-proteinase inhibitor with normal distribution of phenotypes (M1M1, M1M2, M1M3, M2M3). Moreover, serum antitrypsin deficiency has not been reported in association with Behçet's syndrome, and in fact serum levels of this glycoprotein are normal to elevated in patients with Behçet's disease.[14] It is possible that the tissue levels of alpha-1-proteinase inhibitor are more important than the serum concentrations in the pathogenesis of Behçet's syndrome.

Hormonal Factors

According to Yazici et al.,[16] male patients with Behçet's syndrome may have more severe disease as defined by the extent of ocular involvement and the presence of major vascular complications. In one study the mean serum testosterone level was 7.09 ± 1.70 ng/ml in 26 male patients with Behçet's syndrome as compared to 6.70 ± 1.43 ng/ml in 26 age-matched healthy men, while the mean serum estradiol levels were 43.26 ± 15.9 ng/ml and 45.30 ± 26.39 ng/ml in the respective groups. Despite the overlap of the values of serum testosterone and estradiol levels in patients and controls, these investigators postulated that hormonal factors contributed to disease activity.[17] The same group of investigators observed that male patients with Behçet's disease had stronger pathergy reactions compared to female patients of similar age and disease duration; however, there was discordance between the intensity of the pathergy reaction and the severity of disease activity.[18] Ratios of progesterone and estrogen may influence the onset and severity of recurrent oral ulcerations since the onset of aphthous ulcers may commence with puberty or the menarche, and the ulcers often regress during pregnancy. In certain disorders of recurrent aphthous stomatitis, one may observe remissions and exacerbations of the oral lesions during the third trimester of pregnancy and after parturition, respectively. During the third trimester of pregnancy and after parturition, the rates of estrogen secretion are increasing and decreasing, respectively. Also, the development of new oral ulcerations tends to occur during the premenstrual phase, the week starting on the first day of menstruation, and the seven days after ovulation. These intervals also correspond to lower levels of plasma estrogen concentrations. Decreased keratinization of the oral mucosa occurs during these intervals of low estrogen production, thus, perhaps accounting for the increased vulnerability of the oral mucosa to aphthous formation.[19–24] Certain women with Behçet's syndrome have experienced exacerbations of genital ulcerations and uveitis immediately prior to and during menstruation and after delivery or miscarriage, while symptomatic improvement has occurred during pregnancy.[25] Oral contraceptives may also prevent or improve the symptomatology of the acute attacks in Behcet's disease.[20,25] However, complicating these observations have been reports of exacerbations of disease activity during pregnancy including the third trimester.[26,27]

Biochemical and Physiological Responses

Several serum biochemical parameters have been analyzed in patients with Behçet's syndrome, and in these investigations, varying proportions of the study samples had depressed serum histidine and total sulphydryl contentrations while the serum mucoprotein and sialic acid levels were elevated.[28–30] Patients with rheumatoid arthritis may have decreased serum histidine concentrations, probably representing a metabolic response to inflammation[7]; however, Dixon et al.[28] reported that the depressed histidine levels in patients with Behçet's disease were unrelated to the presence of arthritis.

Increased plasma levels of cyclic 3',5'-guanosine monophosphate (cyclic GMP) have been reported in patients with Behçet's disease, especially in those with active clinical symptoms, but such elevated levels may be observed in other systemic inflammatory diseases, including rheumatoid arthritis, systemic lupus erythematosus, and progressive systemic sclerosis. According to Matsumura et al.,[31] plasma cyclic GMP may serve as a useful marker to monitor the activity of Behçet's disease; however, elevated levels have not been shown to correlate with any specific symptom complex. The plasma levels of cyclic 3′,5′-adenosine monophosphate (cyclic AMP) in patients with Behçet's syndrome were comparable to those in normal controls.[31]

Yamada et al.[32] have demonstrated that the collagenolytic activity of neutrophils from patients with Behçet's disease was elevated during the acute phases, and that this enhanced enzymatic activity may be due to activation of intracellular neutral proteases such as elastase and collagenase. These activated neutral proteases may contribute to the tissue destruction characteristic of Behçet's syndrome.

Fujii et al.[33] and Hylton et al.[34] have reported nonstatistically to statistically significant increased levels of 2′,5′-oligoadenylate synthetase activity in the peripheral blood mononuclear leukocytes from patients with Behçet's disease. The induction of this enzyme, which catalyzes the formation of (2′-5′)oligoadenylate from ATP in the presence of double-stranded RNA,[35] is under the influence of interferon, and Hylton et al.[34] have observed an increase in the induced enzyme activity in patients with Behçet's disease as compared to the controls. However, these observations have not been universal,[33] and increased interferon-induced enzyme 2′,5′-oligoadenylate synthetase activity may also occur in the circulating blood lymphocytes from patients with systemic lupus erythematosus, rheumatoid arthritis, Vogt-Koyanagi-Harada disease, sarcoidosis, viral infections, and tuberculous.[34,35]

According to Thomas et al.,[36] the serum concentrations of pregnancy-associated alpha-2-glycoprotein were elevated in a proportion of male patients with Behçet's disease; however, this glycoprotein may also be increased in a variety of malignant and nonmalignant diseases. Only male subjects were studied because of the variations in the levels of this glycoprotein during the menstrual cycle. Pregnancy-associated alpha-2-glycoprotein, unlike alpha-1-acid glycoprotein, is probably not an acute-phase reactant, and its function may involve the modulation of the immune response. This glycoprotein, the source of which may be the membranes of peripheral blood leukocytes, impairs E rosette formation of T lymphocytes, suppresses mitogen and antigen-induced lymphocyte transformation and mixed leukocyte reactions, and prolongs allograft survival in the mouse.[36]

Serum beta-2-microglobulin, which is a small molecular weight protein, is a constituent of the cell surface histocompatibility antigen, and in one study, concentrations of this moiety were significantly elevated in patients with Behçet's syndrome. Increased levels of this protein have also been reported in lymphoproliferative and autoimmune diseases, thus suggesting that these raised concentrations may represent lymphocyte proliferation secondary to altered immune regulation. Serum levels of beta-2-microglobulin may correlate with concentrations of acute-phase reactants, thus representing a marker for disease activity in Behçet's syndrome.[37]

Levels of gamma-aminobutyric acid (GABA), an inhibitory neurotransmitter, have been reported to be decreased in the cerebrospinal fluid from two patients with the neurological complications of Behçet's disease. These low levels may have been secondary to alterations in GABA metabolism, decreased content within the brain tissue, or alterations in the physiological functions of the nervous system. Diminished levels of this neurotransmitter may also occur in patients with Alzheimer's disease, late cortical cerebellar atrophy, olivopontocerebellar atrophy, Huntington's chorea, Parkinson's disease, and cerebral hemorrhage.[38]

Hepatitis B Virus

Since the underlying histopathology of Behçet's disease is an active vasculitis,[39-41] and since immune complex–mediated vasculitis may occur in a variety of infectious diseases,[42] such as the classic association of systemic necrotizing vasculitis and hepatitis B antigenemia,[43,44] several investigators have focused on the incidence of this viral disease in patients with Behçet's disease.[45-48] Although patients with Behçet's syndrome may indeed possess hepatitis B antigenemia, especially if they reside in countries with a high frequency of infection with this agent,[45-48] the role of this virus in the pathogenesis of Behçet's disease remains unknown. Patients with either Behçet's syndrome or hepatitis B virus infection may manifest clinical symptoms owing to vasculitis affecting small, medium, and large vessels,[39-41,43,44,49,50] and there have been anecdotal case reports of patients with both Behçet's disease and hepatitis B antigenemia manifesting unusual features of their illness.[51-54] However, additional prospective studies are needed in order to correlate the clinical and pathological features of Behçet's syndrome with the persistence of hepatitis B viral infection.[45]

Type C RNA Retrovirus

In the sera collected from a limited number of patients with Behçet's disease, Maeda et al.[55] discovered elevated titers of an IgM antibody which reacted with the basal aspect of syncytiotrophoblast of human chorionic villi. This antibody was named anti-BAST and cross-reacted with the subhuman primate type C RNA retrovirus SSV/SSAV (simian sarcoma virus/simian sarcoma-associated virus). However, this antibody may also be detected in the sera of normal controls and in patients with idiopathic thrombocytopenic purpura, autoimmune hemolytic anemia, rheumatoid arthritis, mixed connective-tissue disease, and adult T-cell leukemia.[55]

As is evident from the preceding discussion, investigators have studied various immunological, metabolic, biochemical, and physiological parameters in patients with Behçet's disease; however, not only may these markers represent epiphenomena, but their function in the pathogenesis of this disease remains unknown.

References

1. Ishikawa S, Miyata M, Fujiwara N, et al. Experimental "mucocutaneo-entero-genital syndrome" in pedigreed miniature swine (toxicological study). In Dilşen N, Koniçe M, Övül C, eds: *Behçet's Disease. Proceedings of an International Symposium on Behçet's Disease, Istanbul, 29–30 September 1977.* Amsterdam-Oxford, Excerpta Medica, 1979:53–59.
2. Hori Y, Miyazawa S, Miyata M. et al. Ultrastructural x-ray microanalysis of tissues in Behçet's disease. In Dilşen N, Koniçe M, Övül C, eds: *Behçet's Disease. Proceedings of an International Symposium on Behçet's Disease, Istanbul, 29–30 September 1977.* Amsterdam-Oxford, Excerpta Medica, 1979:66–72.

3. Nishiyama S. Murakami M, Hori Y. The etiological role of organic chloride in Behçet's disease (abstract). In Dilşen N, Koniçe M, Övül C, eds: *Behçet's Disease. Proceedings of an International Symposium on Behçet's Disease, Istanbul, 29–30 September 1977.* Amsterdam-Oxford, Excerpta Medica, 1979:60.

4. O'Duffy JD. Summary of international symposium on Behçet's disease, Istanbul, September 29–30, 1977. *J Rheumatol* 1978; 5:229–233.

5. Shimizu K. Ishikawa S. Miyata M, et al. Relationships between the changes of serum copper levels and ocular attacks in Behçet's disease (an etiological consideration). In Dilşen N, Koniçe M, Övül C, eds: *Behçet's Disease. Proceedings of an International Symposium on Behçet's Disease, Istanbul, 29–30 September 1977.* Amsterdam-Oxford, Excerpta Medica, 1979:61–65.

6. Cengiz K. Serum zinc, copper and magnesium in Behçet's disease (abstract 22). Royal Society of Medicine international conference on Behçet's disease, September 5 and 6, 1985, London, England.

7. Mascioli EA, Blackburn GL. Nutrition and rheumatic disease. In Kelley WN, Harris ED Jr, Ruddy S, Sledge CB, eds: *Textbook of Rheumatology.* Philadelphia, WB Saunders, 1985:352–360.

8. Ohguchi M, Ohno S, Tanaka K, et al. Studies on serum lipids in patients with Behçet's disease. In Inaba G, ed: *Behçet's Disease. Pathogenetic Mechanism and Clinical Future. Proceedings of the International Conference on Behçet's Disease, Tokyo, October 23–24, 1981.* Tokyo, University of Tokyo Press, 1982:177–181.

9. Malloy MJ, Kane JP. Hypolipidemia. *Med Clin North Am* 1982; 66:469–485.

10. Gadek JE, Crystal RG. α_1-antitrypsin deficiency. In Stanbury JB, Wyngaarden JB, Fredrickson DS, et al, eds: *The Metabolic Basis of Inherited Disease.* New York, McGraw-Hill, 1983:1450–1467.

11. Mornex J-G, Chytil-Weir A, Martinet Y, et al: Expression of the alpha-1-antitrypsin gene in mononuclear phagocytes of normal and alpha-1-antitrypsin-deficient individuals. *J Clin Invest* 1986; 77:1952–1961.

12. Brewerton DA, Webley M, Murphy AH, Ward AM. The α_1-antitrypsin phenotype MZ in acute anterior uveitis (letter). *Lancet* 1978; 1:1103.

13. Wakefield D, Breit SN, Clark P, Penny R. Immunogenetic factors in inflammatory eye disease. Influence of HLA-B27 and alpha$_1$-antitrypsin phenotypes on disease expression. *Arthritis Rheum* 1982; 25:1431–1434.

14. Wakefield D, Easter J, Breit SN, et al. α_1-antitrypsin serum levels and phenotypes in patients with retinal vasculitis. *Br J Ophthalmol* 1985; 69:497–499.

15. Colvard DN, Robertson DM, O'Duffy JD. The ocular manifestations of Behçet's disease. *Arch Ophthalmol* 1977; 95:1813–1817.

16. Yazici H, Tüzün Y, Pazarli H, et al. Influence of age of onset and patient's sex on the prevalence and severity of manifestations of Behçet's syndrome. *Ann Rheum Dis* 1984; 43:783–789.

17. Yazici H, Hekim N, Tüzün Y, et al. Sex hormones and Behçet's syn-

drome (abstract 48). Royal Society of Medicine international conference on Behçet's disease, September 5 and 6, 1985, London, England.

18. Yazici H, Tüzün Y, Tanman AB, et al. Male patients with Behçet's syndrome have stronger pathergy reactions. *Clin Exp Rheumatol* 1985; 3:137–141.

19. Cooke BED. Oral ulceration in Behçet's syndrome. In Lehner T, Barnes CG, eds: *Behçet's Syndrome. Clinical and Immunological Features. Proceedings of a Conference Sponsored by the Royal Society of Medicine, February 1979.* London, Academic Press, 1979:143–149.

20. Cooke BED. Recurrent oral ulceration. *Br J Dermatol* 1969; 81:159–161.

21. Francis TC. Recurrent aphthous stomatitis and Behçet's disease. A review. *Oral Surg* 1970; 30:476–487.

22. Lehner T. Oral ulceration and Behçet's syndrome. *Gut* 1977; 18:491–511.

23. Rogers RS III. Recurrent aphthous stomatitis: Clinical characteristics and evidence for an immunopathogenesis. *J Invest Dermatol* 1977; 69:499–509.

24. Ship II, Merritt AD, Stanley HR. Recurrent aphthous ulcers. *Am J Mec* 1962; 32:32–43.

25. Dunlop EMC. Genital and other manifestations of Behçet's disease seen in venereological practice. In Lehner T, Barnes CG, eds: *Behçet's syndrome. Clinical and Immunological Features. Proceedings of a Conference Sponsored by the Royal Society of Medicine, February 1979.* London, Academic Press, 1979:159–175.

26. Hurt WG, Cooke CL, Jordan WP, et al. Behçet's syndrome associated with pregnancy. *Obstet Gynecol* 1979; 53(3, Suppl):31S–33S.

27. Jorizzo JL, Taylor RS, Schmalstieg FC, et al. Complex aphthosis: A forme fruste of Behçet's syndrome? *J Am Acad Dermatol* 1985; 13:80–84.

28. Dixon JS, Yurdakul S, Surrall KE, et al. A study of serum biochemistry in Behçet's syndrome. *Br J Rheumatol* 1984; 23:283–287.

29. Oshima Y, Shimizu T, Yokohari R, et al. Clinical studies on Behçet's syndrome. *Ann Rheum Dis* 1963; 22:36–45.

30. Shimizu T, Katsuta Y, Oshima Y. Immunological studies on Behçet's syndrome. *Ann Rheum Dis* 1965; 24:494–500.

31. Matsumura Y, Hayakawa T. Clinical symptoms and plasma cyclic nucleotide levels in Behçet's disease. In Inaba G, ed: *Behçet's Disease. Pathogenetic Mechanism and Clinical Future. Proceedings of the International Conference on Behçet's Disease, Tokyo, October 23–24, 1981.* Tokyo, University of Tokyo Press, 1982:89–96.

32. Yamada M, Kishida K, Yuasa T, et al. Neutrophil collagenolytic activity in patients with Behçet disease. *Curr Eye Res* 1984; 3:779–782.

33. Fujii N, Kotake S, Hirose S, et al. Oligo-2',5'-adenylate synthetase activity in peripheral blood mononuclear leukocytes in various diseases. *J Clin Microbiol* 1984; 20:1216–1218.

34. Hylton W, Cayley J, Dore C, Denman AM. 2',5'-oligoadenylate synthetase induction in lymphocytes of patients with connective tissue diseases. *Ann Rheum Dis* 1986; 45:220–224.

35. Sugino H, Mitani I, Koike M, et al. Detection of elevated levels of 2-5A synthetase in serum from children with various infectious diseases. *J Clin Microbiol* 1985; 24:478–481.
36. Thomson AW, Lehner T, Adinolfi M, Horne CHW. Pregnancy-associated alpha-2-glycoprotein in recurrent oral ulceration and Behçet's syndrome. *Int Arch Allergy Appl Immunol* 1981; 66:33–39.
37. Scully C. Serum $\beta_2$microglobulin in recurrent aphthous stomatitis and Behçet's syndrome. *Clin Exp Dermatol* 1982; 7:61–64.
38. Kuroda H. Gamma-aminobutyric acid (GABA) in cerebrospinal fluid. *Acta Med Okayama* 1983; 37:167–177.
39. Cupps TR, Fauci AS. Behçet's disease. In: *The Vasculitides*. Philadelphia, WB Saunders, 1981:142–146.
40. Fauci AS. Vasculitis. *J Allergy Clin Immunol* 1983; 72:211–223.
41. Shimizu T, Ehrlich GE, Inaba G, Hayashi K. Behçet disease (Behçet syndrome). *Semin Arthritis Rheum* 1979; 8:223–260.
42. Calabrese LH, Clough JD. Hypersensitivity vasculitis group (HVG). A case-oriented review of a continuing clinical spectrum. *Cleve Clin Q* 1982; 49:17–42.
43. Duffy J, Lidsky MD, Sharp JT, et al. Polyarthritis, polyarteritis and hepatitis B. *Medicine* 1976; 55:19–37.
44. Sergent JS, Lockshin MD, Christian CL, Gocke DJ. Vasculitis with hepatitis B antigenemia; Long-term observations in nine patients. *Medicine* 1976; 55:1–18.
45. Aksungur P. The determination of hepatitis surface antigen and antibody in patients with Behçet's disease. In Dilşen N, Koniçe M, Övül C, eds: *Behçet's Disease. Proceedings of an International Symposium on Behçet's Disease, Istanbul, 29–30 September 1977.* Amsterdam-Oxford, Excerpta Medica, 1979:249–253.
46. Hamza H, Ayed HB. Clinical and histological study of 55 cases of Behçet's disease (abstract). In Dilşen N, Koniçe M, Övül C, eds: *Behçet's Disease. Proceedings of an International Symposium on Behçet's Disease, Istanbul, 29–30 September 1977.* Amsterdam-Oxford, Excerpta Medica, 1979:107.
47. Larsson H, Bengtsson-Stigmar E. Behçet's disease and close contact with pigs. *Acta Med Scand* 1984; 216:541–543.
48. Önes Ü, Urgancioğlu M, Yakacikli S, Yalçin I. Behçet's disease and hepatitis B antigen. In Dilşen N, Koniçe M, Övül C, eds: *Behçet's Disease. Proceedings of an International Symposium on Behçet's Disease, Istanbul, 29–30 September 1977.* Amsterdam-Oxford: Excerpta Medica, 1979:245–248.
49. Gower RG, Sausker WF, Kohler PF, et al. Small vessel vasculitis caused by hepatitis B virus immune complexes. Small vessel vasculitis and HBsAG. *J Allergy Clin Immunol* 1978; 62:222–228.
50. Shusterman N, London WT. Hepatitis B and immune-complex disease. *N Engl J Med* 1984; 310:43–46.
51. Bowles CA, Nelson AM, Hammill SC, O'Duffy JD. Cardiac involvement in Behçet's disease. *Arthritis Rheum* 1985; 28:345–348.
52. Cadman EC, Lundberg WB, Mitchell MS. Pulmonary manifestations

in Behçet syndrome. Case report and review of the literature. *Arch Intern Med* 1976; 136:944–947.

53. Plotkin GR, Patel BR, Shah VN. Behçet's syndrome complicated by cutaneous leukocytoclastic vasculitis. Response to prednisone and chlorambucil. *Arch Intern Med* 1985; 145:1913–1915.

54. Schiff S, Moffatt R, Mandel WJ, Rubin SA. Acute myocardial infarction and recurrent ventricular arrhythmias in Behçet's syndrome. *Am Heart J* 1982; 103:438–440.

55. Maeda S, Yonezawa K, Yachi A. Serum antibody reacting with placental syncytiotrophoblast in sera of patients with autoimmune disease—A possible relation to type C RNA retrovirus. *Clin Exp Immunol* 1985; 60:645–653.

8

PATHOLOGY

Sharad Lakhanpal, J. Desmond O'Duffy, and J. T. Lie

THE TRIPLE SYMPTOM COMPLEX of recurrent oral and genital ulcers and relapsing iritis, that since bears his name, was reported by Hulûsi Behçet, a Turkish dermatologist, in 1937; although similar cases might have been described earlier in the literature.[1] Behçet's syndrome[2] has evolved from the original classic triad into a more recently recognized systemic disease with mucocutaneous, cardiovascular, pulmonary, gastrointestinal, urogenital, ophthalmic, neurological, and musculoskeletal manifestations.[1,3-8] Despite the broadened clinical understanding of this disease, the etiology of Behçet's syndrome remains speculative; viral agents, immunological factors, fibrinolytic defects, genetic causes, bacterial factors, and environmental influences have all been variably implicated in its pathogenecity.[9]

Although the diagnosis of Behçet's syndrome remains essentially a clinical one, many of the manifestations have been well characterized in the literature.[10,11] In the absence of pathognomonic clinical and laboratory findings, various sets of diagnostic criteria have been proposed by different groups of investigators.[12-16] Based upon these accepted criteria, which have been amply reviewed in a previous chapter, the following discussion summarizes the protean features of the pathology of Behçet's syndrome.

From *Behcet's Disease: A Contemporary Synopsis*, edited by Gary R. Plotkin, M.D., John J. Calabro, M.D., and J. Desmond O'Duffy, M.B. © 1988, Futura Publishing Company, Inc., Mount Kisco, NY.

Mucocutaneous Lesions

Aphthous Stomatitis

Recurrent aphthous stomatitis according to certain authorities is a sine qua non of Behçet's syndrome, occurs in virtually all patients with this disorder, and is frequently the first systemic manifestation of the disease.[5,7,10,17,18] The ulcers, which are located on the lips, gingiva, buccal mucosa, tongue, and less commonly on the palate, tonsils, and pharynx, may be single or multiple with some occurring in clusters.[1] The oral lesion usually begins as an erythematous, slightly raised area which ulcerates in one to two days. The ulcer may be 2 to 10 mm in diameter with a central yellow base surrounded by a discrete erythematous halo and may heal in 3 to 30 days[10] (average 7–14 days[1,5]), usually without scarring; however, recurrences are common. Glossitis may also be present in Behçet's syndrome.[8]

Microscopic examination of the oral ulcers resembles that of recurrent aphthae,[10,19,20] that is, an area of the lesion shows eroded epidermis with lymphocytic and monocytic inflammatory infiltrates in the basal and prickle cell layers of the epidermis and the dermis (Fig. 1A).[21] Plasma cells are usually absent during the early stages of ulcer formation. However, as the lesion ages, neutrophils increase in number.[21]

Genital Ulcers

Genital ulcers, similar to oral aphthae in symptomatology, are slightly less common and are reported in 74% to 97% of patients.[5,17,18] Interestingly, genital ulcers were found more commonly than the oral ones in an autopsy series,[8] perhaps reflecting the inadequacy of postmortem examination for oral lesions. In males, the ulcers occur on the urethral orifice, penis, scrotum, and perianal region, while in females, they occur on the vulva, vagina, cervix, and perineum, including the perianal area. As compared to oral ulcers, the genital lesions are fewer, larger, deeper, less recurrent, but more persistent and slower to heal. In addition, vaginal lesions may be asymptomatic unless associated with discharge, and thus

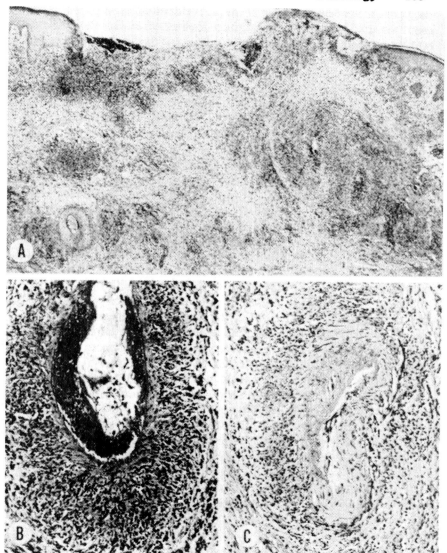

intense mixed-cell inflammatory infiltrate in the dermis. **B** and **C:** photomicrographs of subcutaneous necrotizing vasculitis with polyarteritis-type fibrinoid necrosis of vessel wall. (Hematoxylin-eosin; **A** × 40, **B** × 160)

the patient may be unaware of them.[17] The ulcers in men tend to be more painful than in women, and Huang et al.[17] have reported massive hemorrhage from rupture of a scrotal vein and vaginal wall vein by genital ulcers.

The histology of the genital ulcers is similar to the oral lesions, with edema and inflammatory infiltration of the dermis. Necrotizing vasculitis with fibrinoid necrosis may also be present in the subcutaneous tissue. These inflammatory changes may be accompanied by degeneration of the adjacent connective tissue.

Cutaneous Lesions

A variety of cutaneous lesions have been reported in 88% to 97% of patients with Behçet's syndrome[5,17] and are considered to be manifestations of cutaneous vasculitis (Fig. 1 B and C).[10] However, in another series,[18] cutaneous vasculitis has been reported in only 40% of patients with Behçet's syndrome. This incidence was identical to that of the articular manifestations.[18]

Nodular lesions resembling erythema nodosum macroscopically occur most frequently on the extremities, usually the lower ones, but may also be present on the face, neck, buttocks, or trunk.[1,17] They are considered to be manifestations of cutaneous vasculitis but occasionally may be due to phlebitis of the superficial veins.[10] In contrast to classic erythema nodosum, the nodular lesions in Behçet's syndrome may be grouped, may ulcerate, and after healing, may leave an area of hyperpigmentation.[10,17] Histologically, the lesions consist of vasculitis of venules, arterioles, and capillaries with perivascular lymphocytic and mononuclear cellular infiltration, fibrin deposition in vascular walls, and endothelial cell swelling that may partially obliterate the small vessel lumen, especially of the venules.[1,17,18] Perivascular connective tissue may be seen in the dermis and subcutaneous tissue,[1] and these nodular lesions have been reported to be histologically different from classic erythema nodosum since they lack histiocytic granulomas.[7]

Other cutaneous lesions of Behçet's syndrome, including vesicles and sterile pustules, may evolve into deep, punched-out ulcers.[22] Cutaneous leukocytoclastic vasculitis, which is pathologically characterized by infiltration of the small blood vessel wall with polymorphonuclear leukocytes, destruction of the vessel wall with fibrinoid necrosis, and fragmentation of the infiltrating leukocytes, has characterized these lesions.[22–24] Pustular vasculitis characterized by cutaneous pustular lesions on purpuric bases which histopathologically reveal either leukocytoclastic vasculitis or Sweet's-like vasculitis (neutrophilic vascular reaction), has also been reported in Behçet's syndrome.[23] The skin lesions of Sweet's syndrome are raised, painful plaques that on biopsy reveal neutrophilic infiltration of the dermis which is similar to leukocytoclastic vasculitis except for the absence of fibrinoid necrosis.[23]

The pathergy reaction, which is a characteristic hyperirritability of the skin, occurs commonly in Behçet's syndrome patients, especially those from certain geographic areas.[25] Pathergy may be elicited in 40 to 88% of patients,[7,17] may be induced by aseptic needle prick,[1] acupuncture,[17] and injection of physiological saline,[1,7] saliva,[1,7] or genital ulcer extract,[1,7] and may be demonstrable after 24 to 48 hours as either a tuberculin-like reaction with erythema and edema or as an aseptic pustule. A study of the histologic changes of the pathergy reaction revealed a polymorphonuclear leukocytic inflammatory exudate at 6 and 12 hours without an increase in mast cells.[26] At 24 hours, there was a significant polymorphonuclear infiltration along with mononuclear cells plus an intense mast cell infiltrate demonstrable by the toluidine blue stain. The histology remained unchanged from 24 to 48 hours, and corticosteroids did not alter either the gross appearance or the histology of the pathergy test.[26]

Thrombosis of the subcutaneous venules of the extremities has been reported in Behçet's syndrome and may lead to sclerosis. In addition, the thrombosed vein may be palpable as an area of induration of the subcutaneous tissue with erythema of the overlying skin; rarely, it may resemble obliterative migrating thrombophlebitis.[1] Folliculitis-like lesions with a broad infiltrative base, small pustular top, and wide erythematous halo may occur on the upper trunk, face, scalp, neck, extremities, and perianal region.[17] These may heal with hypertrophic scarring,[17] and some may become pustular in appearance.[1] Other associated cutaneous lesions in Behçet's syndrome include papules, vesicles, abscesses, acne, pyoderma, erythema multiforme, and erythema annulare.[5,7,17]

Cardiovascular Involvement

Cardiovascular involvement has been reported in 7% to 29% of cases of Behçet's syndrome,[17,27] and while vascular manifestations are common and important causes of morbidity and mortality, cardiac involvement has been described less frequently.[1]

Cardiac Pathology

Cardiomegaly was the most common cardiac abnormality found in an autopsy series of 170 cases with Behçet's syndrome, possibly due to primary myocardial disease.[8] However, pericardial and endocardial involvement were noted with equal frequency, and valvular disease affected the aortic, mitral, and tricuspid valves.[8]

Pericardial disease, which is an uncommon feature of Behçet's syndrome, is usually seen during the acute exacerbations of the disease.[27] Acute pericarditis has been documented mainly in isolated case reports,[28-32] and pericardial effusion has been observed at autopsy.[8,33] Mural endocarditis may occur, especially in the right ventricle,[34] and there may be hypertrophy of the right ventricle with thrombotic lesions or focal scars, depending upon disease duration (Fig. 2). Histologically, the lesions consisted of mixed granulocytic and mononuclear cellular infiltrates in vascular granulation tissue (Fig. 3). The inflammatory infiltrates may extend into the myocardium, and the lesions may heal by replacement fibrosis.

The endocardial disease may involve the mitral and aortic valves, producing valvulitis[33] which manifests clinically as valvular regurgitation.[35-37] However, a patient with both mitral stenosis and insufficiency has been reported from China.[17] Depending upon the stage of the disease, the macroscopic appearance of valvular heart disease in Behçet's syndrome may range from small vegetations on the free margins of the valves[33] to scarred structures with perforated leaflets.[36,37] The microscopic appearance also varies with the duration of the lesions; that is, in the acute stage, intense neutrophilic, lymphocytic, and macrophagic infiltration may be seen in association with areas of vascularization, fibrin deposition, and myxoid degeneration.[37] During the later phase, the inflammatory infiltrate is mononuclear with only sparse neutrophils.[33] The infiltrate extends deep to the elastica of the valve approxi-

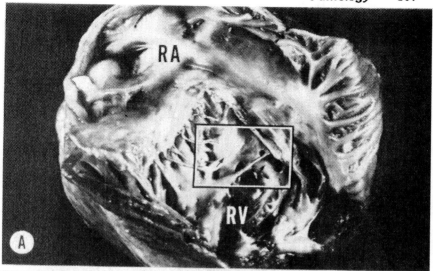

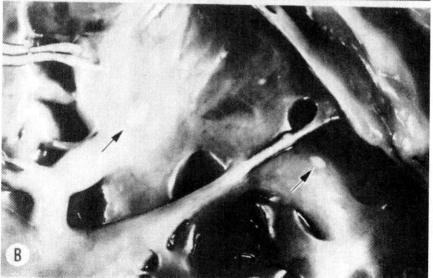

Figure 2—**A:** gross appearance of opened right atrium (RA) and right ventricle (RV) showing mural endocarditis of right ventricular septal wall beneath tricuspid valve. **B:** close-up view of boxed area in **A** with well-demarcated focal scars (arrows).

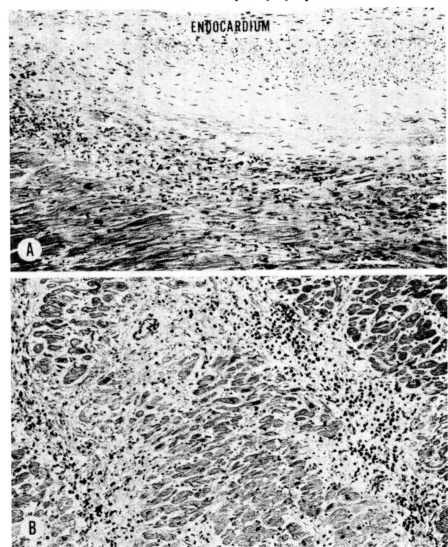

ENDOCARDIUM

A

B

Figure 3—Photomicrographs of endocarditis **(A)** and myocarditis **(B)**. Note early endocardial fibrosis and a predominantly mixed-cell inflammatory infiltrate in granulation tissue that has replaced lost myocardial fibers. (Hematoxylin-eosin; × 160)

mately halfway along the length of the cusp. There may also be focal myocardial fiber degeneration and infiltration of the myocardium and epicardium by mononuclear cells.[33] More chronic cases may show nonspecific fibrosis of the affected valves.[35,36] An aneurysm of the sinus of Valsalva in association with aortic regurgitation has also been described in a patient with Behçet's syndrome.[37]

Myocarditis may be suspected clinically by the presence of a cardiac murmur, gallop rhythm, dilatation of the heart, or electrocardiographic changes.[27,28] In other cases, myocardial disease may not be appreciated clinically and may only be recognized at postmortem examination.[38] Myocardial disease may cause cardiac enlargement[8]; however, the heart also has been reported to be grossly normal on postmortem examination.[38] Histologic examination may show myocardial fiber degeneration with a predominantly mononuclear inflammatory infiltrate.[38,39] Congestive heart failure in one case of Behçet's disease[40] and congestive cardiomyopathy in another[41] have each been attributed to primary myocardial disease of Behçet's syndrome.

Myocardial infarction due to unconfirmed vasculitic coronary artery occlusion in Behçet's syndrome has been reported in the literature.[42,43] In one such case, the autopsy revealed transmural sclerosis of the affected coronary artery which partially destroyed the elastic layer and extended through the adventitia.[42] These changes may represent the resolution phase of old arteritis. Left ventricular aneurysms may also occur secondary to coronary vasculitis in Behçet's syndrome.[32,42]

Conduction defects were among the early cardiac manifestations described in Behçet's syndrome,[4,44] and cardiac dysrhythmias have included sinus node dysfunction, various types of heart block, and atrial and ventricular rhythm disturbances.[4,17,42-45] In some patients the arrhythmias have been attributed to direct extension of the inflammation into the conduction tissue of the heart.[17,45] Histologic examination of the affected tissue has revealed only nonspecific chronic inflammation.[45]

Vascular Pathology

In a nationwide survey of Behçet's syndrome in Japan, vascular symptoms were reported in 7.7% of patients.[1] However, vascular lesions were found in 2.2% of a large series of patients from Tunisia[46] and in 3.6% and 10% in two additional series from Japan.[47,48] There are three categories of vascular lesions which consist of venous and arterial occlusions and aneurysm formation.[47] Venous occlusions are more common than the arterial ones and frequently affect the superior and inferior venae cavae.[1,47] Arterial occlusions are most common in the extremities, and rupture of aneurysms, especially those in the aorta,[47] is a leading cause of death in Behçet's syndrome.[1,47] An association between the presence of anticardiolipin antibodies and vascular pathology in Behçet's syndrome has been suggested in the literature.[49]

Recurrent superficial or deep vein thrombophlebitis is the most common venous lesion and has been reported in 25% to 40% of cases of Behçet's syndrome,[27,48,50] but despite this high incidence, pulmonary embolism secondary to peripheral thrombophlebitis is a rare event.[50] Vena caval obstruction due to spontaneous thrombosis is a frequent venoocclusive lesion, and this is followed, in order of decreasing frequency, by thrombosis of the femoral, subclavian, common iliac, hepatic, and greater saphenous veins.[27,33,51,52] The clinical manifestations depend on the site of venous obstruction and may include the superior vena caval syndrome and Budd-Chiari syndrome. The latter may lead to the development of esophageal varices.[1,8] Pathological examination reveals obstruction of the veins with an inflammatory thrombus which eventually may organize into fibrous cords.[33,51,52]

Histologically, the occluded large and medium-sized veins may show an organized thrombus in the vessel lumen and lymphocytic infiltration in the vessel wall.[33] Some veins may also reveal intimal fibrosis and focal collections of lymphocytes in the organized thrombi. In addition, the dural sinuses may be affected, resulting in certain neurological manifestations characteristic of Behçet's syndrome.

Arterial occlusions occur much less frequently than the venous ones, having been reported with an incidence of 1.3%[46] and 1%,[47] respectively, in two large series of Behçet's syndrome. Diverse clinical presentations are seen depending on the sites of occlusion.[1,27,46,53] Arterial occlusion usually occurs in single vessels with the pulmonary artery being the most often affected, followed by the subclavian, radial, popliteal, femoral, tibial, ulnar, coronary, iliac, carotid, aortic, brachial, renal, and mesenteric arteries.[46] Arterial obstruction may be due to thrombosis or stenosis; however, arteritis including aortitis has also been reported in the literature.[8] Coronary arteritis may cause myocardial ischemia,[8,43] and the mechanical trauma of sigmoidoscopy may lead to arterial thrombosis.[54] Histologically, the healed, occluded vessel shows fibrous · thickening of the intima and media with condensation of the elastic lamina.[1,39,48] Thromboangiitis may be seen involving the systemic arteries with intense cellular infiltration in the organized thrombi (Fig. 4 A and B).

Arterial aneurysm formation is more common than occlusion,[8,46,47] but the two may occur together in some patients.[46,53] The prognosis is better in occlusive disease than with aneurysm formation since the latter may lead to fatal rupture in up to 60% of cases.[17,47] The aneurysm is usually single but multiple lesions may occur,[46] and the aneurysms occur most frequently in the aorta, followed by the pulmonary, femoral, popliteal, brachial, iliac, carotid, coronary, subclavian, axillary, radial, ulnar, renal, and splenic arteries.[46] Although aneurysm formation in Behçet's syndrome is spontaneous and postulated to result from vasculitis,[46,50] arterial puncture from angiography or surgery may lead to formation of an aneurysm at the site of trauma.[27,46] The success rate of surgery for aneurysmal repair in Behçet's syndrome is low because of the recurrence of the lesion, perhaps secondary to the persistence of inflammatory and endarteritic changes in the vessel wall.[55] In addition to aneurysm formation,[55-58] false (pseudo) aneurysms of the aorta[36,53] and coronary arteries[59] have been described in Behçet's syndrome. Macroscopic examination of an aneurysm may show marked intimal roughness and linear wrinkling of the affected vessels,[60] and microscopic analysis has shown thickening of the intima with an inflammatory infiltrate containing lymphocytes, plasma cells, and polymorphonuclear leukocytes. There is disruption of the internal elastic lamina with splitting and loss of the elastic fibers in the media and loss of medial muscle fibers. Adventitial fibrosis and proliferation of the vasa vasorum with perivascular lymphocytic infiltration is present; granulomotous reaction in the adventitia may also be found histologically.[60,61] And since the thoracic aorta of a 16-week-old fetus from a patient with Behçet's syndrome has revealed edema of the

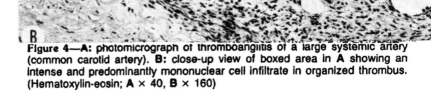

Figure 4—A: photomicrograph of thromboangiitis of a large systemic artery (common carotid artery). **B:** close-up view of boxed area in **A** showing an intense and predominantly mononuclear cell infiltrate in organized thrombus. (Hematoxylin-eosin; **A** × 40, **B** × 160)

intima and the inner part of the tunica media with rarefaction and disarrangement of the smooth-muscle cells, maternal disease may affect the fetal vascular system.[62]

Pulmonary Manifestations

Various pulmonary lesions have been reported in Behçet's syndrome. Pulmonary edema and pulmonary infections are the most common complications observed in autopsy series, suggesting that they most likely represent terminal events.[8,34,63] Clinical pulmonary disease is common in Behçet's syndrome,[1] and there have been reports of chronic obstructive lung disease in a few patients.[64-66] Bronchoscopic examination has shown both narrowing of the bronchial lumens and severe bronchial collapse with normal expiration.[64] Bronchial mucosal biopsies may reveal epithelial cell metaplasia and nonspecific inflammatory cell infiltrates in the submucosa.[64] Autopsy studies have described fibrosis of the small bronchi and bronchioles with narrowing of the bronchial lumens and localized emphysematous changes.[66] These alterations suggest that there may be bronchial stenosis in some cases of Behçet's syndrome secondary to inflammation of the bronchial epithelium.[64]

Vasculitis may affect the pulmonary vessels of all sizes including the arteries, arterioles, veins, and venules. The complications of pulmonary vasculitis may include aneurysm formation with adjacent bronchial erosion, arterial or venous thrombosis, and pulmonary infarcts.[67] Rupture of an arterial aneurysm into pulmonary tissue may cause pulmonary hemorrhage which may heal with fibrosis,[63,68] and rupture into a bronchial lumen may lead to hemoptysis,[50] which may be fatal if massive. Clinically, patients with the pulmonary manifestations of Behçet's syndrome present most often with hemoptysis. Inflammation of a vessel wall may cause aneurysmal dilation leading to thrombus formation, and the thromboangiitis may lead to erosion of the vessel wall with rupture into the adjacent bronchus (Fig. 5 A and B). Thromboangiitis of large branches of the pulmonary artery (Fig. 6 A and B) may result in pulmonary hypertension and right heart failure.[34,69]

Roentgenographically, pulmonary hemorrhages are seen as

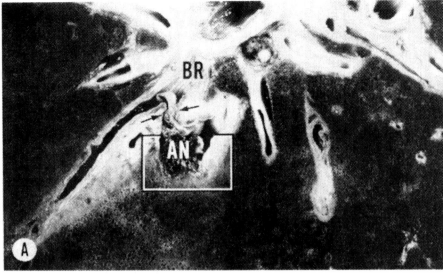

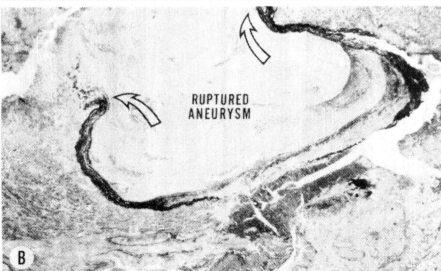

Figure 5—A: gross appearance of aneurysmal dilation of pulmonary artery thromboangiitis (AN) which has ruptured through eroded vessel wall (arrows), discharging blood into adjacent bronchus (BR). **B:** photomicrograph of ruptured aneurysm of pulmonary artery thromboangiitis with hemorrhage through eroded vessel wall (arrows). (Hematoxylin-eosin; **B** × 16)

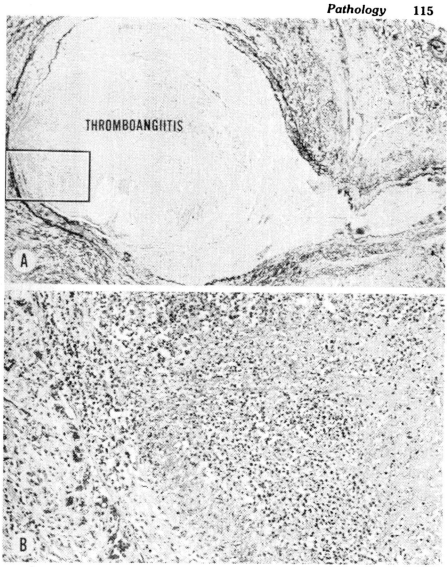

THROMBOANGIITIS

Figure 6—Photomicrograph of thromboangiitis of a large branch of pulmonary artery with intact wall **(A)**. Close-up view of A is seen in **B**, showing an inflammatory thrombus adherent to vessel wall and cell infiltrate in vessel wall. (Hematoxylin-eosin; **A** × 40, **B** × 160)

infiltrates, the necrotic and hemorrhagic pulmonary infarcts usually appear as peripheral opacities, and the proximal opacities may correspond to pulmonary artery aneurysms.[69] Pleural effusions are due to pulmonary infarcts[69] or may precede terminal pulmonary edema.[8] At autopsy, thick-walled pulmonary arteries with aneurysmal dilatation of the lobar and distal branches,[34,70] and pulmonary thrombi of various ages with secondary pulmonary hemorrhages and infarction have been observed by various investigators.[34,70]

Pathologically, the vascular inflammatory response is primarily lymphocytic, but plasma cells, eosinophils, macrophages, and polymorphonuclear leukocytes may also be observed by light microscopy.[34,67] The vasculitis may be transmural, especially in the small vessels, or involve predominantly the inner part of the elastic and large muscular arteries,[67] and in other sections the arterial wall may be necrotic, eroding into the adjacent bronchi.[34] One may observe thromboangiitis at various stages of evolution, and whereas the acute state is characterized by an intense cellular infiltrate, the older lesions show recanalization of organized thrombi[34] (Fig. 7 A–D). Periadventitial fibrosis may bind inflamed pulmonary vessels to adjacent bronchi, and spread of inflammation and collagen necrosis from the fibrous wall of a pulmonary artery aneurysm into an adjacent bronchus may lead to formation of a pulmonary artery–bronchial fistula.[67] Thromboangiitis with transmural inflammation and organization of inflammatory thrombi may also be present in pulmonary veins (Fig. 8 A and B).

Among the various etiologies of the pulmonary vasculitides, aneurysmal formation is characteristic of Behçet's syndrome.[69] Since the syndrome of segmental pulmonary artery aneurysms with peripheral venous thrombosis described by Hughes and Stovin[72] is comparable to Behçet's syndrome clinically, angiographically, and histologically,[67,73] it has been suggested that patients with this syndrome may represent unrecognized or incomplete expressions of Behçet's syndrome.

Gastrointestinal Lesions

Any portion of the gastrointestinal tract may be affected in Behçet's syndrome, and approximately 50% of patients have

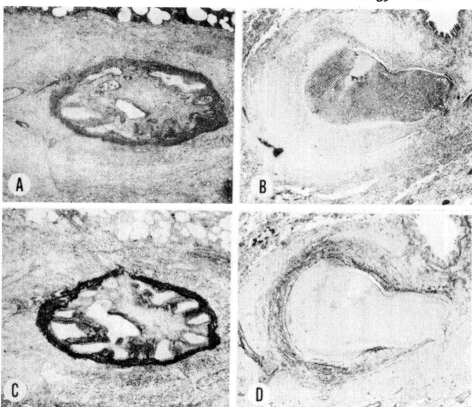

Figure 7.—Photomicrographs of matching hematoxylin-eosin (upper panel) and elastic stain (lower panel) sections of pulmonary artery thromboangiitis of different ages. A and C are old, organized thrombus with recanalization. B and D show an acute stage of thromboangiitis with intense cellular infiltrate. (Original magnification × 16)

symptoms referable to this organ system.[1] Irrespective of whether the fore-, mid-, or hindgut is involved, discrete ulcerations are the primary lesions. Although the oral ulcers are part of the original triple symptom complex described by Behçet,[74] they may occur anywhere in the oral cavity, including the soft and hard palate, and may be multiple and painful.[63] These ulcers have also been reported to cause perforation of the soft palate.[75]

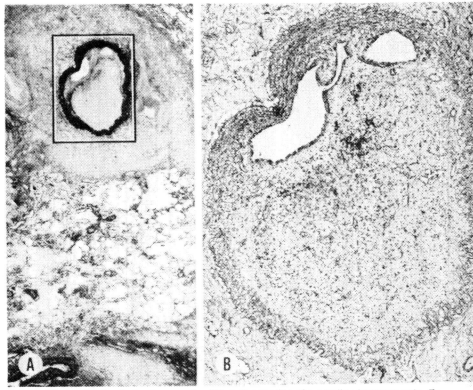

Figure 8—A: photomicrograph of thromboangiitis of a small pulmonary vein. B: close-up view of boxed area in A showing a cellular, recently organized inflammatory thrombus (Hematoxylin-eosin; A × 16, B × 64)

Various morphological forms of esophageal lesions have been described, including esophagitis, erosions, ulcers with or without perforation, healed ulcers, chronic unhealed ulcers with stenosis, and stenosis without ulceration.[76-79] The middle third of the esophagus is the most commonly affected area,[76] and the esophageal ulcers, which may be single or multiple, are discrete with well-demarcated borders (Fig. 9A). The ulcers may be superficial[78] or extend through all layers, leading to perforation.[76,77] Histologically, a typical ulcer shows eroded mucosa with a mixed cellular inflammatory infiltrate of the submucosa (Fig. 9B), and

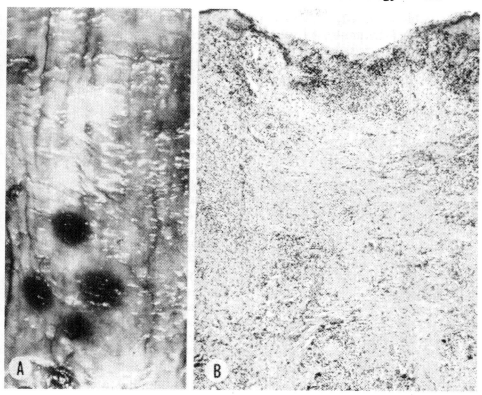

Figure 9—**A:** Gross appearance of multifocal esophageal ulceration, each with a well-demarcated border. **B:** photomicrograph of esophageal ulceration with superficial mucosal erosion and an intense mixed-cell inflammatory infiltrate beneath mucosa. (Hematoxylin-eosin; **B** × 64)

the base of the deeper ulcers may be formed by granulation tissue containing fibroblasts, lymphocytes, polymorphonuclear leukocytes, and plasma cells.[77] Perforation of an esophageal ulcer may lead to the development of an esophagotracheal fistula.[80] Vasculitis at the site of an esophageal erosion has been observed, and inflammation and ulceration may lead to severe esophageal stenosis.[76]

Gastric ulcers may occur in patients with Behçet's syndrome,[8,39,76,81] may be diagnosed by both barium study and endoscopy, and histologically may demonstrate chronic inflammatory infilt-ration of the lamina propria. A single layer of cuboidal epithelial cells infiltrated by polymorphonuclear neutrophils may line the surface of the gastric ulcer, and a fibrous reaction with lymphocy-tic cells may be present below the epithelium.[81] Duodenal ulcers are less frequent than the gastric ones[8,82]; however, both types may result in perforation.[39,82] The margins around a perforated gas-trointestinal ulcer tend to be thin, erosive, and hemmorrhagic,[39] and microscopic examination may reveal necrosis and hemor-rhage with lymphocytes and polymorphonuclear leukocytes around the vessels and in the muscularis.[82] A case of a penetrating duodenal ulcer at the ampulla of Vater causing fatal hemobilia has been reported in a patient with Behçet's syndrome.[82]

Ileal ulcers are more common than the colonic ones, occur on the antimesenteric area,[83–85] and are usually localized, deep, and perforate easily compared to those in the colon which tend to be diffuse and perforate less frequently.[8,83,84] The deep, punched-out ulcers, which are of various sizes, are usually multiple and may perforate during colonoscopy.[85,86] The intestinal ulcers of Behçet's syndrome may be single or multiple, are most common in the ileocecal region where symptoms arising from these may be mis-taken for appendicitis, and tend to recur at the sites of surgical anastomoses where fistulas may also develop postoperatively.[84] Healed ulcers may also appear as reepithelized shallow depres-sions, whereas the open ones can penetrate to reach the muscular or serosal layer. The intestinal ulcers are typically characterized by undermining of the adjacent tissue with edema and crater for-mation around the ulcer margin.[84] In a review of Japanese patients with Behçet's syndrome and intestinal ulcers who underwent laparotomy, postoperative complications were reported in 44% and included reperforation, suture insufficiency, wound dehis-cence, wound sepsis, hematemesis, and melena.[84] Therefore, a con-servative surgical approach may be warranted in certain patients with Behçet's syndrome and intestinal lesions.[87] In addition, pseudopolypous change or bridging formation may occasionally be present in the resected surgical specimens.[85]

Distinguishing Behçet's ulceration from inflammatory bowel disease may be difficult histologically.[84,85] The inflammation of the intestinal ulcer in Behçet's syndrome is transmural, with destruc-tion of the submucous connective tissue and replacement by lym-phocytic infiltration and edema. The muscle layer may be directly covered by regenerated epithelium at the margin of the healed ulcers, and the base of the ulcer may be infiltrated by polymorphonuclear leukocytes, lymphocytes, histiocytes, and plasma cells.[84,85] Pathologically, the intestinal ulcers of Behçet's syndrome have been divided into three types: necrotic, granulomatous and combined. The necrotic type is acute or subacute with necrosis as the primary pathology without either elevation of the muscular layer or thickening of the intestinal wall, while the granulomatous type is composed of granulation tissue with elevation of the muscular layer and thickening of the intestinal wall. The combined type shows both necrotic and granulomatous changes.[88]

Microangiograms of resected intestinal specimens from patients with Behçet's syndrome have demonstrated avascular areas, especially at the base of the ulcers.[61,83,85] The mucosal vessels were slightly increased in the circumference of the ulcers, which may explain the erythema of the ulcer margins seen on colonoscopy, and the microcirculation of the vascular network in the submucosal layer was impaired, thus perhaps contributing to the development of the ulcer.[85] Vasculitis of diverse morphology can affect the arterioles, precapillaries, capillaries, and venules of the gastrointestinal ulcers of Behçet's syndrome (Fig. 10 A and B).[1] The venous changes are more severe than the arterial ones and include intimal proliferation with fibrous thickening, inflammatory cell infiltration, and thrombus formation,[61,63,83,88] while the arterial changes may consist of the disappearance of the internal elastic lumina, degeneration of the media, submucosal edema with inflammatory cell infiltration, and intimal fibrous thickening.[61,83] Perivascular mononuclear cell infiltration is present, and in some areas, vasculitis may be associated with fibrinoid necrosis.[63,85] Intestinal ulcers with pathology similar to that of the ileocecal lesions have been described in the sigmoid colon and rectum in Behçet's syndrome,[8,89,90] and anal ulcerations have been reported extending to the dentate line.[78]

In a series of 170 autopsy cases of Behçet's syndrome from Japan, hepatobiliary pathology was found in 58 patients. The most common changes noted were fatty liver and hepatic congestion; however, the former may have been secondary to corticosteroids which are often used in the therapeutic management of Behçet's syndrome. Histologically, aggregates of inflammatory cells around portal tracts have been reported in a liver biopsy obtained from a Behçet's syndrome patient with firm hepatomegaly and normal

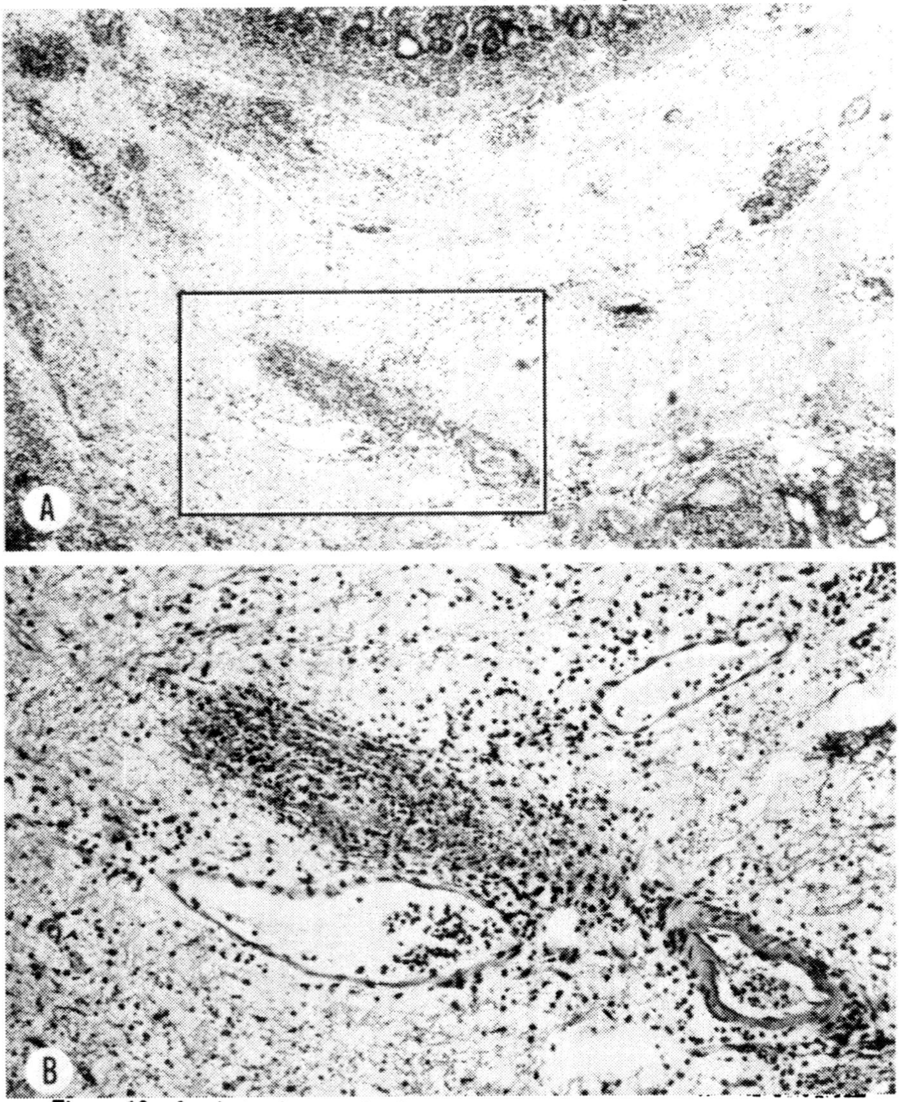

Figure 10—A: photomicrograph of vasculitis in edematous, widened submucosa of small intestine. B: close-up view of boxed area in A showing polyarteritis-type necrotizing vasculitis of submucosal arteriole. (Hematoxylineosin; A × 64, B × 160)

splenic and portal veins by splenoportography.[91] As a result of thrombosis of the hepatic veins, the Budd-Chiari syndrome may develop in patients with Behçet's syndrome, and hemobilia originating in hepatic abscesses has resulted from biliary tract obstruction secondary to a penetrating ulcer at the ampulla of Vater.[82,92]

Splenomegaly has been reported in association with Behçet's syndrome,[8,82,91] and although the splenic histology has usually been normal,[91] splenitis and splenic congestion have been described at autopsy.[882] Acute pancreatitis has been observed both clinically[93] and at autopsy[8,82] in patients with Behçet's syndrome.

Renal Involvement

Although genitourinary involvement has not been commonly reported in those with the triple symptom complex, several renal abnormalities have been thoroughly investigated in Behçet's syndrome. In a series of 170 autopsy cases from Japan, pyelonephritis and cystitis were found in 23 and 10 patients, respectively, followed by nephrosclerosis in 8 and glomerulonephritis in 7.[8] Additionally, epididymoorchitis and urethritis may occur in patients with Behçet's syndrome.[1,94]

Kansu et al.[95] described the first case of acute glomerulonephritis in Behçet's syndrome. Autopsy examination of the kidneys showed focal proliferative and necrotizing glomerulonephritis with patchy acute tubular necrosis. On electron microscopy, epithelial cells and fibrinoid material were seen in the urinary space, in the capillary lumina underlying the endothelium, and in the mesangial areas of the sclerotic capillary loops.[95] A typical renal biopsy showing acute focal necrotizing glomerulonephritis with early crescent formation is illustrated in Figure 11 A and B.

Diffuse proliferative glomerulonephritis with epithelial cell crescent formation has also been reported as a complication of Behçet's syndrome.[96] Light microscopy demonstrated diffusely hypercellular glomeruli compressed by cellular crescents, focal and segmental sclerosis of the mesangium, diffuse interstitial fibrosis, and multiple foci of tubular atrophy. Immunofluorescence revealed IgM, IgG, C3, and fibrinogen deposits along the capillary loops and in the mesangium.[96]

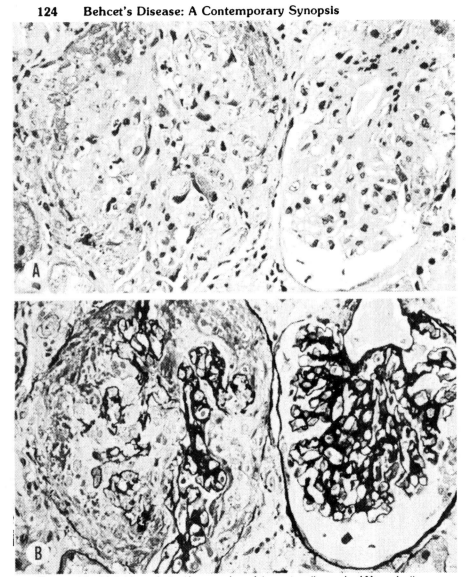

Figure 11—Matching photomicrographs of hematoxylin-eosin **(A)** and silver methenamine **(B)** sections of kidney with focal necrotizing glomerulonephritis. (Original magnification, × 400)

Rapidly progressive glomerulonephritis has been reported in a patient with Behçet's syndrome being treated with transfer factor.[97] The renal biopsy showed extracapillary proliferation with crescent formation and tubular loss associated with lymphocytic and plasma cell interstitial infiltrates. Immunofluorescent studies revealed IgG, IgA, IgM, C3, and fibrinogen deposition in the capillary walls.[97]

Focal necrotizing glomerulonephritis in a patient with Behçet's syndrome prompted a study of renal pathology in 10 patients with Behçet's syndrome with normal renal function and blood pressure.[98,99] Five of these had proteinuria and two had associated leukocyturia. Scattered eosinophilic deposits localized to the mesangium or to the epithelial side of the basement membrane were found in seven of the patients, and interstitial and tubular lesions consisting of areas of fibrosis, edema, and round cell infiltration were noted in two patients. Subendothelial or medial hyaline deposits were present in the arterioles and interlobular arteries of all patients. In two patients the larger vessels were characterized by intimal thickening and reduplication of the internal elastic lamina. Fibrinoid necrosis, thromboses, and vascular or perivascular infiltrates were not present in the tissue specimens. In 10 cases immunofluorescent studies showed C3 deposition in the mesangium and along the capillary basement membrane, and deposits of IgA, IgG, and Clq were observed in four patients.[98,99] Thus, these findings suggested that the renal disease of Behçet's syndrome may be related to immune complex deposition, may be more common than is generally appreciated, and is not invariably detected by an abnormal routine urinalysis.[98,99]

Renal amyloidosis, which has also been reported in Behçet's syndrome, may produce the nephrotic syndrome. Renal biopsy has demonstrated amyloid deposition in the glomerular basal lamina with amyloid fibrils being identified by electron microscopy.[100]

Neuromuscular and Ophthalmic Manifestations

Neuropathology

The frequency of neurological involvement in Behçet's syndrome has been estimated from 10% to 25%.[101] In an autopsy series of Behçet's syndrome, 58 of 170 cases were found to have neurological lesions.[8] Although certain patterns of neurological disease have been described in Behçet's syndrome, any part of the nervous system may be affected, and the disease process may follow a variable course. Anatomically, the site of predilection has been the brain stem, followed by the spinal cord, cerebrum, and cerebellum.[102] Signs and symptoms of meningoencephalitis and cerebellar, pyramidal tract, and extrapyramidal tract involvement were the more common clinical syndromes.[7] Cranial nerve palsies, seizures, organic brain syndrome, altered consciousness, aphasia, coma, hemi- or quadriparesis, pseudobuler palsy, spastic paraplegia, Brown-Séquard syndrome, papilledema, and subarachnoid and intracranial hemorrhages have all been reported in Behçet's syndrome.[101-104] The onset of neurological disease may be sudden or gradual, and although usually seen in established Behçet's syndrome, the neurological symptoms or signs may be the presenting manifestations of disease.[101,105] A pleocytosis of the cerebrospinal fluid, either lymphocytic or neutrophilic, has been the predominant laboratory finding, while the cerebrospinal fluid pressure and protein may be elevated and the glucose normal.[16, 101,105] Cultures of the cerebrospinal fluid and oral-genital lesions for bacteria, fungi, and viruses have been negative, and selected serologies of serum and cerebrospinal fluid for viruses and of serum for fungi have been nondiagnostic or negative.[101,103]

On gross pathological examination, there are no pathognomonic findings, and although the brain may appear swollen at autopsy,[105] it is more commonly atrophic.[102] The meninges may be opacified by fibrous thickening, the ventricles are mildly dilated, and the brain stem, optic nerves, and spinal cord may be atrophic histologically.[102] The pathological lesions may affect the cerebral cortex, cerebral white matter, caudatum, putamen, globus pallidus, striatum, internal capsule, thalamus, hypothalamus, hippocampus, midbrain, pons, medulla oblongata, cerebellum, spinal cord, and the optic tracts.[105-107] Since the brain histology in Behçet's syndrome has been reported almost exclusively from autopsy specimens, the nature of the earliest lesions is not well established. Focal leukocytic infiltration is considered to be the initial lesion,[105] and perivascular leukocytic infiltration may be associated with fibrinoid necrosis of the small blood vessels.[61] The chronic lesions may reveal perivascular and meningeal infiltration by lymphocytes, histiocytes, plasma cells, and macrophages.[101,105] Small-vessel vasculitis (Fig. 12 A and B) may cause thrombotic arteritis or phlebitis leading to areas of infarction and softening in the perivascular regions,[102] and on histopathology one may observe perivascular fibrosis, foamy cell proliferation in the parenchyma, and destruction of the nerve fibers and myelin sheaths with resultant axonal degeneration and demyelination. Inflammation of the arterioles and venules is occasionally associated with diapedesis, glial nodules, and fatty granular cells. Proliferation of microglial and glial cells and mesenchymal fibers may also be demonstrated microscopically with secondary degeneration occurring in the spinal cord, inferior olivary cells, and dentate nuclear cells of the cerebellum.[102]

Intracranial venous thrombosis of the sigmoid, dural, superior sagittal, and transverse sinuses may occur in Behçet's syndrome.[108–112] Some of these affected patients may present with symptoms and signs of raised intracranial tension without any localizing neurological findings,[109,110] and the diagnosis has been established by digital subtraction angiography.[111,112] The syndrome of intracranial hypertension may be an early feature in Behçet's syndrome.[111] Autopsy of a patient with Behçet's syndrome and a dural arteriovenous malformation also revealed findings consistent with anoxic encephalopathy including an edematous brain with multiple small hemorrhages.[108]

Inner-ear involvement has been described in Behçet's syndrome,[113] and both cochlear and vestibular systems may be affected, resulting in hearing acuity deficits and vertigo. During the ensuing years, there may be continued and gradual deterioration in the hearing difficulties; however, the episodes of vertigo, despite increasing in frequency, may become less severe in intensity and duration. Pathologically, vascular inflammation has been postulated to explain these inner-ear complications.[113]

During certain exacerbations of the neurological deficits, contrast-enhancing central nervous system lesions visualized by computerized tomography have been reported in Behçet's syndrome. These roentgenographic findings may be due to the extravasation of contrast material dye into the cerebral parenchyma resulting from increased vascular permeability secondary to vasculitis.[114] Since patients with Behçet's syndrome and neurological disease may have received corticosteroids systemically, one must

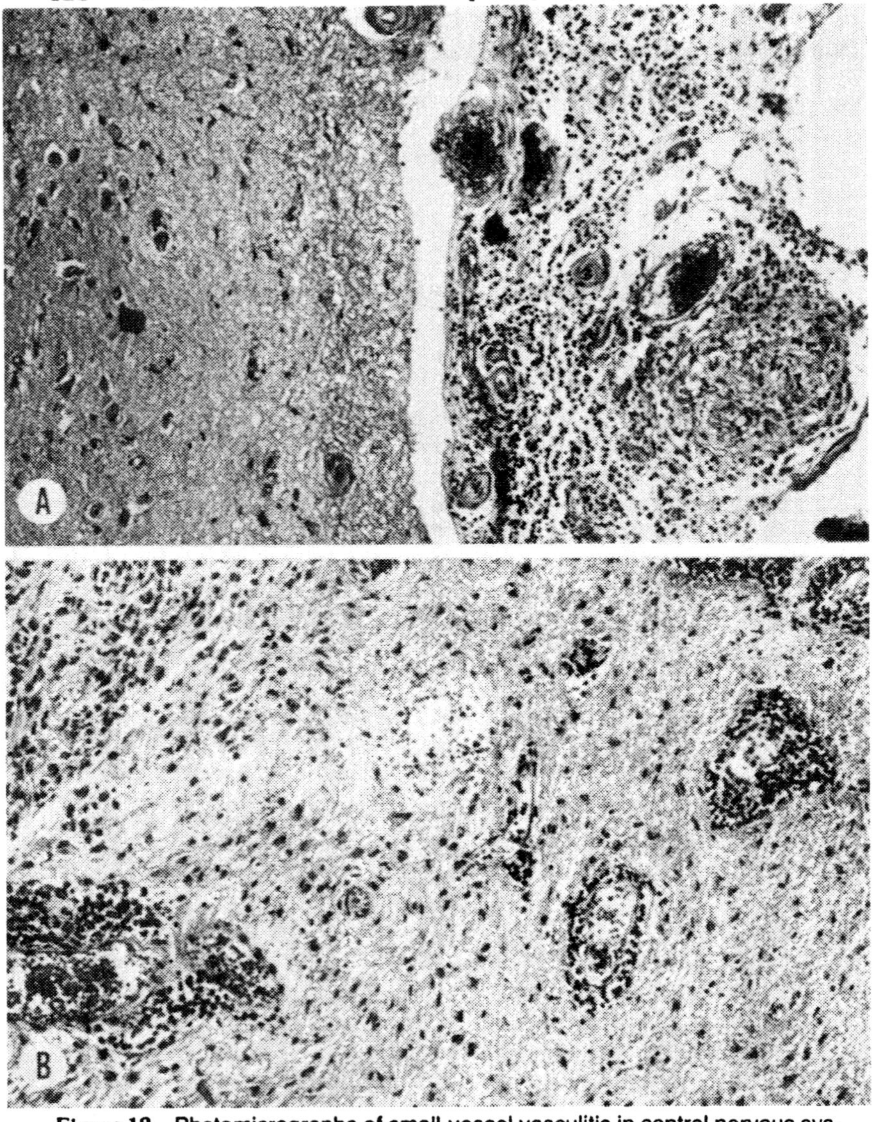

Figure 12—Photomicrographs of small-vessel vasculitis in central nervous system involvement of Behçet's syndrome, affecting leptomeningeal **(A)** and intracerebral **(B)** blood vessels. (Hematoxylin-eosin; × 160)

be cautious in ascribing all contrast-enhancing nervous system lesions to the basic disease process; and thus one must consider other etiologic factors, both infectious and noninfectious, in the differential diagnosis.

Muscle Pathology

Three types of muscle pathology have been described in association with Behçet's syndrome. Although the muscle enzymes may be serologically elevated in some patients, myositis is rarely suspected clinically since there may be only minimal muscle weakness on physical examination.[38,115-117] Muscle biopsies have revealed inflammation and necrosis, and the muscle fibers which varied in size had evidence of degeneration histologically. Both mononuclear and polymorphonuclear cellular infiltrations have been reported and were most prominent in the perivascular areas[116]; vasculitis may also be demonstrable pathologically in tissue sections.[117]

The second type of muscle pathology reported in Behçet's syndrome is neurogenic muscular atrophy.[8,118] The muscle fibers are small, angulated, and atrophic, with perivascular cellular infiltrates, and a predominance of type II fiber atrophy is seen histologically. Electron microscopy has shown small muscle fibers with disorganized myofibrillar architecture and dilatation of the sarcoplasmic reticulum profiles. The mitochondria, which are rather sparse, demonstrate vacuolization, myelin formation, and decreased number of cristae. Additionally, thickening of the capillary basement membrane and subendothelial proliferation may result in luminal occlusion.[118]

The third variety of myopathy has been reported in seven patients with Behçet's syndrome, five of whom had no evidence of neuromuscular disease clinically while two had evidence of peripheral neuropathy on physical examination.[119] Light microscopy was normal in six; however, there was variation in muscle fiber size with increase in the sarcolemmal nuclei in a biopsy from one patient. Despite normal histochemical profiles in all muscle-tissue specimens, electron microscopy revealed abnormalities including thickening of the capillary basement membrane with reduction in capillary lumen, disorganization of the myofilaments, and loss of the myofibrils with their sarcomeral structure. Other findings included massive subsarcolemmal aggregates of mitochondria and glycogen, abundant lysosomal profiles, and excessive amounts of lipid droplets within some fibers. An unusual discovery in all cases was cytoplasmic inclusions in subsarcolemmal sites. In addition, the structure of the cytoplasmic inclusions varied in different fibers and included filament-like, cristae-like, paracrystalline, and circular inclusions. Virus-like particles were not found in any of the tissue specimens.[119]

Ophthalmic Pathology

Ocular involvement is a common feature of Behçet's syndrome and is usually the most serious in light of its potential to produce blindness. In Japan, 10 to 25% of all cases of uveitis are due to Behçet's syndrome,[120] with the severity of visual loss being related to the duration of ocular disease.[121] Recurrent attacks of anterior and posterior uveitis produce irreversible changes with posterior segment inflammation being ultimately responsible for most of the visual loss in Behçet's syndrome. The initial ocular lesion may affect only isolated areas in the eye, but with subsequent inflammatory attacks, multiple ocular tissues are involved in the inflammatory process.[17]

The external eye lesions include conjunctivitis, subconjunctival hemorrhage, episcleritis, scleritis, corneal ulceration, keratitis, and skin lesions affecting the eyelids.[8,17,121] Inflammation of the anterior segment of the eye may manifest as either granulomatous or nongranulomatous iridocyclitis[5,7,121]; however, hypopyon formation, which was frequently reported in the earlier literature, is now less common, perhaps reflecting the use of corticosteroids in the treatment of Behçet's syndrome.[121]

Posterior segment uveal inflammation produces cellular infiltration of the vitreous body. Other manifestations include retinal, macular, and optic disc edema, retinal pigmentary changes, chorioretinitis, choroiditis, optic papillitis, vitreous hemorrhage, necrotizing retinitis, retinal vessel phlebitis or arteritis, and retinal detachment.[5,7,121] Chronic sequelae of ocular involvement include the development of cataracts, glaucoma,[5,7] optic atrophy, and phthisis bulbi.[121] Papilledema, in the absence of uveitis, may also occur as a manifestation of intracranial hypertension in Behçet's syndrome.[109,110,122]

The major inflammatory components of the ocular complications are concentrated in the vitreous humor and around the retinal vessels, and patches of white exudates due to choroiditis or choriocapillaritis may be seen in the fundus.[120] Perivascular sheathing of the retinal vessels and less commonly fulminating vasoocclusive retinitis may occur in Behçet's syndrome.[120,121] Fluorescein fundus angiography has demonstrated that the early and main feature of ocular involvement is a retinal vasculitis which causes increased permeability of the retinal vessels.[123] Based on fluorescein angiography, the retinal vascular disorders in Behçet's syndrome have been classified into six main categories which consist of the papillary, peripapillary, retinal venous branch occlusion, papillomacular, retinal, and retinal vascular obliteration types.[123]

The histopathology data of the ocular lesions in Behçet's syndrome are relatively sparse since seldom is the eye enucleated for complete examination in a routine autopsy. The enucleated eye is usually atrophic with aggregation and scarification of all intraocular tissues.[1,39] Lymphocytic infiltration is present in the iris, vitreous, ciliary body, and the perivascular region,[39,105] while tubular structures have been reported in the vascular endothelial fibroblasts of the bulbar conjunctiva.[1] Microscopic examination of the retina may reveal inflammation, hemorrhage, and infiltration in almost all layers of the retina; however, retinal ganglion cells can also be identified in the inner retinal layer.[124] The axonal portions of the optic nerve may be replaced by fibrous astrocytes, and axonal degeneration may cause atrophy of the optic nerves.[105,124] The central retinal artery may also be extremely narrowed; however, a capillary network may still exist in the optic nerve.[124]

Synovial Involvement

Joint disease has been reported in 5% to 75% of patients with Behçet's syndrome,[5] and synovitis may affect approximately half the patients during the course of their disease.[1,7] The synovitis may be asymmetric,[1] and the arthritis, which is usually of the oligo- or monoarticular, nondeforming type, most commonly affects the knees.[125] However, symmetric polyarthritis resembling rheumatoid arthritis[125] and perhaps sacroiliitis[126] can occur in Behçet's syndrome. Although the arthritis is usually nondestructive, erosive changes have been reported,[125,126] and the synovial fluid may be an inflammatory type with an elevated polymorphonuclear leukocyte count.[125]

Synovial biopsies have revealed acute inflammatory reactions with dilated venules, fibrin thrombi, and mononuclear cell infiltration.[1] Perivascular collections of lymphocytes, histiocytes, and neutrophils, thrombophlebitis, capillaritis, and fibrinoid degeneration of the vessel wall and synovial surface have also been recorded in the histologic examinations of synovial tissue.[39] Also, the superficial cell layer of the synovium may be destroyed and replaced by inflammatory granulation tissue composed of lymphocytes, macrophages, vascular elements, fibroblasts, and neutrophils (Fig. 13). Plasma cell infiltration of the synovium is rare;

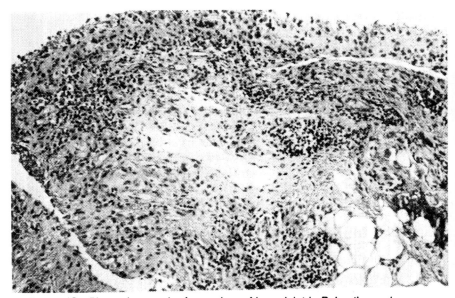

Figure 13—Photomicrograph of synovium of knee joint in Behçet's syndrome. Nonspecific synovitis with a predominantly mixed-cell infiltrate and small-vessel vasculitis is morphologically indistinguishable from synovitis of rheumatoid arthritis and other collagen vascular disease. (Hematoxylin-eosin; × 160)

however, lymphoid follicles may be present and pannus formation may be responsible for cartilage destruction.[125,127] In a study comparing synovial tissue from patients with either Behçet's syndrome or early rheumatoid arthritis, light and electron microscopic examinations failed to demonstrate any distinguishing features. Hypertrophy and hyperplasia of synovial-lining cells with subsynovial cellular accumulations were seen in both types of arthritides; however, immunofluorescent studies indicated that the consistent deposition of IgG in the synovium may be characteristic in Behçet's syndrome.[128]

In Behçet's syndrome, acute synovial rupture has been reported in patients with synovitis of the knees, and it is obviously important to distinguish this from deep venous thrombosis since there are major differences in the treatment and prognosis.[129,130] Atlantoaxial subluxation, which is more common in rheumatoid arthritis, has been described in a case of Behçet's syndrome, and radiographically there was anterior subluxation of one centimeter of the atlantoaxial joint. Despite the presence of a spur at the anterior undersurface of the second cervical vertebra, the authors postulated that trauma was not a factor in the pathogenesis of the subluxation.[131]

Miscellaneous Lesions

The occurrence of epididymitis in patients with Behçet's syndrome has been described,[1,5,7,17] but it is usually transient, only to recur at variable intervals.[1,5] Relapsing urethritis,[5] lymphoid thyroiditis, and pathological changes in the thymus have also been reported, and histologically, the thymus gland may reveal lymphoid follicles with germinal centers and hyperplasia of the epithelial cells.[39] Also, the occurrence of a benign lymphoproliferative disorder with mixed cryoglobulinemia[132] or various types of malignancy[39,133,134] have been described in Behçet's syndrome; and in an autopsy series of 170 cases of Behçet's syndrome, neoplastic lesions were noted in 13 patients.[8] In light of the sparsity and diversity of these malignancies and the frequent use of immunosuppressive therapy, the occurrence of hematologic or solid malignancies may be completely independent of the underlying pathogenetic mechanisms of Behçet's syndrome.

Conclusion

In recent years the emphasis on the clinical findings, epidemiology, and immunology of Behçet's syndrome has surpassed that of the reported pathological findings.[1-10] In part, this is due to the distribution of the lesions since one seldom biopsies the oral and genital ulcers, uveitic eyes, and inflamed joints. Also, many of the lesions are transient and thus are not amenable to pathological study. In light of the existence of several diverse arbitrary sets of diagnostic criteria and the lack of pathognomonic histologic findings, the diagnosis of Behçet's syndrome remains a clinical one.[12-16] Thus, this chapter has reviewed the pathology of Behçet syndrome in the context of the associated clinical manifestations. Despite the apparent diversity of the histologic changes observed in the different organ systems, vasculitis is perceived as the basic pathological process in Behçet's syndrome although its expression may vary considerably, being modulated perhaps by host susceptibility, environmental influences, and other undefined factors.

References

1. Shimizu T, Ehrlich GE, Inaba G, Hyashi K. Behçet disease (Behçet syndrome). *Semin Arthritis Rheum* 1979; 8:223–260.
2. Behçet H: Über Rezidivierende, Aphthöse, durch ein Virus Verursachte Geschwüre am Mund, am Auge und an den Genitalien. *Dermat Wchnschr* 1937; 105:1152–1157.
3. Strachan RW, Wigzell FW. Polyarthritis in Behçet's multiple symptom complex. *Ann Rheum Dis* 1963; 22:26–35.
4. Oshima Y, Shimizu T, Yokohari R, et al. Clinical studies on Behçet's syndrome. *Ann Rheum Dis* 1963; 22:36–45.
5. Chajek T, Fainaru M. Behçet's disease. Report of 41 cases and a review of the literature. *Medicine* (Baltimore) 1975; 54:179–196.
6. Chamberlain MA. Behçet's syndrome in 32 patients in Yorkshire. *Ann Rheum Dis* 1977; 36:491–499.
7. Wong RC, Ellis CN, Diaz LA. Behçet's disease. *Int J Dermatol* 1984; 23:25–32.
8. Lakhanpal S, Tani K, Lie JT, et al. Pathologic features of Behçet's syndrome: A review of Japanese autopsy registry data. *Hum Pathol* 1985; 16:790–795.

9. Haim S. Pathogenesis of Behçet's disease. *Int J Dermatol* 1983; 22:101–102. .
10. O'Duffy JD. Behçet's disease. In Kelly WN, Harris ED Jr, Ruddy S, Sledge CB, eds: *Textbook of Rheumatology.* Philadelphia, WB Saunders, 1985:1174–1178.
11. O'Duffy JD. Summary of international symposium on Behçet's disease, Istanbul, September 29–30, 1977. *J Rheumatol* 1978; 5:229–233.
12. Curth HO. Recurrent genito-oral aphthosis and uveitis with hypopyon (Behçet's syndrome). Report of two cases. *Arch Dermatol Syphilol* 1946; 54:179–196.
13. Mason RM, Barnes CG. Behçet's syndrome with arthritis. *Ann Rheum Dis* 1969; 28:95–103.
14. Yamamoto S, Toyokoma H, Matsubra J, et al. A nationwide survey of Behçet's disease in Japan. *Jpn J Ophthalmol* 1974; 18:282–290.
15. Behçet's Disease Research Committee of Japan. Behçet's disease: Guide to diagnosis of Behçet's disease. *Jpn J Ophthalmol* 1974; 18:291–294.
16. O'Duffy JD, Goldstein NP. Neurologic involvement in seven patients with Behçet's disease. *Am J Med* 1976; 61:170–178.
17. Huang Z-J, Lido K-H, Xu L-Y, et al. Study of 310 cases of Behçet's syndrome. *Chinese Med J* 1983; 96:483–490.
18. Gustafson RO, McDonald TJ, O'Duffy JD, Goellner JR. Upper aerodigestive tract manifestations of Behçet's disease: Review of 30 cases. *Otolaryngol Head Neck Surg* 1981; 89:409–413.
19. Graykowski EA, Barile MF, Lee WB, Stanley HR Jr. Recurrent aphthous stomatitis. Clinical, therapeutic, histopathologic, and hypersensitivity aspects. *JAMA* 1966; 196:637–644.
20. Rogers RS III. Recurrent aphthous stomatitis: Clinical characteristics and evidence for an immunopathogenesis. *J Invest Dermatol* 1977; 69:499–509.
21. Müller W, Lehner T. Quantitative electron microscopical analysis of leukocyte infiltration in oral ulcers of Behçet's syndrome. *Br J Dermatol* 1982; 106:535–544.
22. Plotkin GR, Patel BR, Shah VN. Behçet's syndrome complicated by cutaneous leukocytoclastic vasculitis. Response to prednisone and chlorambucil. *Arch Intern Med* 1985; 145:1913–1915.
23. Jorizzo JL, Schmalstieg FC, Solomon AR, et al. Thalidomide effects in Behçet's syndrome and pustular vasculitis. *Arch Intern Med* 1986; 146:878–881.
24. Jorizzo JL, Solomon AR, Cavallo T. Behçet's syndrome. Immunopathologic and histopathologic assessment of pathergy lesions is useful in diagnosis and follow-up. *Arch Pathol Lab Med* 1985; 109:747–751.
25. Yazici H, Chamberlain MA, Tuzun Y, et al. A comparative study of the pathergy reaction among Turkish and British patients with Behçet's disease. *Ann Rheum Dis* 1984; 43:74–75.
26. Tüzün Y, Altaç M, Yazici H, et al. Nonspecific skin hyperreactivity in Behçet's disease. Iperreattivita' cutanea aspecifica nel di Behçet. *Haematologica* 1980; 65:395–398.

27. James DG, Thomson A. Recognition of the diverse cardiovascular manifestations in Behçet's disease. *Am Heart J* 1982; 103:457–458.
28. Lewis PD. Behçet's disease and carditis. *Br Med J* 1964; 1:1026–1027.
29. Sigel N, Larson L. Behçet's syndrome. A case with benign pericarditis and recurrent neurological involvement treated with adrenal steroids. *Arch Intern Med* 1965; 115:203–207.
30. Godeau P, Herreman G, Ismail MB, et al. Syndrome de Behçet. Atteintes péricardique et pulmonaire. *Nouv Presse Med* 1972; 1:391–395.
31. Scarlett JA, Kistner ML, Yang LC. Behçet's syndrome. Report of a case associated with pericardial effusion and cryoglobulinemia treated with indomethacin. *Am J Med* 1979; 66:146–148.
32. Binak K, Ucak D, Yalcin B, et al. Left ventricular aneurysm and acute pericarditis in a case of Behçet's disease (letter). *J Rheumatol* 1980; 7:578–580.
33. McDonald GSA, Gad-Al-Rab J. Behçet's disease with endocarditis and the Budd-Chiari syndrome. *J Clin Pathol* 1980; 33:660–669.
34. Davies JD. Behçet's syndrome with haemoptysis and pulmonary lesions. *J Pathol* 1973; 109:351–356.
35. Pèna JM, Garcia-Alegria J, Garcia-Fernandez F, et al. Mitral and aortic regurgitation in Behçet's syndrome. *Ann Rheum Dis* 1985; 44:637–639.
36. Rae SA, Vandenburg M, Scholtz CL. Aortic regurgitation and false aortic aneurysm formation in Behçet's disease. *Postgrad Med J* 1980; 56:438–439.
37. Comess KA, Zibelli LR, Gordon D, Fredrickson SR. Acute, severe, aortic regurgitation in Behçet's syndrome. *Ann Intern Med* 1983; 99:639–640.
38. Arkin CR, Rothschild BM, Florendo NT, Popoff N. Behçet syndrome with myositis. A case report with pathologic findings. *Arthritis Rheum* 1980; 23:600–604.
39. Kaneko H, Nakajima H, Okamura A, et al. Histopathology of Behçet disease. Review of the literature with a case report. *Acta Pathol Jpn* 1976; 26:765–769.
40. Shoida Y, Ueda A, Matsuzaki S, et al. A case of Behçet's disease with myocarditis and gastrointestinal bleeding. *Naika (Intern Med)* 1976; 38:695–700 (in Japanese).
41. Higashihara M, Mori M, Takeuchi A, et al. Myocarditis in Behçet's disease—A case report and review of the literature. *J Rheumatol* 1982; 9:630–633.
42. Schiff S, Moffatt R, Mandel WJ, Rubin SA. Acute myocardial infarction and recurrent ventricular arrhythmias in Behçet's syndrome. *Am Heart J* 1982; 103:438–440.
43. Bowles CA, Nelson AM, Hammill SC, O'Duffy JD. Cardiac involvement in Behçet's disease. *Arthritis Rheum* 1985; 28:345–348.
44. Stucchi C, Vollenweider A. Maladie de Behçet et manifestations atypiques. *Ophthalmologica* 1958; 135:573–578.
45. Nojiri C, Endo M, Koyanagi H. Conduction disturbance in Behçet's

disease. Association with ruptured aneurysm of the sinus of Valsalva into the left ventricular cavity. *Chest* 1984; 86:636–638.
46. Hamza M. Large artery involvement in Behçet's disease. *J Rheumatol* 1987; 1 4:554–559.
47. Urayama A, Sakuragi S, Sakai F, et al. Angio-Behçet syndrome. In Inaba G, ed: *Behçet's Disease. Pathogenetic Mechanism and Clinical Future. Proceedings of the International Conference on Behçet's Disease, Tokyo, 1981.* Tokyo, University of Tokyo Press, 1982:171–176.
48. Shimuzu T. Behçet's disease: A systemic inflammatory disease. In Shiokawa Y, ed: *Vascular Lesions of Collagen Diseases and Related Conditions. Proceedings of the International Workshop on Vascular Lesions of Collagen Diseases and Related Conditions, Tokyo, 1976.* Tokyo, University Park Press, 1977:201–211.
49. Hull RG, Harris EN, Gharavi AE, et al. Anticardiolipin antibodies: Occurrence in Behçet's syndrome. *Ann Rheum Dis* 1984; 43:746–748.
50. Adler OB, Rosenberger A. Vascular aspects of Behçet disease. Case presentations and review of literature. *Ann Radiol* (Paris) 1984; 27:371–375.
51. Enoch BA, Castillo-Olivares JL, Khoo TCL, et al. Major vascular complications in Behçet's syndrome. *Postgrad Med J* 1968; 44:453–459.
52. Kansu E, Özer FL, Akalin E, et al. Behçet's syndrome with obstruction of the venae cavae. *Q J Med* 1972; 41:151–168.
53. Park JE, Han MC, Bettmann MA. Arterial manifestations of Behçet disease. *AJR* 1984; 143:821–825.
54. Gruber HE, Weisman MN. Aortic thrombosis during sigmoidoscopy in Behçet's disease. *Arch Intern Med* 1983; 143:343–345.
55. Rosenthal T, Rubenstein Z, Adar R, Gafni J. Major vessel arteritis with aortic aneurysm in Behçet's disease. *VASA* 1982; 11:124–127.
56. Hills EA. Behçet's syndrome with aortic aneurysms. *Br Med J* 1967; 4:152–154.
57. Little AG, Zarins CK. Abdominal aortic aneurysm and Behçet's disease. *Surgery* 1982; 91:359–362.
58. Dündar-Kaldirimci SV, Ates KB, Akpolat T, Nazli N. Iliac artery aneurysm in Behçet's disease: A case report. *Angiology* 1985; 36:549–551.
59. Kaseda S, Koiwaya Y, Tajimi T, et al. Huge false aneurysm due to rupture of the right coronary artery in Behçet's syndrome. *Am Heart J* 1982; 103:569–571.
60. Murakami T. Pathological changes in the large blood vessels caused by Behçet's disease, especially by neuro-Behçet's disease. In Shiokawa Y, ed: *Vascular Lesions of Collagen Diseases and Related Conditions. Proceedings of the International Workshop on Vascular Lesions of Collagen Diseases and Related Conditions, Tokyo, 1976.* Tokyo, University Park Press, 1977:229–234.
61. Fukuda Y, Sakuma Y, Sumita M. Pathological studies of vascular changes in Behçet's disease. In Shiokawa Y, ed: *Vascular Lesions of Collagen Diseases and Related Conditions. Proceedings of the Interna-*

tional Workshop on Vascular Lesions of Collagen Diseases and Related Conditions, Tokyo, 1976. Tokyo, University Park Press, 1977:212–225.

62. Clausen J, Bierring F. Fetal arterial involvement in Behçet's disease: An electron microscope study. *Acta Pathol Microbiol Immunol Scand* [A] 1983; 91:133–136.

63. Bøe J, Dalgaard JB, Scott D. Mucocutaneous-ocular syndrome with intestinal involvement. A clinical and pathological study of four fatal cases. *Am J Med* 1958; 25:857–867.

64. Ahonen AV, Stenius-Aarniala BSM, Viljanen BC, et al. Obstructive lung disease in Behçet's syndrome. *Scand J Resp Dis* 1978; 59:44–50.

65. Evans WV, Jenkins RM. Pulmonary function in Behçet's syndrome. *Scand J Resp Dis* 1979; 60:314–316.

66. Gibson JM, O'Hara MD, Beare JM, Stanford CF. Bronchial obstruction in a patient with Behçet's disease. *Eur J Resp Dis* 1982; 63:356–360.

67. Slavin RE, de Groot WJ. Pathology of the lung in Behçet's disease. Case report and review of the literature. *Am J Surg Pathol* 1981; 5:779–788.

68. Cadman EC, Lundberg WB, Mitchell MS. Pulmonary manifestations in Behçet syndrome. Case report and review of the literature. *Arch Intern Med* 1976; 136:944–947.

69. Grenier P, Bletry O, Cornud F, et al. Pulmonary involvement in Behçet disease. *AJR* 1981; 137:565–569.

70. Bank H. Thrombotic pulmonary manifestations in Behçet's syndrome. *Isr J Med Sci* 1973; 9:955.

71. Decroix AG. Thoracic manifestations of Behçet's syndrome. *Thorax* 1969; 24:380.

72. Hughes JP, Stovin PGI. Segmental pulmonary artery aneurysms with peripheral venous thrombosis. *Br J Dis Chest* 1959; 53:19–27.

73. Durieux P, Bletry O, Huchon G, et al. Multiple pulmonary arterial aneurysms in Behçet's disease and Hughes-Stovin syndrome. *Am J Med* 1981; 71:736–741.

74. Behçet H. Some observations on the clinical picture of the so-called triple symptom complex. *Dermatologica* 1940; 81:73–83.

75. Lavalle C, Gudiño J, Reinoso SR, et al. Behçet's syndrome and palate perforation (letter). *Arthritis Rheum* 1979; 22:308.

76. Mori S, Yoshihira A, Kawamura H, et al. Esophageal involvement in Behçet's disease. *Am J Gastroenterol* 1983; 78:548–553.

77. Brodie TE, Ochsner JL. Behçet's syndrome with ulcerative esophagitis: Report of the first case. *Thorax* 1973; 28:637–640.

78. Lockhart JM, McIntyre W, Caperton EM Jr. Esophageal ulceration in Behçet's syndrome. *Ann Intern Med* 1976; 84:572–573.

79. Griffin JW Jr, Harrison HB, Tedesco FJ, Mills LR IV. Behçet's disease with multiple sites of gastrointestinal involvement. *South Med J* 1982; 75:1405–1408.

80. Levack B, Hanson D. Behçet's disease of the oesophagus. *J Laryngol Otol* 1979; 93:99–101.

81. Hyman NM, Sagar HJ. Behçet's syndrome: Unusual multisystem in-

volvement and immune complexes. *Postgrad Med J* 1980; 56:182–184.
82. Good AE, Mutchnick MG, Weatherbee L. Duodenal ulcer, hepatic abscesses, and fatal hemobilia with Behçet's syndrome: A case report. *Am J Gastroenterol* 1982; 77:905–909.
83. Baba S, Morika S. Treatment of intestinal Behçet's disease. In Inaba G, ed: *Behçet's Disease. Pathogenetic Mechanism and Clinical Future. Proceedings of the International Conference on Behçet's Disease, Tokyo 1981.* Tokyo, University of Tokyo Press, 1982:559–570.
84. Kasahara Y, Tanaka S. Nishino M, et al. Intestinal involvement in Behçet's disease: Review of 136 surgical cases in the Japanese literature. *Dis Colon Rectum* 1981; 24:103–106.
85. Baba S, Maruta M, Ando K, et al. Intestinal Behçet's disease: Report of five cases. *Dis Colon Rectum* 1976; 19:428–440.
86. Reuben A, Jones RR, Lovell D. Behçet's syndrome with colonic involvement and arterial thrombosis. *J R Soc Med* 1980; 73:520–524.
87. Ketch LL, Buerk CA, Liechty RD. Surgical implications of Behçet's disease. *Arch Surg* 1980; 115:759–760.
88. Fukuda Y, Watanabe I. Pathological studies on intestinal Behçet's (entero-Behçet's) disease. In Dilşen N, Koniçe M, Övül C, eds: *Behçet's Disease. Proceedings of an International Symposium on Behçet's Disease, Istanbul, 29–30 September 1977.* Amsterdam-Oxford, Excerpta Medica, 1979:90–95.
89. Thach BT, Cummings NA. Behçet syndrome with "aphthous colitis." *Arch Intern Med* 1976; 136:705–709.
90. Yim CW, White RH. Behçet's syndrome in a family with inflammatory bowel disease. *Arch Intern Med* 1985; 145:1047–1050.
91. Kiernan TJ, Gillan J, Murray JP, McCarthy CF. Behçet's disease and splenomegaly. *Br Med J* 1978; 2:1340–1341.
92. Karam JH, Jacobs T. Hemobilia. Report of a case of massive gastrointestinal bleeding originating from a hepatic abscess. *Ann Intern Med* 1961; 54:319–326.
93. O'Duffy JD, Carney JA, Deodhar S. Behçet's disease. Report of 10 cases, 3 with new manifestations. *Ann Intern Med* 1971; 75:561–570.
94. Vordermark JS II, Hudson LD. Behçet disease with genitourinary involvement treated with colchicine. *Urology* 1984; 23:290–292.
95. Kansu E, Deglin S, Cantor RI, et al. The expanding spectrum of Behçet syndrome. A case with renal involvement. *JAMA* 1977; 237:1855–1856.
96. Olsson PJ, Gaffney E, Alexander RW, et al. Proliferative glomerulonephritis with crescent formation in Behçet's syndrome. *Arch Intern Med* 1980; 140:713–714.
97. Landwehr DM, Cooke CL, Rodriguez GE. Rapidly progressive glomerulonephritis in Behçet's syndrome. *JAMA* 1980; 244:1709–1711.
98. Beaufils H, Cassou B, Auriol M, et al. Kidney involvement in Behçet's syndrome. A report of 11 cases studied by optic, ultrastructural and immunopathological techniques. *Virchows Arch A Path Anat and Histol* 1980; 388:187–198.

99. Herreman G, Beaufils H, Godeau P, et al. Behçet's syndrome and renal involvement: A histological and immunofluorescent study of eleven renal biopsies. *Am J Med Sci* 1982; 284:10–17.

100. Dilşen N, Koniçe M, Övül C, et al. Three cases of Behçet's disease with amyloidosis. In Inaba G, ed: *Behçet's Disease. Pathogenetic Mechanism and Clinical Future. Proceedings of the International Conference on Behçet's Disease, Tokyo, 1981.* Tokyo, University of Tokyo Press, 1982:449–457.

101. Wolf SM, Schotland DL, Phillips LL. Involvement of nervous system in Behçet's syndrome. *Arch Neurol* 1965; 12:315–325.

102. Totsuka S, Hattori T, Yazaki M, Nagao K. Clinicopathology of neuro-Behçet's disease. In Inaba G, ed: *Behçet's Disease. Pathogenetic Mechanism and Clinical Future. Proceedings of the International Conference on Behçet's Disease, Tokyo, 1981.* Tokyo, University of Tokyo Press, 1982:183–196.

103. Feagin OT. Behçet's disease: The Ochsner experience, 1979 to 1982. *South Med J* 1984; 77:442–446.

104. Nagata K. Recurrent intracranial haemorrhage in Behçet disease (letter). *J Neurol Neurosurg Psychiatry* 1985; 48:190–192.

105. Fukuda Y, Hayashi H, Kuwabara N. Pathological studies on neuro-Behçet's disease. In Inaba G, ed: *Behçet's Disease. Pathogenetic Mechanism and Clinical Future. Proceedings of the International Conference on Behçet's Disease, Tokyo, 1981.* Tokyo, University of Tokyo Press, 1982:137–143.

106. Matsumoto K, Matsumoto H, Murofushi K. The clinico-electroencephalographical correlation to the underlying neuropathology in neuro-Behçet's syndrome. In Inaba G, ed: *Behçet's Disease. Pathogenetic Mechanism and Clinical Future. Proceedings of the International Conference on Behçet's Disease, Tokyo, 1981.* Tokyo, University of Tokyo Press, 1982:219–231.

107. Hayashi H, Fukuda Y, Kuwabara N. Pathological studies on neuro-Behçet's disease: With special reference to leukocytic reaction. In Inaba G, ed: *Behçet's Disease. Pathogenetic Mechanism and Clinical Future. Proceedings of the International Conference on Behçet's Disease, Tokyo, 1981.* Tokyo, University of Tokyo Press, 1982:197–211.

108. Imaizumi M, Nukada T, Yoneda S, Abe H. Behçet's disease with sinus thrombosis and arteriovenous malformation in brain. *J Neurol* 1980; 222:215–218.

109. Bank I, Weart C. Dural sinus thrombosis in Behçet's disease. *Arthritis Rheum* 1984; 27:816–818.

110. Ben-Itzhak J, Keren S, Simon J. Intracranial venous thrombosis in Behçet's syndrome. *Neuroradiology* 1985; 27:450.

111. Harper CM Jr, O'Neill BP, O'Duffy JD, Forbes GS. Intracranial hypertension in Behçet's disease: Demonstration of sinus occlusion with use of digital subtraction angiography. *Mayo Clin Proc* 1985; 60:419–422.

112. Brissaud P, Laroche L, de Gramont A, Krulik M. Digital angiography for the diagnosis of dural sinus thrombosis in Behçet's disease (letter). *Arthritis Rheum* 1985; 28:359–360.

113. Brama I, Fainaru M. Inner ear involvement in Behçet's disease. *Arch Otolaryngol* 1980; 106:215–217.
114. Dobkin BH. Computerized tomographic findings in neuro-Behçet's disease. *Arch Neurol* 1980; 37:58–59.
115. Hamza M, Zribi A, Chadi A, Benayed H. La maladie de Behçet. Etude de 22 cas. *Nouv Press Med* 1975; 4:563–566.
116. Yazici H, Tüzüner N, Tüzün Y, Yurdakul S. Localized myositis in Behçet's disease (letter). *Arthritis Rheum* 1981; 24:636.
117. Di Giacomo V, Carmenini G, Meloni F, Valesini G. Myositis in Behçet's disease (letter). *Arthritis Rheum* 1982; 25:1025.
118. Frayha RA, Afifi AK, Bergman RA, et al. Neurogenic muscular atrophy in Behçet's disease. *Clin Rheumatol* 1985; 4:202–211.
119. Afifi AK, Frayha RA, Bahuth NB, Tekian A. The myopathology of Behçet's disease. A histochemical, light-, and electron-microscopic study. *J Neurol Sci* 1980; 48:333–342.
120. BenEzra D, Nussenblatt R. Ocular manifestations of Behçet's disease. *J Oral Pathol* 1978; 7:431–435.
121. Colvard DM, Robertson DM, O'Duffy JD. The ocular manifestations of Behçet's disease. *Arch Ophthalmol* 1977; 95:1813–1817.
122. Kalbian VV, Challis MT. Behçet's disease. Report of twelve cases with three manifesting as papilledema. *Am J Med* 1970; 49:823–829.
123. Matsuo N, Ojima M, Kumashiro O, et al. Fluorescein angiographic disorders of the retina and the optic disc in Behçet's disease. In Inaba G, ed: *Behçet's Disease. Pathogenetic Mechanism and Clinical Future. Proceedings of the International Conference on Behçet's Disease, Tokyo, 1981.* Tokyo, University of Tokyo Press, 1982:161–170.
124. Uga S, Ishikawa S, Wakakura M. Histopathology of the optic nerve and retina in Behçet's disease. In Dilşen H, Koniçe M, Övül C, eds: *Behçet's Disease. Proceedings of an International Symposium on Behçet's Disease, Istanbul 29–30 September 1977.* Amsterdam-Oxford, Excerpta Medica, 1979:85–89.
125. Yurdakul S, Yazici H, Tüzün Y, et al. The arthritis of Behçet's disease: A prospective study. *Ann Rheum Dis* 1983; 42:505–515.
126. Caporn B, Higgs ER, Dieppe PA, Watt I. Arthritis in Behçet's syndrome. *Br J Radiol* 1983; 56:87–91.
127. Vernon-Roberts B, Barnes CG, Revell PA. Synovial pathology in Behçet's syndrome. *Ann Rheum Dis* 1978; 37:139–145.
128. Gibson T, Laurent R, Highton J, et al. Synovial histopathology of Behçet's syndrome. *Ann Rheum Dis* 1981; 40:376–381.
129. Dawes PT, Raman D, Haslock I. Acute synovial rupture in Behçet's syndrome. *Ann Rheum Dis* 1983; 42:591–592.
130. Hanly JG, Molony J, Bresnihan B. Acute synovial rupture in Behçet's syndrome. *Ir J Med Sci* 1984; 153:286–287.
131. Koss JC, Dalinka MK. Atlantoaxial subluxation in Behçet's syndrome. *AJR* 1980; 134:392–393.
132. Huston KA, O'Duffy JD, McDuffie FC. Behçet's disease associated with a lymphoproliferative disorder, mixed cryoglobulinemia, and an immune complex mediated vasculitis. *J Rheumatol* 1978; 5:217–223.

133. Kaneko H, Hōjō Y, Nakajima H, et al. Behçet syndrome associated with nasal malignant lymphoma. Report of an autopsy case. *Acta Pathol Jpn* 1974; 24:141–150.
134. Tamaoki N, Habu S, Yoshimatsu H, et al. Thymic change in Behçet's disease. *Keio J Med* 1972; 21:201–213.

9

TRIPLE SYMPTOM COMPLEX (CLASSIC TRIAD)

Gary R. Plotkin

TRADITIONALLY DESCRIBED AS A DISTINCT triple symptom complex in 1937 by Professor Hulûsi Behçet, a Turkish professor of dermatology, Behçet's disease consists of recurrent aphthous stomatitis, genital ulcerations, and uveitis.[1] Since this description, which emphasized the occurrence of an independent mucocutaneous-ocular syndrome, Behçet's syndrome has become recognized as a systemic illness that may present predominantly with cardiac, vascular, renal, gastrointestinal, hepatic, pulmonary, rheumatologic, neuropsychiatric, or cutaneous manifestations. This chapter reviews the triple symptom complex; however, this should not detract from the importance of the other protean manifestations which may be the presenting complaints of patients with Behçet's disease.[2-15]

Professor Behçet[1] described the triple symptom complex as "an illness which lasts many years and in which the three following types of symptoms are prominent: firstly transient aphthous changes in the mouth; secondly ulcerations on the genitalia, and thirdly attacks of iritis, although the latter symptom is not always present. Each of these three symptoms tends, according to its degree of severity at any one time, to simulate a number of other

From *Behcet's Disease: A Contemporary Synopsis*, edited by Gary R. Plotkin, M.D., John J. Calabro, M.D., and J. Desmond O'Duffy, M.B. © 1988, Futura Publishing Company, Inc., Mount Kisco, NY.

better-known diseases, and this makes the differential diagnosis somewhat complicated." Despite the passage of 50 years, this original description remains most relevant in terms of our understanding of the clinical manifestations of the disease.

The usual age of onset of Behçet's disease is between 20 and 30 years; however, the syndrome has been desribed in neonates and in patients over 70.[9,16] Lewis et al.[16] have reported the onset of Behçet's disease in an eight-day-old infant whose mother had an eight-year history of Behçet's disease and who was receiving prednisone therapy during her pregnancy. The neonate developed destructive ulcerations of the oral mucosa, periungual ulcerations, and pustulonecrotic skin lesions. The child continued to have recurrent oral ulcerations at the age of nine months.[16]

Patients with Behçet's disease may have generalized symptoms occurring especially just prior to the onset of the acute attack; these include malaise, anorexia, weight loss, generalized weakness, headache, perspiration, decreased or elevated temperature, lymphadenopathy, and pain of the substernal and temporal regions.[8,10,17] Often there is a history of repeated sore throats or tonsillitis, and myalgias and migratory arthralgias without overt arthritis may be present, to be followed by erythema nodosum-like eruptions. These constitutional signs and symptoms, which may be recurrent, may also precede the onset of the mucosal membrane ulcerations by an average of six months to five years.[8,13] The presence of fever in Behçet's disease was probably first reported by Hippocrates in his *Third Book of Endemic Diseases*.[18] The febrile episodes usually last from two or three days to a month, may recur at intervals of two months, and may be unaffected by treatment.[8,9] Fever is usually observed during periods of active disease, especially when Behçet's disease is complicated by arthritis, thrombophlebitis, or meningoencephalitis[3]; however, fever may occur rarely between the acute attacks. In addition, Gotfried et al.[19] and Pines et al.[20] have reported two patients with a fever of unknown origin preceding the development of Behçet's disease. Only after 12 weeks and 16 months, respectively, were the more classic manifestations of Behçet's syndrome observed in these patients.[19,20] The lymphadenopathy of Behçet's disease may be generalized, and the histologic examination may reveal normal or hyperplastic nodes.[3,21-23]

Exacerbations of the generalized symptoms may occur during the premenstrual phase of the menstrual cycle,[24] and symptoms of active disease may subside during pregnancy and the immediate postpartum period.[3,17,25] However, Hurt et al.[26] have reported a patient who developed the new onset of Behçet's disease during pregnancy, and parturition may herald the acute exacerbations of disease activity. Amenorrhea may also occur in untreated patients with Behçet's disease; however, this observation does not necessarily imply a cause and effect relationship.[28]

One of the most important characteristics of Behçet's syndrome is the recurrent nature of the remissions and exacerbations of disease activity. The average interval between recurrences may be two months, with four to five recurrences per year; however, remissions may be as short as one week or persist for years. As the duration of the syndrome lengthens, the intervals between the attacks may become longer, eventually leading to spontaneous resolution but with permanent sequelae including blindness. The average acute attack in Behçet's disease abates within 11 days, but there may be wide variation with resolution occurring from several days to one month later. Of the triple symptom complex, aphthous stomatitis is usually the initial manifestation, followed by genital lesions and then ocular complications. The average interval between the onset of the oral ulcerations and the occurrence of the complete triad is four to five years; however, this range may vary from less than one month to over 15 years.[9] Moreover, only one facet of the triad may be present at a specific time, and even years may separate the onset of the genital and the oral lesions.[15,17]

A variety of neoplastic processes have been reported in patients with Behçet's disease, including sarcoma, lymphoma, lymphosarcoma, acute and chronic myeloid leukemia, carcinoma of the thyroid, larynx, lung, and esophagus, and hepatic angioma.[1,12,29-33] Since many immunological abnormalities have been reported in untreated patients with Behçet's disease, and since patients with Behçet's syndrome have also received immunosuppressive agents including corticosteroids, chlorambucil, and azathioprine, there may obviously be complex interrelationships between the occurrence of neoplasia and Behçet's disease. Only additional prospective studies will enable these variables to be better defined.

Oral Manifestations

According to the Behçet's Disease Research Committee of Japan,[34] recurrent aphthous ulcerations of the oral mucous membranes are listed as a major criterion in the diagnosis of Behçet's disease. These ulcers may frequently be painful, are usually small and sharply circumscribed, are located in the labial, buccal, gingival and lingual areas, usually heal within 7 to 10 days without scarring, and may recur after variable intervals.[34] The oral lesions may also occur on the alveolar ridges, hard and soft palates, tonsils, tonsillar fossae, pharynx, larynx, and epiglottis with extension into the esophagus. The oral ulcers may be discrete or irregular, superficial or deep, single or multiple, and range in size from 2 to 12 mm in diameter. The intervening mucosa may be normal. The oral lesions may bleed readily, and since they may be painful, the patient may have difficulty in speaking, chewing, and swallowing, with resultant dehydration and weight loss. Other signs and symptoms include recurrent sore throats, tonsillitis, oral fetor, perlèche, hoarseness, referred otalgia, odynophagia, dysphagia, and dyspnea.[2-4,6,8,9,13,14,17,35-45] The recurrent oral ulcers in Behçet's disease are virtually identical to those characteristic of the common clinical entity of recurrent idiopathic aphthous stomatitis (ulcerations): that is, the ulcers may be minute, superficial, and heal without scar formation. However, the ulcers in Behçet's syndrome may often be more invasive and numerous, larger and deeper, affect a more extensive area, and heal with scarring and circumoral contractures.[36,46-49]

The same three varieties of oral ulcers that occur in recurrent aphthous ulcerations may occur in patients with Behçet's disease; these include the minor aphthous ulcers (recurrent aphthae of Mikulicz and Kümmel, 1898), the major aphthous ulcers (periadenitis mucosa necrotica recurrens, Sutton 1911), and the herpetiform ulcers (Cooke, 1960).[50] The minor aphthous ulcers consist of one to five small (less than 10 mm in diameter), recurrent, moderately painful lesions affecting the nonkeratinized oral mucosa of the lips, cheeks, sulci, tongue, and floor of the mouth. They persist usually for 4 to 14 days, 8% may heal with scar tissue, there is a high incidence of hemagglutinating antibodies to oral mucosa, and lymphocyte transformation to oral mucosa and immunofluorescent binding of IgG or IgM are positive. The major aphthous ulcers consist of 1 to 10 very painful lesions that measure 10 to 30 mm in diameter, recur at frequent intervals, affect fauces, pharynx, and the soft palate in addition to the sites of the minor aphthous ulcers, last up to six weeks, and leave a scar on healing in 64% of patients. There is a high incidence of hemagglutinating antibodies to oral mucosa, serum IgG and IgA are statistically increased, and lymphocyte transformation to oral mucosa and immunofluorescent binding of IgG or IgM are positive. The herpetiform ulcers are recurrent crops of up to 100 small (1 to 2 mm in diameter), shallow, painful ulcers which may involve any part of the oral mucosa. They may persist for 7 to 10 days, may coalesce into large plaques, and result in scar tissue in 32% of patients. There is also a low incidence of hemagglutinating antibodies to oral mucosa, lymphocyte transformation to oral mucosa may or may not be detectable, and immunofluorescent binding of IgG or IgM is negative.[46,50-54] Although serum antibodies and cellular immune responses to oral epithelial antigens occur in Behçet's disease, they may also be present in recurrent idiopathic oral ulcerations and thus cannot completely distinguish between these two disorders.[55]

In Behçet's disease the oral ulcers can also be intractable, indolent, persist for months, recur at the same site, result in thickening of the mucosa with significant tissue destruction, and form erosions or large areas of necrotic slough. Pain may be less severe in Behçet's disease as compared to patients with recurrent aphthous ulcerations; however, this may be due to the ulcers occurring at the sites of scar tissue. Fibrosis is more frequent among those ulcers that fuse.[9,46,56] The majority of patients with Behçet's disease and oral ulcerations may have the major aphthous type[46]; however, in a series[57] of 20 patients, the frequency of oral lesions was: minor ulcerations 45%, herpetiform ulcers 40%, and major aphthous ulcers 15%. However, not all oral ulcerations in Behçet's disease can be readily classified into one of the three main types described above.[57]

Aphthous stomatitis has been divided into four clinical stages with the first or premonitory phase occurring during the first 24 hours of the process. Within this period, there may be tingling, tenseness, hyperesthesia, pain or a burning sensation, and a feeling of a roughened or a raw sensation of the oral mucosa. There may be no obvious physical findings, and this stage is not invariably present. The preulcerative or second stage lasts 18 hours to 3 days and is characterized by the appearance of a small localized area of redness, specifically a macule or papule which is indurated on examination. The lesion gradually develops a superficial membrane which may extend for 20 mm, the erythema evolves into a dusky red inflammatory halo, and the pain is of moderate intensity. The ulcerative or third stage persists for 1 to 16 days. During this phase, the central superficial membrane undergoes blanching necrosis, and as a result of the sloughing of this layer, a discrete ulcer is formed. Subsequently, the floor of the ulcer is covered by a gray-white or yellowish fibrinous exudate or clot, and the persisting erythematous halo is responsible for the raised margins of the ulcer. Initially, the ulcer is small and shallow; however, it may enlarge for four to six days. The ulcer is very painful and several of them may coalesce to form large lesions 1 cm or more in diameter. After an additional two to three days, the pain begins to decrease immediately after the ulcer attains its maximal size, probably thus reflecting cessation of further tissue destruction. The ulcer is next covered by a fibromembranous slough or fibrinous clot which protects the underlying tissue from surface irritation. The last stage is one of resolution or healing and lasts 4 to 35 days. The small and superficial ulcers tend to resolve uneventfully; however, the larger ones may heal with scar formation.[35,37,46,58-62]

Although oral ulcerations may be the most common initial manifestation of Behçet's disease,[3] Koniçe et al.[63] have reported almost one-third of patients presenting without oral aphthae. Their initial signs included erythema nodosum, thrombophlebitis, or arthritis, and this preaphthous phase persisted for 6 months to 27 years with a mean duration of 5 years. Jorizzo et al.[64] have reported a patient with an 18-year history of recurrent oral and genital aphthae or complex aphthosis who on laboratory investigation had circulating immune complexes and biopsy-confirmed cutaneous Sweet's-like vasculitis (neutrophilic vascular reaction) 24 hours after intradermal histamine injection. This patient evolved clinically into classic Behçet's disease one year after her immunological evaluation, thus emphasizing that complex aphthosis in association with immune complex–mediated tissue injury may indicate a group of patients who are at high risk of developing the complete triple symptom complex of Behçet's syndrome.[64]

Firestein et al.[65] described five patients with features of coexistent relapsing polychondritis and Behçet's disease. Their patients had cartilage inflammation, oral and genital ulcers, arthritis, ocular inflammation, thrombosis, gastrointestinal manifestations, audiovestibular dysfunction, and vasculitis in various combinations. This constellation of findings was named the "mouth and genital ulcers with inflamed cartilage (MAGIC) syndrome," and the authors postulated that there may be a common mechanism of pathogenesis. Specifically, autoimmunity to components of cartilage including proteoglycans or elastic tissue (elastin) but not type II collagen may be responsible for this disorder.[65]

Iron deficiency may also be associated with atrophic glossitis and recurrent oral ulcerations, and in one study,[66] 15% of patients with Behçet's disease and oral lesions had iron deficiency based on decreased serum ferritin levels. However, the decreased ferritin levels apparently did not affect the incidence or the specific type of oral ulceration. Also, the influence of supplemental iron therapy on the oral ulcerations in Behçet's disease remains unknown.[66]

Various investigators have reported a relationship between aphthous stomatitis and the ovarian cycle. Recurrent oral ulcers may be more prominent or severe during the seven days preceding menstruation, immediately after ovulation, and during the week starting on the first day of menstruation. The week after menstruation and the week starting on the 14th day preceding the next cycle may exhibit the least activity. There may also be an increased severity of oral ulcerations during pubescence or menarche. These periods of increased activity are associated with increasing progesterone and decreasing estrogen plasma levels, and the degree of keratinization or cornification of the oral mucosa is also diminished, thus perhaps increasing the vulnerability of the mucous membrane to naturally occurring stimuli.[24,46,47,54,60,67,68] Remission of oral aphthous stomatitis may occur during pregnancy[47,68]; however, Hurt et al.[26] and Jorizzo et al.[64] have reported exacerbations of the oral lesions during pregnancy, while Chamberlain[36] noticed that recurrent oral ulcers may lack any relationship to the ovarian cycle. Thus, hormonal factors do not entirely explain the severity or periodicity of the oral aphthous ulcerations of Behçet's disease.

Since patients with Behçet's disease may experience oral aphthous ulcers after local trauma, pathergy has been demonstrated in the oral mucosa by the injection of physiological saline or the application of a needle prick. The clinical course of these experimentally induced oral ulcerations was similar to those that occurred spontaneously; that is, they may either regress rapidly or extend widely and deeply and may be accompanied by intense pain and systemic symptoms. In addition, the histology of the naturally occurring and experimentally induced oral aphthae was similar.[69]

As sequelae of the recurrent episodes of oral ulcerations, there may be cicatricial contraction of the mouth with decreased range of motion, fusion of the base of the tongue with the soft palate, and pharyngeal stenosis at the junction of the oropharynx and hypopharynx with resultant dysphagia, odynophagia, and dyspnea.[36,70–72] Brookes[70] reported a patient with dysphagia due to severe pharyngeal stenosis resulting from recurrent episodes of multiple ulcerations of the mouth and pharynx, and indirect laryngoscopy showed a scarred pharynx at the junction of the oropharynx and hypopharynx. The flow volume loop respiratory function test showed extrathoracic obstructive upper airway disease, and the patient, who also had clubbing of the fingernails on physical examination, required endoscopic dilatation for control of his symptoms.[70] Kobayashi et al.[73] reported two patients with Behçet's disease and ulcerative lesions of the hypopharynx, one of whom developed severe stenosis of the hypopharyngeal mucosa with resultant dyspnea. Moreover, the epiglottis was markedly deformed and diminished in size, frontal tomography of the larynx revealed obliteration of the pyriform sinuses, and the flow volume loop similarly showed extrathoracic upper airway obstruction.[73] Scarring with adhesion formation in the pharynx and fusion of the soft palate to the base of the tongue with scar tissue have been reported in an occasional patient with Behçet's disease, and these anatomical abnormalities have resulted in difficulties in nasotracheal and oropharyngeal intubation.[71,72] Recurrent ulcerations of the mouth and throat may result in fistulas among the oral and nasal pharynx, larynx, trachea, and esophagus, strictures of the nasopharynx, uvula area, and mucous membranes of the mouth and esophagus, and decreased range of motion of the mouth due to cicatricial changes.[36,45,74] Ulcerations in Behçet's disease may also affect the arytenoid, aryepiglottic folds, piriform fossa, and the epiglottis.[10,17,62]

Other less common oral physical findings in patients with

Behçet's disease include leukoplakia or plaque-like lesions, furred tongue, absent or sparse lingual fungiform papillae as determined by the use of the ocular slit lamp microscope, and soft palate perforation.[5,10,15,42,75-77] Absent or decreased lingual fungiform papillae, which is due to their replacement by filiform papillae, is not pathognomonic for Behçet's disease since this physical finding may occur in Riley-Day syndrome (familial dysautonomia) and certain other medical conditions that were not described by Davis and Melzer.[76] Patients with either isolated aphthous stomatitis or uveitis but without other evidence of Behçet's disease had normal distribution of the lingual fungiform papillae.[76]

Shuttleworth et al.[78] reported a patient with neuro-Behçet's disease with palatal myoclonus secondary to brain-stem disease with involvement of the dentatoolivary system. On examination there were rhythmic contractions of the muscles of the soft palate. Associated with palatal myoclonus, other structures derived from the branchial arches including the pharynx, larynx, tongue, mouth, face, orbicularis oculi, diaphragm, and extraocular and neck muscles may also undergo synchronous contractions due to brain-stem lesions of various origins.[78]

Histology of Oral Lesions

The histology of the oral lesions in Behçet's disease resembles that observed in recurrent idiopathic aphthous ulcerations.[50,79] Pathologically, there is initially an intense monocytic and lymphocytic infiltration of the lamina propria which is followed by a mixed response with polymorphonuclear leukocytes and plasma cells. Mast cells, which may also be present, are frequently increased in quantity.[50,53,54] Mast cells which may be present in the cutaneous lesions of Behçet's disease have been quantified in spontaneous and localized trauma-induced (reactive) skin lesions and in apparently normal skin. Based upon the histologic studies of biopsy specimens, there was a significant increase in the number of mast cells in the reactive and spontaneous skin lesions as compared with the apparently uninvolved skin of patients during the active stage of Behçet's disease. The uninvolved skin revealed either normal or slightly elevated numbers of mast cells. In addition, the histamine content was increased twofold in the reactive or pathergic lesions, and the percentage of degranulating mast cells was markedly increased in both the pathergic and spontaneously occurring skin lesions, thus implying an active role for the mast cell in the pathogenesis of the mucocutaneous lesions. Mechanisms similar to cutaneous basophil hypersensitivity may enable the mast cell to contribute to the production of the mucocutaneous lesions in Behçet's disease, and many patients may also have elevated serum IgE levels.[80-83]

The inflammatory infiltrates in the oral lesions in Behçet's disease are often perivascular in location, affecting primarily the small blood vessels, especially the venules. There may also be vascular endothelial proliferation, destruction of the intimal elastic lamina, thrombosis, fibrinoid necrosis, and obliteration of the lumen.[8,48,50,84-86] According to Nazzaro,[69] the oral lesions histologically may reveal swelling and proliferation of the endothelial cells of the small blood vessels consistent with an obliterating vasculitis. There are perivascular infiltrations with lymphocytes, monocytes, polymorphonuclear leukocytes, some characterized by karyorrhexis, and plasma cells followed by an acute necrotizing vasculitis.[69] The histopathological examination of an aphthous ulcer in Behçet's disease may reveal either Sweet's-like (neutrophil vascular reaction) or leukocytoclastic vasculitis.[87-91] Pathological findings in leukocytoclastic vasculitis consist of endothelial swelling of dermal blood vessels, perivascular neutrophilic infiltration with degeneration of the leukocytes (leukocytoclasis), invasion of walls of arterioles, capillaries, and venules by neutrophils, fibrinoid necrosis, and extravasation of erythrocytes. In Sweet's-like vasculitis vascular necrosis, leukocytoclasia and extravasation of erythrocytes are not prominent features.[88-90]

Correlation of Oral Histology with Immunology

According to Lehner,[50] mononuclear cells may play an important primary role in the pathogenesis of aphthous ulcers in Behçet's disease since the histologic appearance resembles a delayed hypersensitivity reaction; that is, light microscopy shows an early intense infiltration with lymphocytes and monocytes, and electron microscopy suggests damage to epithelial cells by the mononuclear leukocytes. There is also significant lymphocyte transformation induced by the oral mucosal cells. The polymorphonuclear leukocyte reaction with fibrinoid necrosis and the presence of peripheral immune complexes are consistent with a type III Arthus reaction, but it is not known if this reaction is secondary to the epithelial damage of the oral lesion or is responsible for the development or progression of the ulceration.[48,50] Immunofluorescent microscopy has demonstrated Clq and C3 deposition in the perivascular precipitates, thus suggesting that an immune complex Arthus reaction may be involved in the pathogenesis of the oral aphthous ulcerations in Behçet's disease.[91] According to Reimer et al.,[92] immunofluorescence microscopy has revealed deposition of C3 and IgM in the vessel walls of the papillary and/or subepithelial connective tissue in the oral ulcers of Behçet's disease. Although immune complex deposition was not demonstrable and examinations for IgG, IgA, Clq, and C4 were negative, the authors postulated an immune complex–mediated vasculitis to explain the pathogenesis of the oral lesions in Behçet's syndrome. Since the presence of immune complexes may be transient and thus not detected in all biopsy specimens, their absence did not mitigate the concept of an immune complex–mediated vasculitis.[92] Sanders[93] has also demonstrated complement, specifically C3 and C9, deposition within the vessel walls of the oral ulcers. The immunofluorescent results in recurrent idiopathic aphthous ulcers and in the oral ulcers of Behçet's disease may be similar.[92] In summary, the histologic studies of the oral ulcers in patients with Behçet's disease have revealed evolution from a Type IV delayed hypersensitivity or cell-mediated immune reaction during the early phase to a Type III immune complex–mediated Arthus response in the later phase of the ulceration.[84,94]

The pathological features of the oral lesions have also been described as a function of the four clinical stages of ulcer formation: during the premonitory and preulcerative stages (up to 72 hours) of aphthous stomatitis, the primary pathological features are in the lamina propria and consist of "chronic" inflammatory foci containing mononuclear or lymphoid cells. As the reaction progresses, there may be subepithelial edema, liquefication degeneration of the basal and prickle cell layers, and degenerative changes of the epithelial cells. Subsequently, neutrophils begin to appear and increase in the immediate ulcerated area in the ulcerative stage (1–16 days). Mononuclear cells are still present, and the inflammatory infiltrates are significantly perivascular in location. Thus, the main pathology of the active ulcerative phase is predominantly a polymorphonuclear leukocyte infiltration at the base of the ulcer and a lymphocytic reaction at a deeper level. As the neutrophilic inflammatory process intensifies, the architecture of the lamina propria is severely altered with sloughing of the overlying epithelium. Plasma cells, eosinophils, and mast cells are also present. After three to ten days, the number of neutrophils decreases concomitantly with stabilization in the size of the ulcer, and plasma cells and the eosinophils increase in intensity.[61] According to Schroeder et al.,[86] biopsies from three-day-old oral ulcers have also shown foci of intense extravascular erythrocyte accumulation. During the healing stage (4–35 days), granulation tissue appears beneath the fibropurulent covering and contains capillaries and fibrous tissue. Subsequently, the granulation tissue undergoes collagenization with regeneration of the epithelium and continued decrease in the inflammatory infiltrates.[61]

According to Rapidis et al.,[95] the immunological responses observed in the oral ulcerations in patients with Behçet's disease may be divided into four phases: the initiating phase is characterized by a gradual rise in sensitized lymphocytes occurring one to three days before the ulceration. During the ulcerative phase there is an influx of lymphocytes around the ulcer, and during the healing phase there is significant decline in the sensitized lymphocytes within the oral lesion. The fourth or resting phase represents remission of the clinical manifestations.[95]

Based upon electron microscopic studies, dark cells have been observed in the basal cell layer of the epidermis of skin from normal individuals, and since this cell may manifest degenerative characteristics with shrinkage of the cell nucleus and cytoplasm and the formation of contraction vacuoles, these changes were considered to represent the physiological phenomenon of apoptosis or apoptotic degeneration. In patients with either recurrent idiopathic aphthous ulcerations or Behçet's disease and oral lesions, this contracted cell is located not only in the basal cell layer of the apparently normal oral mucosa but also in the prickle cell layer. These intraepithelial apoptotic cells fragment into debris containing a variety of cytoplasmic organelles and nuclear fragments, which not only attracts mononuclear cells but is phagocytized at the preulcerative stage by the increasing number of macrophages or reticuloid cells within the prickle cell layer. Histologically, degeneration of the prickle cell layer is observed, with an early intense perivascular mononuclear cell infiltration.[96] Macrophages predominate in the oral lesions of Behçet's disease, while the reticuloid cell, which differs from the macrophage in that its nucleus is homogeneous and lacks heterochromatin, is more numerous in recurrent idiopathic aphthous stomatitis.[79,96] According to Saito et al.,[97] three types of macrophages can be identified by electron microscopy in association with the degenerated prickle cells within areas adjacent to the ulcerations: type I macrophages had prominent cytoplasmic organelles and phagocytized material liberated from the degenerated prickle cells; type II macrophages with sparse endoplasmic reticulum were in contact with small lymphocytes and may have been responsible for them to undergo blastoid transformation (lymphoblast) with resultant immunoglobulin production; and type III macrophages had Birbeck granules and may be regarded as Langerhans cells of the thymus-dependent type.[97] Langerhans cells are normally located in the midepidermis of the skin as well as in the lymph nodes, spleen, tonsils, thymus, dermis, and the epithelia of the oral and genital mucous membranes.[98-101] These cells originate from the bone marrow mesenchymal precursors and, like macrophages, have cell surface Ia antigens and membrane receptors for the C3b complement component and the Fc portion of IgG. These markers participate in the recognition of antigens and in the interactions with T lymphocytes, thus enabling the Langerhans cells to participate in cell-mediated reactions.[100] The Langerhans cells probably process foreign antigen for presentation to the T lymphocytes possessing identical Ia antigens; and as a result, these activated T lymphocytes react with foreign antigen bearing Ia antigen compatible Langerhans cells in the epidermis, causing the Langerhans cells to produce an interleukin-1-like molecule named epidermal cell-derived thymocyte-activating factor (ETAF) and to release lyososomal enzymes, thus contributing to the production of inflammation, especially T-cell-dependent immune responses including syngeneic and allogeneic T-cell activation and epidermal cell-induced cytotoxic T-cell responses.[99-102] Skin biopsies from erythema nodosum-like lesions in patients with Behçet's disease have revealed the Langerhans cells to possess more prominent rough endoplasmic reticulum and granules, thus indicating a more active metabolic state.[103] In addition, during the preulcerative stage of the aphthous ulcer in Behçet's disease, macrophages phagocytizing the degenerating prickle cells may also be in contact with lymphocytes in the epithelium, and on electron microscopy these lymphocytes may possess nuclei with deep indentations resembling Sézary cells.[104] The apoptotic debris in the prickle cell layer also attracts neutrophilic leukocytes, and these neutrophils may undergo phagocytosis by large mononuclear cells.[96,105] In summary, it has been postulated that aphthous ulcerations in Behçet's disease are initiated by the phagocytosis of degenerating dark cells by intraepithelial mononuclear cells. This may result in the interaction of macrophages and lymphocytes with the production of immunoglobulins which form immune complexes with the subsequent activation of complement and the acceleration of the infiltration by polymorphononuclear leukocytes with resultant ulcer formation.[84,86,94,96,105]

Autoimmunity has been consistently implicated in the pathogenesis of the oral lesions in Behçet's disease, as demonstrated by the presence of polyclonal B-cell activation, elevated serum immunoglobulin levels, oral mucosal bound immunoglobulin, circulating immune complexes and antibodies to fetal oral mucosal cells, cell-mediated immunity to mucosal antigens as shown by lymphocyte transformation by human oral epithelial cells and inhibition of leukocyte migration, reduced T-suppressor cell function during the active phase of Behçet's disease, deficient interleukin-2 activity, macrophage migration inhibitory factor production by mucosal antigen-stimulated T cells, antibody-dependent cell-mediated cytotoxicity to oral epithelial cells, and diminished peripheral blood natural killer (NK) cell activation.[106–112] According to Kaneko et al.,[108] cytologic analysis has demonstrated the infiltration of the aphthous ulcers by activated T cells and macrophages in association with NK cells, thus supporting the pathogenetic role of delayed hypersensitivity reactions, especially antibody-dependent cell-mediated cytotoxicity. Poulter et al.,[113,114] investigating immunohistologically the oral ulcers of Behçet's disease, have shown a cell-mediated immune response with conversion of the normal Ia– to the Ia+ state of epithelium adjacent to the ulcer. Based upon monoclonal antibody studies, Poulter et al.[113] have also demonstrated the infiltrating cellular elements in the oral lesions to consist of T helper-inducer (T4) and

T cytotoxic-suppressor (T8) cells, T2 blast cells, B lymphocytes, D7+ macrophages, and Langerhans cells. The T-helper-inducer cell may be the predominant cell.[87]

Various studies have been performed to determine the role, if any, of the Herpes Simplex virus in the pathogenesis of the oral ulcers in Behçet's disease.[115–119] Using autoradiograph techniques, Eglin et al.[117] have shown greater hybridization between Herpes Simplex virus type 1 DNA and the complementary RNA present in the peripheral mononuclear cells in patients with Behçet's syndrome and minor aphthous ulcers than in patients with the major ulcers. Denman et al.[115] have demonstrated decreased activity of Herpes Simplex virus type 1 to grow in phytohemagglutinin-stimulated lymphocyte cultures obtained from patients with Behçet's disease. Specific antibody production and proliferative responses of lymphocytes to Herpex Simplex virus type 1 and varicella-zoster virus were also studied in patients with Behçet's disease. There was definite impairment of antibody and proliferative responses against Herpes Simplex virus type 1 and varicella-zoster virus.[116] Other investigators have shown hyporeactivity of the T4 helper-inducer cells and a hyperreactivity of T8 cytotoxic-suppressor cells to Herpes Simplex virus type 1[119] and the presence of Herpes Simplex virus type 1 specific IgG1 subclass circulating immune complexes and anti-Herpes Simplex virus type 1 antibodies in polyethylene glycol precipitable complexes.[118,120] However, the latter complexes were also demonstrable in patients with rheumatoid arthritis, systemic lupus erythematosus, and ankylosing spondylitis.[118] Since these immunological results were also reported in a percentage of patients with Behçet's disease who lacked oral ulcers and additionally were not present in some patients with Behçet's syndrome with oral lesions, the role of Herpes Simplex virus type 1 in the pathogenesis of aphthous stomatitis in Behçet's disease remains undefined.

Genital Ulcers

Genital ulcerations, which may affect various parts of the external genitalia including the scrotum and vulva, are described by the Behçet's Disease Research Committee of Japan[34] as being painful, punched-out ulcers which often heal with scar formation. The aphthous ulcers of the genitalia usually appear after the oral lesions; however, they may be the first manifestation of Behçet's disease, may resemble the oral ones in appearance and clinical course, and may recur as often as every two weeks.[3,7,9,12,17] In addition to the scrotum and vulva (labia majora and minora, mons pubis), the affected areas may include the prepuce, glans penis, shaft of the penis, vagina, introitus vaginae, fourchette (frenulum labiorum pudendi), cervix, clitoris, urethra, anus, perineum, groin, buttocks, genitocrural folds, and the cutaneous areas of the inner thighs.[9,17,26,27,39,95,121] The genital lesions, besides being characterized by recurrent painful aphthous ulcerations, may consist of vesicles, erythematous macules, papules, nodules, folliculitis, and sterile pustules involving the skin or mucous membranes of the affected structures.[2,17,39,75,122] The initial papular lesions may form pustules in 24 to 48 hours followed by aphthous ulcers which may have apparently normal intervening cutaneous areas.[62,69] The genital ulcers, which may heal within 10 days to 4 weeks with or without scar formation, may consist of a single or as many as 15 or more lesions at any one time, ranging in size from a few millimeters to several centimeters; these ulcers may have a white, yellow, or grayish-red base covered by an eschar or by a whitish-gray exudate or slough, may form large grayish necrotic areas, may be distributed in a linear fashion along the course of vessels, and may be accompanied by systemic symptoms including rigors and fever and by regional lymphadenopathy which may be tender.[4,6-9,11,13,39,62,69,75] Compared to the oral aphthous ulcers of Behçet's disease, the genital ones are less painful, may be deeper with indurated and very prominent margins, are larger and persist longer, may result in a greater degree of scar formation with tissue loss, and may have less frequent recurrences.[6,8,9,11,14,17,27,44,75,95] However, the genital ulcers may also be superficial, with distinct margins and minimal surrounding induration, transient, and painless, may heal rapidly without scarring, and because of minimal symptoms, especially if they involve the cervix and vagina, may be unnoticed by the patient. Therefore, routine pelvic examination may be necessary to detect these asymptomatic ulcers.[5,7,9,13,27,62,121,122] The vaginal and cervical ulcers, which are more painful upon palpation or if accompanied by a discharge, may be complicated by bleeding and dyspareunia.[11,15,36] Compared to herpes progenitalis, the genital ulcers in Behçet's disease are larger, deeper, and persist for longer periods of time.[123]

The genital ulcers in Behçet's disease may result in destruction of the vulva with scarring, tissue loss, and fenestration of the labia minora or labial perforation.[4,11,13,27,36,39,122,124] Curth[4] described a 21-year-old woman with Behçet's disease with an extensive, indurated, atrophic, and destructive process of the vulva resulting in extensive scarring of the labia majora and multiple fenestrations of the labia minora. O'Duffy et al.[12] reported a patient with Behçet's disease who had a deep cicatricial penile ulcer which was extremely chronic and because of its progression and inability to heal, necessitated penile amputation seven years after its onset.

The genital ulcers are more prominent and frequent during the premenstrual and menstrual phases of the ovarian cycle and immediately after delivery, and are usually less active during pregnancy; however, the genital lesions may be independent of the menstrual cycle, and acute exacerbations of Behçet's disease with genital ulcers may occur during pregnancy.[4,7,17,26,27,64] The Behçetin reaction refers to pathergy or mucocutaneous hyperreactivity induced by the injection of an aseptic, autogenous, genital ulcer extract, and the skin and mucous membranes of the genitalia may manifest this phenomenon.[14,17,69,125] The features of these experimentally induced lesions mimic those that occur spontaneously: they may initially form papules followed by pustules, then ulcers, may regress rapidly or spread diffusely and deeply, and may be accompanied by intense pain.[69] In light of the probable association of trauma with the initiation of ulcerations in Behçet's disease, coitus has been reported to precipitate genital lesions.[7,69,126]

In 1923 Lipschütz described ulcus vulvae acutum which consisted of acute ulcerations of the female external genitalia. Since these ulcers have also been reported in association with acute and recurrent oral ulcerations, the relationship of Lipschütz's ulcers vulvae and Behçet's disease is unknown.[127,128] In addition, the genital ulcers may be part of the MAGIC (mouth and genital ulcers with inflamed cartilage) syndrome which has been previously described in this chapter.[65] Other manifestations referable to the genitalia, described in subsequent chapters, include hematuria, epididymitis, orchitis, thrombosis of the penile vein, urethral, trigonal, and bladder ulcers, neurogenic bladder, fissure-in-ano, and perirectal, rectovesical, and rectovaginal fistulas.[3,9,14,15,129-135]

Pathology

Histologically, a biopsy from a preulcerative scrotal nodule has demonstrated perivascular and interstitial edema, an interstitial infiltration of small mononuclear cells especially around the capillaries and venules with relatively sparse polymorphonuclear leukocytes, and an intact epidermis. Sections from a fully, developed scrotal ulcer, however, have revealed more prominent inflammatory changes especially in the upper dermis. These changes were characterized by an influx of polymorphonuclear leukocytes, endothelial cell swelling, mural and periadventitial edema, infiltration of the vessel wall with mononuclear cells, and fibrinoid necrosis.[6] According to another study,[69] the pathological examination of a spontaneously appearing aphthous ulcer of the genitalia has shown endothelial swelling of the vessel wall with obliteration of its lumen, endothelial proliferation indicative of an obliterating vasculitis, thickened vessel walls, and perivascular infiltration with lymphocytes, monocytes, polymorphonuclear leukocytes with karyorrhexis, and plasma cells. Biopsies of early-appearing pathergic lesions of the scrotum have revealed inflammation of the dermis with edema and perivascular infiltration by lymphocytes, monocytes, polymorphonuclear leukocytes with karyorrhexis, and eosinophils. Subsequently, the epithelium ulcerated, and histologic examination revealed thickening of the vessel wall, endothelial swelling, obliteration of the vessel lumen, and perivascular inflammatory infiltrates, especially around the small vessels. In summary, the spontaneously appearing and trauma-induced genital ulcerations histologically were characterized by a vasculitis, often necrotizing, affecting mainly the capillaries and the smaller arterial and venous vessels.[69] However, the genital ulcers may also show nonspecific inflammatory changes with infiltrates consisting of lymphocytes, histiocytes, and polymorphonuclear leukocytes.[14,136]

Uveitis

The ocular symptoms which usually occur after the aphthous ulcers of the mouth and genitalia may not commence until six years or longer after the first manifestation of Behçet's disease; however, they may be the presenting symptom or begin during the quiescent stage of the disease. Historically, the main ocular complication of the triple symptom complex of Behçet's disease was described as anterior segment involvement, that is, recurrent anterior uveitis or iridocyclitis with hypopyon; however, iridocyclitis may also occur without hypopyon and this may be of the serous or fibrinous type. Ocular involvement in Behçet's disease may also affect and even begin in the posterior segment, with inflammation of the posterior uvea or chorioretinitis. Although ocular involvement may be initially unilateral, progression to bilateral disease may begin at the second attack or may not occur for six years or longer. However, blindness has also been reported to occur within four to five years from the onset of the ocular symptoms.[1,2,11,41,137-141] The ocular manifestations are recurrent, with episodes occurring every several weeks to months or years, and attacks of iridocyclitis with hypopyon may occur regularly during menses.[137] The ocular signs and symptoms of Behçet's disease may start with minimal to intense periorbital pain, photophobia, erythema of the eye with miosis, and lacrimation of variable intensity.[6,95,142] Each ocular attack may result in diminution in visual acuity eventually leading to blindness.[6,13,140,143] In one study, binocular visual acuity of 6/60 or less developed in 43% of 30 patients with Behçet's disease at an average of 3.2 years from the onset of ocular symptoms.[138]

According to the criteria established by the Behçet's Disease Research Committee of Japan in 1972, ocular manifestations constitute one major criterion in the diagnosis of Behçet's disease.[34] These criteria list iridocyclitis and chorioretinitis as the main ocular findings. Recurrent hypopyon-iritis may be common, usually disappearing within several days; however, in other patients, serous iritis may occur unaccompanied by hypopyon. During periods of apparent disease inactivity, posterior synechiae, iris atrophy, and keratic precipitates indicative of previous iritis may be appreciated on physical examination. The posterior uveal tract may also be involved as manifested by the presence of chorioretinitis which may be characterized by edematous opacification of the retina, macular exudates, hemorrhages and retinal angiitis. These manifestations may be recurrent and may coexist with iridocyclitis. Vitreous opacities due to exudates may also be observed, and sequelae of iridocyclitis and chorioretinitis have included diffuse retinal atrophy, optic nerve atrophy, cataract, secondary glaucoma, and phthisis bulbi.[34] The ocular complications of Behçet's syndrome may be categorized into three main clinical presentations consisting of pain and photophobia secondary to anterior uveitis, blurred vision due to vitreous opacities, and markedly decreased visual acuity resulting from retinal vasculitis.[114]

The Mayo Clinic reported the ocular findings in 32 patients with Behçet's disease.[144] Twenty-one patients had uveitis, and once established, it tended to be chronic, bilateral, and involved both the anterior and posterior segments. Hypopyon was not common, and involvement of the anterior segment in most patients consisted of nongranulomatous iritis with fine keratic precipitates; however, one patient had granulomatous uveitis with abundant "mutton-fat" keratic precipitates and Koeppe nodule. Posterior segment involvement, which was the leading cause of blindness in Behçet's disease, consisted of vitreous cellular infiltration, edema of the macula, retina, and disc, necrotizing retinitis with perivascular sheathing and venous and arterial occlusions including thrombosis of the central and branch retinal arteries, and retinal exudation, detachment, and pigmentary changes. Neuroophthalmologic abnormalities occurred in six patients and consisted of sixth nerve and seventh nerve palsies secondary to brain-stem involvement, papillitis with central scotoma, and homonymous hemianopia due to an intraccranial lesion. Other ocular findings in Behçet's disease reported by the Mayo Clinic included conjunctivitis, episcleritis, keratitis, optic atrophy, and phthisis bulbi. The eyelids can manifest the same typical cutaneous lesions characteristic of Behçet's syndrome, including papules, pustules, and nodules.[144]

Despite the experience of the Mayo Clinic, predominantly isolated anterior segment disease has been recently reaffirmed in Behçet's disease.[145] However, according to Pazarli et al.,[146] among

104 Turkish patients with Behçet's disease and ocular complications, 58% had uveoretinitis, 22% retinal vasculitis unaccompanied by anterior uveal changes,11% anterior uveitis, and 8% vitreous cellular infiltrates. In the series reported by Chajek and Fainaru,[3] posterior segment involvement was complicated by cataracts, glaucoma, and blindness, while those patients with isolated anterior segment involvement (iridocyclitis with hypopyon) had only recurrent attacks without complications. Blindness occurred in 40% of patients after four to eight years from the first ocular manifestation of posterior segment involvement.[3] Anterior uveitis with hypopyon clinically may be transient and regress rapidly often without sequelae, while the cloudiness of the vitreous and posterior segment involvement, which often last longer, may not resolve completely and therefore may be associated with progressive impairment in visual acuity.[9,41,44,56,141,147] Behçet's disease of the eye may progress from the anterior segment with iridocyclitis toward the posterior segment with chorioretinitis followed by sclerosis and atrophy of the globe or phthisis bulbi in the final stages.[14,137,141] However, ocular lesions may begin in the retina and optic nerve with resultant progression of posterior uveal disease, or the inflammatory process may spread from the uvea to the optic nerve (uveopapillitis).[9,140,148,149] Because of the aggressive use of corticosteroids both topically and systemically in the treatment of the ocular complications of Behçet's disease, the incidence of anterior uveitis with hypopyon may be decreasing, while posterior uveitis may be the predominant ocular complication and the main cause of vision loss in Behçet's disease.[11,13,37,41]

In summary, essentially all parts of the ocular structures may be affected in Behçet's disease, and these various manifestations and complications have included panophthalmitis; endophthalmitis; hemophthalmia; hemosiderosis bulbi; sclerosis of the globe; panuveitis; nongranulomatous uveitis; chorioretinitis; circumscribed or diffuse choroiditis; retinal atrophy, edema, exudates, degeneration, pigmentation, hemorrhages, and microaneurysms involving the arteriolar end of the capillaries; retinal vasculitis with periphlebitis, periarteritis, endarteritis, attenuation of the retinal arteries, capillary closure, dilatation of the retinal veins, and venous and arterial occlusions including thrombosis of the central retinal vein or its branches (branch retinal vein occlusion) and central or branch retinal artery occlusions; macular hole, edema, hemorrhage, or degeneration; uveopapillitis; optic neuritis (papillitis) and optic atrophy; central and paracentral scotomata; vitreous inflammation or hemorrhage complicated by proliferating retinopathy and retinal detachment; vitreous cellular infiltrates; posterior ring abscess; complicated cataract; atrophy of the lens; iris bombé; rubeosis iridis; iridocyclitis with or without hypopyon; iritis; depigmentation of the iris; cyclitis; ciliary muscle myopathy; hyphema; scleritis including episcleritis; corneal edema, opacity, cloudiness, dystrophy, ulcerations, and punctate infiltrations; cellular veil on Descemet's membrane; secondary glaucoma due to diminution in the chamber angle; keratitis of the fascicular or filamentous type; keratic precipitates; keratoconjunctivitis; chemosis; subconjunctival hemorrhages; conjunctivitis; pseudomembranous conjunctivitis; conjunctivitis sicca; symblepharon; irregularity of the pupil; occlusion and seclusion of the pupil; cholinomimetic miotic pupil secondary to autonomic abnormality; paresis or paralysis of the extrinsic ocular muscles with diplopia and ptosis due to central nervous system involvement (cranial nerves III to VII); anterior and posterior synechiae; blepharospasm, blepharitis; and hordeolum.[2-6,8,9,13-15, 29,37,41,44,56,95,114,121,122,134,140,141,144,146,150-162] Since these various ocular diagnoses were occasionally mentioned without adequate clinical and pathological descriptions, some of them may indeed represent identical complications; however, they have been listed for the purpose of completeness. In diabetic retinopathy, the microaneurysms usually occur on the venous end of the capillaries.[161] The cornea has been shown to demonstrate pathergy in Behçet's disease, and photocoagulation applied to the fundus has produced chorioretinitis after 48 hours with the clinical course of these experimentally evoked lesions being similar to the spontaneously or naturally occurring ones.[137,163]

Of the vascular ocular lesions in Behçet's disease, the preocclusive phase of retinal vein occlusion may be characterized by diffuse venous dilation of the retinal veins, optic disc hyperemia due to slight papilledema, and retinal hemorrhage, while central retinal vein occlusion may result in vitreous hemorrhages, macular edema with a cystoid structure, neovascularization of the optic disc, and macular hole or dystrophy of the macular pigmented epithleium.[150] Fundus fluorescein angiography in Behçet's disease has been shown to represent an extremely sensitive method of detecting even subtle changes in the permeability of the choroidal and retinal vasculature.[150,157,164] According to Matsuo et al.,[164] there are six types of papillary and retinal vascular disorders in Behçet's syndrome based upon fluorescein angiography. In the papillary type, the fluorescein dye escapes from the papillary superficial racemose capillaries and their collector venules located within the optic disc; in the peripapillary type, the dye leaks out of the radial epipapillary capillaries and their collector venules plus the vessels described in the papillary type. In the retinal venous branch occlusion type, the occluded regions of the branches of the retinal veins are affected. In the papillomacular type, the dye escapes from both the papillary and macular capillaries and cystoid macular edema is also present. In the retinal type, the papillary and the retinal vessels, such as the radial peripapillary capillaries, other retinal capillaries, and the retinal veins, reveal diffuse prominent leakages on both the disc and retina. And in the retinal vascular obliteration type, there isn't any leakage of dye; however, one can observe a window defect appearance with hyperfluorescence due to retinochoroidal degeneration and areas of hypofluorescence due to retinal pigmentation. Some of these angiographic abnormalities may be present in the absence of clinical symptoms, and the papillary and the retinal venous branch occlusion types have been associated with the most favorable and worst prognoses, respectively.[164] Based upon fluorescein angiographic features, Sanders[93] has divided the fundoscopic findings into four groups which consisted of perivenous and capillary leakage with predominant involvement of the retinal capillaries in the optic disc, macula, and periphery; venous occlusion complicated by capillary closure or neovascularization; retinal inflammatory infiltration; and the optic atrophic stage with destructive changes in the retina, choroid, and the optic disc.

Visual defects in Behçet's disease may also be of intracranial origin with resultant bitemporal hemianopia or uniocular field loss.[137,144,155,157] Papilledema, besides resulting from active uveitis, may be due to the syndrome of benign intracranial hypertension (pseudotumor cerebri) which may present with headaches and vomiting accompanied by elevated cerebrospinal fluid pressure.[7,165-169] This syndrome, which may be caused by thrombosis of the intracranial dural venous sinuses, had been diagnosed in the past by standard cerebral arteriography, but more recently has been detected by venous digital subtraction angiography.[166,167,169] The natural history of cerebral sinus thrombosis is unknown; however, the occluded sinuses may remain thrombosed with persistently increased intracranial pressure, recanalize, stimulate alternate drainage pathways, or develop into a dural arteriovenous malformation.[167,170]

Pathology and Immunology of Ocular Lesions

The underlying histopathological feature of the ocular disease of Behçet's disease is an inflammatory necrotizing obliterative vasculitis, probably immune complex–mediated, affecting both arteries and veins of all sizes including arterioles, capillaries, venules, and vasa nervorum and vasorum with vascular and perivascular infiltration by varying proportions of polymorphonuclear leukocytes, mononuclear cells, and plasma cells. The inflammatory cells are initially polymorphonuclear leukocytes followed by lymphocytes and monocytes.[4,11,13,29,41,93,126,134,141,148,159,171–177] Mast cells have also been observed in the iris.[172] In light of the presence of a vasculitis, the ocular complications of Behçet's disease may be dependent on or at least influenced by immune complex deposition within the vessel walls in association with activation of complement by the classic pathway. Indeed, there may be a diminution in the various complement components in the sera immediately prior to the onset of the ocular attack with the return to normal or elevated levels by three days after apparent resolution of the acute episode.[106,174] In addition, Chan et al.[178] have found antibodies against the outer segments of retinal photoreceptors and Müller cells in the sera of patients with Behçet's disease; however, these antibodies were also present in patients with the Vogt-Koyangi-Harada syndrome and in those with uveitis due to other etiologies. Patients with Behçet's disease and retinal vasculitis may have elevated titers of serum immune complexes detected by Clq binding assay, absolute peripheral lymphopenia (<1,500 cells/mm³), and decreased peripheral blood T and B cells with a normal T4 helper to T8 suppressor ratio.[179] However, the significance of these immunological abnormalities is not entirely known.

The aqueous humor obtained two to three days before the

onset of the ocular attack has demonstrated enhanced chemotactic activity for polymorphonuclear leukocytes, and this activity has been found in the protein and prostaglandin fractions of the aqueous humor. Prostaglandins E and F have been isolated from the aqueous humor of patients with Behçet's disease and have been shown to activate random neutrophil movement. This chemotactic activity decreases two to three days after the appearance of the hypopyon.[141] Namba and Masuda[180] studied the activities of the lysosomal enzymes of peripheral polymorphonuclear leukocytes from patients with Behçet's disease and ocular complications. There was no correlation between the attacks and the activities of acid phosphatase or beta-glucuronidase. However, the myeloperoxidase activity was significantly decreased in those patients with anterior or posterior uveitis with the more pronounced diminution being in the posterior type of ocular disease. During periods of remission, myeloperoxidase activity increased; however, absolute levels were normal or elevated in patients with anterior uveitis while still slightly depressed in those with posterior segment involvement.[180] In another study, Takeuchi et al.[181] have shown increased beta-glucuronidase release from neutrophils obtained from a limited number of patients with Behçet's disease and active ocular disease.

Alpha-1-proteinase inhibitor (antitrypsin), which is a glycoprotein and an acute-phase reactant, is the major alpha-1-globulin in human serum, and its main function is to inhibit various serine proteases including plasmin, thrombin, Factor XI, Factor XIII, neutrophil proteases elastase and cathepsin G, and pancreatic elastase, trypsin, and chymotrypsin.[182] This serum protease inhibitor, which is primarily of hepatic origin, and to a lesser extent mononuclear phagocytes may be detected on the ocular serosal surface,[182,183] and its deficiency in human sera has been reported in patients with idiopathic anterior uveitis.[184–186] Wakefield et al.[186] have reported eight patients with Behçet's syndrome and retinal vasculitis, all of whom possessed normal to elevated serum levels of alpha-1-antitrypsin with normal distribution of phenotypes (M1M1, M1M3, M3M3). Serum antitrypsin deficiency has not been reported in association with Behçet's syndrome, and in fact serum levels of this glycoprotein have been normal or elevated in Behçet's disease.[186] Perhaps the tissue levels of this alpha-1-proteinase inhibitor are more important than serum concentrations in the pathogenesis of the ocular complications of Behçet's syndrome.

The next series of chapters will continue the clinical review of Behçet's disease, focusing on those organ systems that have received the most attention in the recent literature.

References

1. Behçet H. Some observations on the clinical picture of the so-called triple symptom complex. *Dermatologica* 1940; 81:73–83.
2. Berlin C. Behçet's disease as a multiple symptom complex. Report of ten cases. *Arch Dermatol* 1960; 82:73–79.
3. Chajek T, Fainaru M. Behçet's disease. Report of 41 cases and a review of the literature. *Medicine* 1975; 54:179–196.
4. Curth HO. Recurrent genito-oral aphthosis and uveitis with hypopyon (Behçet's syndrome). Report of two cases. *Arch Dermatol Syphilol* 1946; 54:179–196.
5. Ehrlich GE. Intermittent and periodic arthritic syndromes. In McCarty DJ, ed: *Arthritis and Allied Conditions. A Textbook of Rheumatology.* Philadelphia, Lea and Febiger, 1985:883–900.
6. France R, Buchanan RN, Wilson MW, Sheldon MR Jr. Relapsing iritis with recurrent ulcers of the mouth and genitalia (Behçet's syndrome). Review: With report of additional case. *Medicine* 1951; 30:335–355.
7. Kalbian VV, Challis MT. Behçet's disease. Report of twelve cases with three manifesting as papilledema. *Am J Med* 1970; 49:823–829.
8. Mamo JG, Baghdassarian A. Behçet's disease. A report of 28 cases. *Arch Ophthalmol* 1964; 71:4–14.
9. Mavioğlu H. Behçet's recurrent disease. Analytical review of the literature. *Mo Med* 1958; 55:1209–1222.
10. Morrison AW. Behçet's syndrome. *J Laryngol Otol* 1959; 73:833–837.
11. O'Duffy JD. Behçet's disease. In Kelly WN, Harris ED Jr, Ruddy S, Sledge CB, eds: *Textbook of Rheumatology.* Philadelphia, WB Saunders, 1985:1174–1178.
12. O'Duffy JD, Carney TA, Deodhar S. Behçet's disease. Report of 10 cases, 3 with new manifestations. *Ann Intern Med* 1971; 75:561–570.
13. Price CA. Behçet's syndrome—A distressing, intriguing malady. *J R Coll Gen Pract* 1969; 18:38–45.
14. Shimizu T, Ehrlich GE, Inaba G, Hayashi K. Behçet disease (Behçet syndrome). *Semin Arthritis Rheum* 1979; 8:223–260.
15. Strachan RW, Wigzell FW. Polyarthritis in Behçet's multiple symptom complex. *Ann Rheum Dis* 1963; 22:26–35.
16. Lewis MA, Priestley BL, Ward AM, Bleehen SS. Neonatal and familial Behçet's disease (abstract 57). Royal Society of Medicine international conference on Behçet's disease, September 5 and 6, 1985, London, England.

17. Marchionini A, Müller E. The dermatological view of Morbus Hulsi Behçet. In Monacelli M, Nazzaro P, eds. *Behçet's Disease. International Symposium on Behçet's Disease, Rome, 1964.* Basel, S. Karger, 1966:6–14.
18. Feigenbaum B. Description of Behçet's syndrome in the Hippocratic third book of endemic diseases. *Br J Ophthalmol* 1956; 40:355–357.
19. Gotfried M, Jutrin H, Ravid M. Behçet's disease preceded by fever of unknown origin (letter). *Arch Intern Med* 1985; 145:1329.
20. Pines A, Kaplinsky N, Olchovsky D, et al. Fever of undetermined origin as the presenting symptom of Behçet's disease: A favorable response to colchicine. *South Med J* 1984; 77:802–803.
21. Davies JD. Behçet's syndrome with haemoptysis and pulmonary lesions. *J Pathol* 1973; 109:351–356.
22. Haim S, Barzilai D, Hazani E. Involvement of veins in Behçet's syndrome. *Br J Dermatol* 1971; 84:238–241.
23. Kansu E, Ozer FL, Akalin E, et al. Behçet's syndrome with obstruction of the venae cavae. A report of seven cases. *Q J Med* 1972; 41:151–168.
24. Ramalho PS, Rodrigo FG, Magalhães AS, et al. Behçet's disease in Portugal. A review of 17 cases. In Dilşen N, Koniçe M, Öuül C, eds: *Behçet's Disease. Proceedings of an International Symposium on Behçet's Disease, Istanbul, 29–30 September 1977.* Amsterdam-Oxford, Excerpta Medica, 1979:108–113.
25. Yim CW, White RH. Behçet's syndrome in a family with inflammatory bowel disease. *Arch Intern Med* 1985; 145:1047–1050.
26. Hurt WG, Cooke CL, Jordan WP, et al. Behçet's syndrome associated with pregnancy. *Obstet Gynecol* 1979; 53(3 Suppl):31S–33S.
27. Dunlop EMC. Genital and other manifestations of Behçet's disease seen in venereological practice. In Lehner T, Barnes CG, eds: *Behçet's Syndrome. Clinical and Immunological Features. Proceedings of a Conference Sponsored by the Royal Society of Medicine, February 1979.* London, Academic Press, 1979:159–175.
28. Aksungur L, Çayhan A, Şentut Z. A clinical and histopathological study of 35 patients with Behçet's Disease. In Dilşen N, Kouiçe M, Övül C, eds: *Behçet's Disease. Proceedings of an International Symposium on Behçet's Disease, Istanbul, 29–30 September 1977.* Amsterdam-Oxford, Excerpta Medica, 1979:114–119.
29. Lakhanpal S, Tani K, Lie JT, et al. Pathologic features of Behçet's syndrome: A review of Japanese autopsy registry data. *Hum Pathol* 1985; 16:790–795.
30. Huston KA, O'Duffy JD, McDuffie FC. Behçet's disease associated with a lymphoproliferative disorder, mixed cryoglobulinemia, and an immune complex mediated vasculitis. *J Rheumatol* 1978; 5:217–223.
31. Kaneko H, Hojo Y, Nakajima H, et al. Behçet syndrome associated with nasal malignant lymphoma—Report of an autopsy case. *Acta Pathol Jpn* 1974; 24:141–150.

32. McDonald GSA, Gad-Al-Rab J. Behçet's disease with endocarditis and the Budd-Chiari syndrome. *J Clin Pathol* 1980; 33:660–669.
33. Tamaoki N, Habu S, Yoshimatsu H, et al. Thymic change in Behçet's disease. *Keio J Med* 1972; 21:201–213.
34. Behçet's Disease Research Committee of Japan. Behçet's disease: guide to diagnosis of Behçet's disease. *Jpn J Ophthalmol* 1974; 18:291–294.
35. Ammann AJ, Johnson A, Fyfe GA, et al. Behçet's syndrome. *J Pediatr* 1985; 107:41–43.
36. Chamberlain MA. Behçet'a syndrome in 32 patients in Yorkshire. *Ann Rheum Dis* 1977; 36:491–499.
37. Fife RS. Behçet's disease. *Clin Rheumatol Pract* 1983; 1:249–254.
38. Gustafson RO, McDonald TJ, O'Duffy JD, Goellner JR. Upper aerodigestive tract manifestations of Behçet's disease: Review of 30 cases. *Otolaryngol Head Neck Surg* 1981; 89:409–413.
39. Held BL, Knox JM. Behçet's syndrome. *Clin Obstet Gynaecol* 1972; 15:1017–1022.
40. James DG. Behçet's syndrome. *N Engl J Med* 1979; 301:431–432.
41. Michelson JB, Chisari FV. Behçet's disease. *Surv Ophthalmol* 1982; 26:190–203.
42. Ramsay CA. Behçet's syndrome with large bowel involvement. *Proc R Soc Med* 1967; 60:185–186.
43. Rapport PN, Duckert LG, Boies LR Jr. Behçet's disease. *Ear Nose Throat J* 1979: 58:168–172.
44. Wong RC, Ellis CN, Diaz LA. Behçet's disease. *Int J Dermatol* 1984; 23:25–32.
45. Wright MI. Behçet's disease in the mouth, pharynx, and larynx: An underdiagnosed disease? (abstract 56). Royal Society of Medicine international conference on Behçet's disease, September 5 and 6, 1985, London, England.
46. Cooke BED. Oral ulceration in Behçet's syndrome. In Lehner T, Barnes CG, eds: *Behçet's Syndrome. Clinical and Immunological Features. Proceedings of a Conference Sponsored by the Royal Society of Medicine, February 1979*. London, Academic Press, 1979:143–149.
47. Francis TC. Recurrent aphthous stomatitis and Behçet's disease. A review. *Oral Surg* 1970; 30:476–487.
48. Lehner T. Immunological aspects of recurrent oral ulceration and Behçet's syndrome. *J Oral Pathol* 1978; 7:424–430.
49. Wray D. Recurrent aphthous stomatitis and Behçet's syndrome. In Hooks JJ, Jordan GW, eds: *Viral Infections in Oral Medicine*. New York, Elsevier North Holland, 1982:279–289.
50. Lehner T. Pathology of recurrent oral ulceration and oral ulceration in Behçet's syndrome: Light, electron and fluorescence microscopy. *J Pathol Bacteriol* 1969; 97:481–494.
51. Bell GF, Royers RS III. Observations on the diagnosis of recurrent aphthous stomatitis. *Mayo Clin Proc* 1982; 57:297–302.
52. Cohen L. Etiology, pathogenesis and classification of aphthous stomatitis and Behçet's syndrome. *J Oral Pathol* 1978; 7:347–352.

53. Lehner T. Immunologic aspects of recurrent oral ulcers. *Oral Surg* 1972; 33:80–85.
54. Lehner T. Oral ulceration and Behçet's syndrome. *Gut* 1977; 18:491–511.
55. Levinsky RJ, Lehner T. Circulating soluble immune complexes in recurrent oral ulceration and Behçet's syndrome. *Clin Exp Immunol* 1978; 32:193–198.
56. Venkatasubramaniam KV, Swinehart DR. Behçet's syndrome: Case report and literature review. *Henry Ford Hosp Med J* 1981; 29:153–159.
57. Lehner T. Behçet's syndrome and autoimmunity. *Br Med J* 1967; 1:465–467.
58. Burns RA, Davis WJ. Recurrent aphthous stomatitis. *Am Fam Physician* 1985; 32:99–104.
59. Hersh SP, Grimes CD Jr, Harrison W, Nonkin P. Behçet's syndrome. An overlooked entity in otolaryngology. *Arch Otolaryngol* 1982; 108:250–252.
60. Rogers RS III. Recurrent aphthous stomatitis: Clinical characteristics and evidence for an immunopathogenesis. *J Invest Dermatol* 1977; 69:499–509.
61. Stanley HR. Aphthous lesions. *Oral Surg* 1972; 33:407–416.
62. Yassin A, Girgis IH. Behçet's disease. *J Laryngol Otol* 1966; 80:481–494.
63. Koniçe M, Dilşen N, Aral O. The preaphthous phase (PAP) of Behçet's disease (BD), abstract 47. Royal Society of Medicine international conference on Behçet's disease, September 5 and 6, 1985, London, England.
64. Jorizzo JL, Taylor RS, Schmalstieg FC, et al. Complex aphthosis: A forme fruste of Behçet's syndrome? *J Am Acad Dermatol* 1985; 13:80–84.
65. Firestein GS, Gruber HE, Weisman MN, et al. Mouth and genital ulcers with inflamed cartilage: MAGIC syndrome. Five patients with features of relapsing polychondritis and Behçet's disease. *Am J Med* 1985; 79:65–72.
66. Challacombe ST, Scully C, Keevil B, Lehner T. Serum ferritin in recurrent oral ulceration. *J Pathol* 1983; 12:290–299.
67. Cooke BED. Recurrent oral ulceration. *Br J Dermatol* 1969; 81:159–161.
68. Ship II, Merritt AD, Stanley HR. Recurrent aphthous ulcers. *Am J Med* 1962; 32:32–43.
69. Nazzaro P. Cutaneous manifestations of Behçet's disease. Clinical and histopathological findings. In Monacelli M, Nazzaro P, eds: *Behçet's Disease. International Symposium on Behçet's Disease, Rome, 1964.* Basel, S. Karger, 1966:15–41.
70. Brookes GB. Pharyneal stenosis in Behçet's syndrome. The first reported case. *Arch Otolaryngol* 1983; 109:338–340.
71. Screech G. An unusual cause of respiratory obstruction during anaesthesia. A case report. *Br J Anaesth* 1965; 37:978–979.

72. Turner ME. Anaesthetic difficulties associated with Behçet's syndrome. Case report. *Br J Anaesth* 1972; 44:100–102.
73. Kobayashi T, Kikawada T, Shima K, Fukuda O. Ulceration and stenosis of the hypopharynx and its surgical management. *Head Neck Surg* 1982; 5:65–69.
74. Fromer JL. Behçet's syndrome. *Arch Dermatol* 1970; 102:116–117.
75. Ayers MA. Behçet's syndrome. Report of a case and review of the literature. *Obstet Gynecol* 1965; 26:575–579.
76. Davis E, Melzer E. A new sign in Behçet's syndrome. Scanty fungiform papillae in tongue. *Arch Intern Med* 1969; 124:720–721.
77. Lavalle C, Gudiño J, Reinoso SR, et al. Behçet's syndrome and palate perforation (letter). *Arthritis Rheum* 1979; 22:308.
78. Shuttleworth EC, Voto S, Sahar D. Palatal myoclonus in Behçet's disease. *Arch Intern Med* 1985; 145:949–950.
79. Honma T. Electron microscopic study on the pathogenesis of recurrent aphthous ulceration as compared to Behçet's syndrome. *Oral Surg* 1976; 41:366–377.
80. Haim S. The pathogenesis of lesions in Behçet's disease. *Dermatologica* 1979; 158:31–37.
81. Hain S, Sobel JD, Friedman-Birnbaum R, Lichtig C. Histological and direct immunofluorescence study of cutaneous hyperreactivity in Behçet's disease. *Br J Dermatol* 1976; 95:631–636.
82. Lichtig C, Haim S, Gilhar A, et al. Mast cells in Behçet's disease: Ultrastructural and histamine content studies. *Dermatologica* 1981; 162:167–174.
83. Lichtig C, Haim S, Hammel I, Friedman-Birnbaum R. The quantification and significance of mast cells in lesions of Behçet's disease. *Br J Dermatol* 1980; 102:255–259.
84. Lehner T. Immuno-pathology of Behçet's syndrome. In Lehner T, Barnes CG, eds: *Behçet's Syndrome. Clinical and Immunological Features. Proceedings of a Conference Sponsored by the Royal Society of Medicine, February 1979.* London, Academic Press, 1979:127–139.
85. Lever WF, Schaumburg-Lever G. Systemic diseases with cutaneous manifestations. In: *Histopathology of the Skin.* Philadelphia, JB Lippincott, 1983:190–197.
86. Schroeder HE, Müller-Glauser W, Sallay K. Stereologic analysis of leukocyte infiltration in oral ulcers of developing Mikulicz aphthae. *Oral Surg* 1983; 56:629–640.
87. Jorizzo JL. Behçet's disease. An update based on the 1985 international conference in London. *Arch Dermatol* 1986; 122:556–558.
88. Jorizzo JL. Behçet's syndrome: Pathogenesis, diagnosis, and treatment. *Cutis* 1983; 32:441–442, 444–445, 448.
89. Jorizzo JL, Schmalstieg FC, Solomon AR Jr, et al. Thalidomide effects in Behçet's syndrome and pustular vasculitis. *Arch Intern Med* 1986; 146:878–881.
90. Jorizzo JL, Solomon AR, Cavallo T. Behçet's syndrome. Immunopathologic and histopathologic assessment of pathergy lesions is useful in diagnosis and follow-up. *Arch Pathol Lab Med* 1985; 109:747–751.

91. Schroeder HE, Müller-Glauser W, Sallay K. Pathomorphologic features of the ulcerative stage of oral aphthous ulcerations. *Oral Surg* 1984; 58:293–305.
92. Reimer G, Luckner L, Hornstein OP. Direct immunofluorescence in recurrent aphthous ulcers and Behçet's disease. *Dermatologica* 1983; 167:293–298.
93. Sanders MD. Ophthalmic features of Behçet's disease. In Lehner T, Barnes CG, eds: *Behçet's Syndrome. Clinical and Immunological Features. Proceedings of a Conference Sponsored by the Royal Society of Medicine, February 1979.* London, Academic Press, 1979:183–189.
94. Müller W, Lehner T. Quantitative electron microscopial analysis of leukocyte infiltration in oral ulcers of Behçet's syndrome. *Br J Dermatol* 1982; 106:535–544.
95. Rapidis AD, Langdon JD, Patel MF. Recurrent oral and oculogenital ulcerations (Behçet's syndrome). *Oral Surg* 1976; 457–466.
96. Honma T, Saito T, Fujioka Y. Possible role of apoptotic cells of the oral epithelium in the pathogenesis of aphthous ulceration. *Oral Surg* 1985; 59:379–387.
97. Saito T, Honma T, Sato T, Fujioka Y. Auto-immune mechanisms as a probable aetiology of Behçet's syndrome, an electron microscopic study of the oral mucosa. *Virchows Arch [A]* 1971; 353:261–272.
98. Hammar S, Bockus D, Remington F, Bartha M. The widespread distribution of Langerhans cells in pathologic tissues: An ultrastructural and immunohistochemical study. *Hum Pathol* 1986; 17:894–905.
99. Holbrook KA, Wolff K. The structure and development of skin. In Fitzpatrick TB, Eisen AZ, Wolff K, et al, eds: *Dermatology in General Medicine.* New York, McGraw-Hill, 1987:93–131.
100. Jakubovic HR, Ackerman AB. Structure and function of skin. Sect 1. Development, morphology, and physiology. In Moschella SL, Hurley HJ, eds: *Dermatology.* Philadelphia, WB Saunders, 1985:1–74.
101. Stingl G, Wolff K. Langerhans cells and their relation to other dendritic cells and mononuclear phagocytes. In Fitzpatrick TB, Eisen AZ, Wolff K, et al, eds. *Dermatology in General Medicine.* New York, McGraw-Hill, 1987:410–426.
102. Dinarello CA. Interleukin-1. *Rev Infect Dis* 1984; 6:51–95.
103. Kohn S, Haim S, Gilhar A, et al. Epidermal Langerhans' cells in Behçet's disease. *J Clin Pathol* 1984; 37:616–619.
104. Honma T, Saito T, Fujioka P. Intraepithelial atypical lymphocytes in oral lesions of Behçet's syndrome. *Arch Dermatol* 1981; 117:83–85.
105. Honma T. Electron microscopic observation of infiltrating neutrophils in aphthous ulceration in Behçet's disease. *Acta Derm Venereol* (Stockh) 1980; 60:521–524.
106. Gupta RC, O'Duffy JD, McDuffie FC, et al. Circulating immune complexes in active Behçet's disease. *Clin Exp Immunol* 1978; 34:213–218.
107. Kaneko F, Takahashi Y, Muramatsu R, et al. Natural killer cell numbers and function in peripheral lymphoid cells in Behçet's disease. *Br J Dermatol* 1985; 113:313–318.

108. Kaneko F, Takahushi Y, Muramatsu Y, Miura Y. Immunological studies on aphthous ulcer and erythema nodosum-like eruptions in Behçet's disease. *Br J Dermatol* 1985; 113:303–312.
109. Michelson JB, Chisari FV, Kansu T. Antibodies to oral mucosa in patients with ocular Behçet's disease. *Ophthalmology* 1985; 92:1277–1281.
110. Sakane T, Suzuki N, Ueda Y, et al. Analysis of interleukin-2 activity in patients with Behçet's disease. Ability of T cells to produce and respond to interleukin-2. *Arthritis Rheum* 1986; 29:371–378.
111. Suzuki N, Sakane T, Ueda Y, Tsunematsu T. Abnormal B cell function in patients with Behçet's disease. *Arthritis Rheum* 1986; 29:212–219.
112. Williams BD, Lehner T. Immune complexes in Behçet's syndrome and recurrent oral ulceration. *Br Med J* 1977; 1:1387–1389.
113. Poulter LW, Lehner T, Duke O. Immunohistological investigation of recurrent oral ulcers and Behçet's disease (abstract 31). Royal Society of Medicine international conference on Behçet's disease, September 5 and 6, 1985, London, England.
114. Hames DG. Silk route disease. *Postgrad Med J* 1986; 62:151–153.
115. Denman AM, Fialkow PJ, Pelton BK, et al. Lymphocyte abnormalities in Behçet's syndrome. *Clin Exp Immunol* 1980; 42:175–185.
116. Efthimiou J, Harikumar MK, Knight PA, Snaith ML. Inappropriate peripheral blood lymphocyte responses to herpes virus in patients with Behçet's syndrome. *Immunol Lett* 1984; 8:317–318.
117. Eglin RP, Lehner T, Subak-Sharpe JH. Detection of RNA complementary to herpes-simplex virus in mononuclear cells from patients with Behçet's syndrome and recurrent oral ulcers. *Lancet* 1982; 2:1356–1361.
118. Hasain L, Ward R, Lehner T, Barnes CG. Herpes simplex virus IgG, IgM, IgA and IgG subclass antibodies in polyethelene glycol precipitable complexes from sera of patients with Behçet's disease and controls (abstract 19). Royal Society of Medicine international conference on Behçet's disease, September 5, and 6, 1985, London, England.
119. Pugh CJ, Lehner T. The proliferative responses of separated and reconstituted T4+ and T8+ cells to herpes simplex virus in Behçet's disease (abstract 10). Royal Society of Medicine international conference on Behçet's disease, September 5 and 6, 1985, London, England.
120. Lehner T. The role of a disorder in immunoregulation in the development of Behçet's disease (abstract 8). Royal Society of Medicine international conference on Behçet's disease, September 5 and 6, 1985, London, England.
121. Katzenellenbogen I. Behçet's syndrome. *Arch Dermatol Syphilol* 1950; 61:481–484.
122. Wright VA, Chamberlain MA. Behçet's syndrome. *Bull Rheum Dis* 1978–79; 29:972–977.
123. Corey L. Genital herpes. In Holmes KK, Mårdh P-A, Sparling PF,

Wiesner PJ, eds: *Sexually Transmitted Diseases*. New York, McGraw-Hill, 1984:449–474.

124. Dowling GB. Behçet's disease. *Proc R Soc Med* 1961; 54:101–104.
125. Shimizu T, Katsuta Y, Oshima Y. Immunological studies on Behçet's syndrome. *Ann Rheum Dis* 1965; 24:494–500.
126. Fishof FE. Behçet's syndrome: Report of two cases. *J Int Coll Surg* 1960; 34:213–229.
127. Phillips DL, Scott JS. Recurrent genital and oral ulceration with associated eye lesions. Behçet's syndrome. *Lancet* 1955; 1:366–371.
128. Whitewell GPB. Recurrent buccal and vulval ulcers with associated embolic phenomena in the skin and eye. *Br J Dermatol* 1934; 46:414–419.
129. Baba S, Maruta M, Ando K, et al. Intestinal Behçet's disease: Report of five cases. *Dis Colon Rectum* 1976; 19:428–440.
130. Empey DW, Hale JE. Rectal and colonic ulceration in Behçet's disease. *Proc R Soc Med* 1972; 65:163–164.
131. Goldstein SJ, Crooks DJM. Colitis in Behçet's disease. Two new cases. *Radiology* 1978; 128:321–323.
132. Ketch LL, Buerk CA, Liechty D. Surgical implications of Behçet's disease. *Arch Surg* 1980; 115:759–760.
133. O'Connell DJ, Courtney JV, Riddell RH. Colitis of Behçet's syndrome—Radiologic and pathologic features. *Gastrointest Radiol* 1980; 5:173–179.
134. Sezer N. Further investigations on the virus of Behçet's disease. *Am J Ophthalmol* 1956; 41:41–55.
135. Smith GE, Kime LR, Pitcher JL. The colitis of Behçet's disease: A separate entity? Colonscopic findings and literature review. *Dig Dis Sci* 1973; 18:987–1000.
136. Stolz E, Menke HE, Uvzerski VD. Nonveneral genital dermatosis. In Holmes KK, Mårdh P-A, Sparling PF, Wiesner PJ, eds: *Sexually Transmitted Disease*. New York, McGraw-Hill 1984:714–736.
137. Bietti GB, Bruna F. An ophthalmic report on Behçet's disease. In Monacelli M, Nazzaro P, eds: *Behçet's Disease. International Symposium on Behçet's Disease*, Rome, 1964. Basel, S Karger, 1966:79–110.
138. Dinning WJ. Behçet's disease and the eye: Epidemiological considerations. In Lehner T, Barnes CG, eds: *Behçet's Syndrome. Clinical and Immunological Features. Proceedings of a Conference Sponsored by the Royal Society of Medicine, February 1979*. London, Academic Press, 1979:177–181.
139. Katzenellenbogen I. Recurrent aphthous ulceration of oral mucous membrane and genitals associated with recurrent hypopyon iritis (Behçet's syndrome). Report of three cases. *Br J Dermatol* 1946; 58:161–172.
140. Mamo JG. The rate of visual loss in Behçet's disease. *Arch Ophthalmol* 1970; 84:451–452.
141. Mishima S, Masuda K, Izawa Y, et al. The eighth Frederick H. Verhoeff lecture presented by Saiichi Mishima, MD, Behçet's disease in

Japan: Ophthalmologic aspects. *Trans Am Ophthalmol Soc* 1979; 77:225–279.

142. Rosenbaum JT, Nozik RA. Uveitis: Many diseases, one diagnosis. *Am J Med* 1985; 79:545–547.

143. Pezzi PP, Gasparri V, DeLiso P, Catarinelli G. Prognosis in Behçet's disease. *Ann Ophthalmol* 1985; 17:20–25.

144. Colvard DM, Robertson DM, O'Duffy JD. The ocular manifestations of Behçet's disease. *Arch Ophthalmol* 1977; 95:1813–1817.

145. Dining WJ. Ocular disease—An overview (abstract 58). Royal Society of Medicine conference on Behçet's disease, September 5 and 6, 1985, London, England.

146. Pazarli H, Özyazgan Y, Bahcecioĝlu H, et al. Ocular involvement in Behçet's (BS) in Turkey (abstract 59). Royal Society of Medicine, international conference on Behçet's disease, September 5 and 6, 1985, London, England.

147. BenEzra D, Nussenblatt R. Ocular manifestations of Behçet's disease. *J Oral Pathol* 1978; 7:431–435.

148. Cotticelli L, Apponi-Battini G, Federico A, et al. Behçet's disease: An unusual case with bilateral obliterating retinal panarteritis and ischemic optic atrophy. *Ophthalmologica* 1980; 180:328–332.

149. Scouras J, Koutroumanos J. Ischaemic optic neuropathy in Behçet's syndrome. *Ophthalmologica* 1976; 173: 11–18.

150. Bonamour G, Grange JD, Bonnet M. Retinal vein involvement in Behçet's disease. In Dilşen N, Koniçe M, Övül C, eds: *Behçet's Disease. Proceedings of an International Symposium on Behçet's Disease, Istanbul, 29–30 September 1977.* Amsterdam-Oxford, Excerpta Medica, 1979:142–144.

151. Calin A. Seronegative spondyloarthritides. *Med Clin North Am* 1986; 70:323–326.

152. Clausen J, Bierring F. Involvement of post-capillary venules in Behçet's disease: An electronmicroscopic study. *Acta Derm Venereol* (Stockh) 1983; 63:181–197.

153. Fenton RH, Easom HA. Behçet's syndrome. A histopathologic study of the eye. *Arch Ophthalmol* 1964; 72:71–81.

154. Green WR, Koo BS. Behçet's disease. A report of the ocular histopathology of one case. *Surv Ophthalmol* 1967; 12:324–332.

155. Harfitt R, Lehner T. Ocular findings in patients with Behçet's syndrome and recurrent oral ulcers. In Lehner T, Barnes CG, eds: *Behçet's Syndrome. Clinical and Immunological features. Proceedings of a Conference Sponsored by the Royal Society of Medicine, February 1979.* London, Academic Press, 1979:191–198.

156. Hong C. Clinical observations of Behçet's disease (abstract 53). Royal Society of Medicine international conference on Behçet's disease. September 5 and 6, 1985, London, England.

157. James DG, Spiteri MA. Behçet's disease. *Ophthalmology* 1982; 89:1279–1284.

158. Lowder CY, Char DH. Uveitis. A review. *West J Med* 1984; 140:421–432.

159. Michelson JB, Michelson PE, Chisari FV. Subretinal neovascular membrane and disciform scar in Behçet's disease. *Am J Ophthalmol* 1980; 90:182–185.
160. O'Duffy JD, Goldstein NP. Neurologic involvement in seven patients with Behçet's disease. *Am J Med* 1976; 61:170–178.
161. Smith RB, Prior IAM, Sturman D. Behçet's disease with retinal vascular lesions. *Br Med J* 1967; 2:220–221.
162. Tabuchi S, Ishikama S. Pupillary study of Behçet's disease (abstract 65). Royal Society of Medicine international conference on Behçet's disease, September 5 and 6, 1985, London, England.
163. Urayama A, Takahashi N, Sakai F. The position of ocular symptoms in Behçet's disease. In Inaba G, ed: *Behçet's Disease. Pathogenetic Mechanism and Clinical Future. Proceedings of the International Conference on Behçet's Disease, Tokyo, October 23–24, 1981.* Tokyo, University of Tokyo Press, 1982; 153–160.
164. Matsuo N, Ojima M, Kumashiro O, et al: Fluorescein angiographic disorders of the retina and the optic disc in Behçet's disease. In Inaba G, ed: *Behçet's Disease. Pathogenetic Mechanism and Clinical Future. Proceedings of the International Conference on Behçet's Disease, Tokyo, October 23–24, 1981.* Tokyo, University of Tokyo Press, 1982:161–170.
165. Bank I, Weart C. Dural sinus thrombosis in Behçet's disease. *Arthritis Rheum* 1984; 27:816–818.
166. Brissaud P, Laroche L, de Gramont A, Krulik M. Digital angiography for the diagnosis of dural sinus thrombosis in Behçet's disease (letter). *Arthritis Rheum* 1985; 28:359–360.
167. Harper CM Jr, O'Neill BP, O'Duffy JD, Forber GS. Intracranial hypertension in Behçet's disease: Demonstration of sinus occlusion with use of digital subtraction angiography. *Mayo Clin Proc* 1985; 60:419–422.
168. Pamir MN, Kansu T, Erbengi A, Zileli T. Papilledema in Behçet's syndrome. *Arch Neurol* 1981; 38:643–645.
169. Wechsler B, Bousser MG, Du LTH, et al. Central venous sinus thrombosis in Behçet's disease (letter). *Mayo Clin Proc* 1985; 60:891.
170. Houser OW, Campbell JK, Campbell RJ, Sundt TM Jr. Arteriovenous malformation affecting the transverse dural venous sinuses—An acquired lesion. *Mayo Clin Proc* 1979; 54:651–661.
171. Mullaney J, Collum LMT. Ocular vasculitis in Behçet's disease. A pathological and immunohistochemical study. *Int Ophthalmol* 1985; 7:183–191.
172. Nii S, Yasuda I, Mimura Y, et al. Ultrastructure of mast cells in the iris of cases of Behçet's disease. *Biken J* 1971; 17:121–125.
173. Ohno S. Clinical and immunological studies on ocular lesions in Behçet's disease. In Inaba G, ed: *Behçet's Disease. Pathogenetic Mechanism and Clinical Future. Proceedings of the International Conference on Behçet's Disease, Tokyo, October 23–24, 1987.* Tokyo, University of Tokyo Press, 1982:127–136.
174. O'Connor GR. Epidemiology and pathogenesis of the ocular and cerebral forms of Behçet's disease. In Inaba G, ed: *Behçet's Disease.*

Pathogenetic Mechanism and Clinical Future. Proceedings of the International Conference on Behçet's Disease, Tokyo, October 23–24, 1987. Tokyo, University of Tokyo Press, 1982:115–126.

175. Shikano S. Ocular pathology of Behçet's syndrome. In Monacelli M, Nazzaro P, eds: *Behçet's Disease. International Symposium on Behçet's Disease, Rome, 1964.* Basel, S Karger, 1966:111–136.

176. Shimizu K. Fluorescein fundus angiography in Behçet's syndrome. *Mod Probl Ophthalmol* 1972; 10:224–228.

177. Winter FC, Yukins RE. The ocular pathology of Behçet's disease. *Am J Ophthalmol* 1966; 62:257–262.

178. Chan C-C, Palestine AG, Nussenblatt RB, et al. Anti-retinal auto-antibodies in Vogt-Koyanagi-Harada syndrome, Behçet's disease, and sympathetic ophthalmia. *Ophthalmology* 1985; 92:1025–1028.

179. Wakefield D, Easter J, Penny R. Immunological abnormalities in patients with untreated retinal vasculitis. *Br J Ophthalmol* 1986; 70:260–265.

180. Namba K, Masuda K. Types of ocular attacks and lysosomal enzymes in Behçet's disease. *Jpn J Ophthalmol* 1984; 28:80–88.

181. Takeuchi A, Kobayashi K, Mori M, Hashimoto A. Nonphagocytic beta-glucuronidase release in Behçet's disease. *Clin Exp Rheumatol* 1986; 4:3–7.

182. Gadek JE, Crystal RG. α_1-antitrypsin deficiency. In Stanbury JB, Wyngaarden JB, Fredrickson DS, et al, eds. *The Metabolic Basis of Inherited Disease.* New York, McGraw-Hill, 1983:1450–1467.

183. Mornex J-F, Chytil-Weir A, Martinet Y, et al. Expression of the alpha-1-antitrypsin gene in mononuclear phagocytes of normal and alpha-1-antitrypsin-deficient individuals. *J Clin Invest* 1986; 77:1952–1961.

184. Brewerton DA, Webley M, Murphy AH, Ward AM. The α_1-antitrypsin phenotype MZ in acute anterior uveitis (letter). *Lancet* 1978; 1:1103.

185. Wakefield D, Breit SN, Clark P, Penny R. Immunogenetic factors in inflammatory eye disease. Influence of HLA-B27 and alpha$_1$-antitrypsin phenotypes on disease expression. *Arthritis Rheum* 1982; 25:1431–1434.

186. Wakefield D, Easter J, Breit SN, et al. α_1-antitrypsin serum levels and phenotypes in patients with retinal vasculitis. *Br J Ophthalmol* 1985; 69:497–499.

10

MUSCULOSKELETAL MANIFESTATIONS

John J. Calabro

WHILE THE TURKISH DERMATOLOGIST HULUSI BEHÇET, described a chronic relapsing syndrome characterized by the clinical triad of aphthous stomatitis, genital ulceration, and uveitis in 1937,[1] in 1938, he reported that "rheumatoid pains" might also be a component of the disorder.[2] Since then, numerous reports have focused on the musculoskeletal manifestations of this complex and highly protean entity. Because they are central to an understanding of rheumatologic features, the prevalence and classification of Behçet's syndrome will be briefly reviewed.

Prevalence and Classification

Prevalence

The prevalence of Behçet's syndrome varies widely from one part of the world to another (Table 1). Initially, the syndrome was believed to be an extremely rare disorder, limited to countries neighboring the Mediterranean Sea and to Japan. Cases are now recognized worldwide, although Japan continues to have the highest prevalence. In fact, the syndrome affects 1 per 1,000 of the

From *Behcet's Disease: A Contemporary Synopsis*, edited by Gary R. Plotkin, M.D., John J. Calabro, M.D., and J. Desmond O'Duffy, M.B. © 1988, Futura Publishing Company, Inc., Mount Kisco, NY.

Table 1

Prevalence of Behçet's Syndrome by Geographic Areas	
Geographic Area	cases/100,000
Japan	100
Worcester County, Massachusetts	5
Olmsted County, Minnesota	4
Yorkshire County, England	0.6

Japanese population in certain localities, constituting one of the leading causes of blindness.[3,4]

In Worcester County, Massachusetts, the prevalence is much less than that of Japan (Table 1).[5] However, it is comparable to that of Olmsted County,[3] Minnesota, but considerably higher than the prevalence of Behçet's syndrome in Yorkshire, England.[6] Although the reason for this wide discrepancy is unclear, it must be related in some way to the pathogenesis of Behçet's syndrome.

Classification

Behçet's syndrome is currently classified as a form of vasculitis.[7] In England, however, it is included as a member of the seronegative spondyloarthropathies, a group of rheumatic disorders that also includes ankylosing spondylitis, Reiter's syndrome, enteric arthritis, and psoriatic arthritis.[8] As a group, the seronegative spondyloarthropathies share a number of clinical, roentgenographic, serologic, and genetic features (Table 2).[8-16] These disor-

Table 2

Unifying Features of the Seronegative Spondyloarthropathies
• Negative tests for IgM rheumatoid factor (latex fixation) and antinuclear antibodies
• Absence of subcutaneous (rheumatoid) nodules
• Inflammatory peripheral arthritis, often asymmetric
• Roentgenographic evidence of sacroiliitis, with or without spondylitis
• Overlap of mucocutaneous, ocular, genital, and gastrointestinal manifestations
• High frequency of enthesopathy, characterized clinically by heel pain or other localized tender areas from inflammation of ligaments, tendons, or fascia, and roentgenographically by osseous proliferation and/or erosions at these sites
• Tendency to cluster in families
• Striking association with the inherited antigen HLA-B27

ders have little in common with Behçet's syndrome, although each of them, and especially Reiter's syndrome, may occasionally mimic it. Moreover, sacroiliitis, the hallmark of the seronegative spondyloarthropathies, is not a feature of Behçet's syndrome.[17-19] Nevertheless, Dilşen et al.[20] from Istanbul have noted an increased incidence of sacroiliitis and ankylosing spondylitis in association with HLA-B27 in patients with Behçet'ş disease. It is possible that either regional and genetic factors are responsible for these differences or that the reported patients are afflicted with two separate disease processes.

In order to emphasize the recurrent nature of the syndrome, Ehrlich includes Behçet's syndrome in the intermittent and periodic arthritis syndromes, a group that also includes intermittent hydrarthrosis (periodic arthrosis), palindromic rheumatism, familial Mediterranean fever, and the Stevens-Johnson syndrome.[21] The only common factor among these disorders is their intermittency, that is, the propensity to recur after having apparently completed their course.

To differentiate between clinical involvement of diverse organs, the terms "oculo-Behçet," "neuro-Behçet," "orogenital Behçet," and others are in common use. Above all, they serve to remind us that in the natural history of the syndrome, there may be a delay for many years between orogenital manifestations and neuroocular involvement.

Musculoskeletal Manifestations

Arthropathy in the form of arthritis and/or arthralgia is an important feature of Behçet's syndrome.[6,22-27] The mean frequency of arthritis is approximately 50%.[6,22-24] However, the incidence varies widely (Table 3), probably a reflection of interest and referral so that the highest rates are reported by rheumatology centers.[6,22-29]

Arthritis

Articular involvement may occur first in Behçet's syndrome, although oral ulceration is the most frequent initial feature. In

Table 3

Frequency of Arthritis in Nine Series Reported after 1960*

Series	Specialty	No. of Cases	Arthritis
Mason & Barnes (1969)	Rheumatology	25	76%
Calabro (1987)†	Rheumatology	30	73%
Oshima et al. (1963)	Rheumatology/ Internal Medicine	85	64%
Gow et al. (1979)	Rheumatology/. Internal Medicine	25	56%
Dilşen et al. (1979)	Rheumatology	106	54%
Chamberlain (1977)	Rheumatology	32	47%
Yurdakul et al. (1983)	Multidisciplinary‡	184	39%
Chajek & Fainaru (1975)	Internal Medicine	41	29%
Haim (1968)	Dermatology	23	26%

*Modified after Barnes.[22]
†Series not reported previously.
‡Outpatient clinic attended by two rheumatologists, two hematologists, two dermatologists, and two ophthalmologists.

fact, joint manifestations may antedate other Behçet features by years.[22] However, arthritis usually evolves with other features or develops at variable times after the onset of the syndrome. Other clinical features of Behçet's syndrome do not differ in patients either with or without arthritis, except that erythema nodosum and the HLA-B5 tissue antigen occur more frequently in those with joint involvement.[27]

The inflammatory nature of the arthritis is documented by the history of pain, swelling, and morning stiffness, by the presence of joint swelling, by synovial fluid analysis, by synovial histology, and by concomitant elevation of the erythrocyte sedimentation rate (ESR) and presence of other acute-phase reactants with recurrent flares of synovitis. Affected joints are usually warm and swollen, but redness of the overlying skin is unusual except when associated with erythema nodosum. The severity of joint involvement may range from intermittent mild arthralgia with tenderness and stiffness of the fingers to chronic arthritis and articular destruction.

Early morning stiffness of joints may also occur, but it rarely lasts more than one hour. Consequently, the duration of morning stiffness with few exceptions is rarely prolonged to three or four hours, as it is in rheumatoid arthritis. Limitation of joint motion may occur and is usually confined to one or two joints. In fact, progressive deformity of multiple joints is distinctly uncommon in Behçet's syndrome.

The onset of arthritis is variable.[22] It may begin acutely with fever and florid joint swelling, suggesting septic arthritis; however, it may also begin insidiously with mild joint swelling misdiagnosed as seronegative rheumatoid arthritis. Essentially, any presentation between these two extremes may occur in Behçet's syndrome.

The pattern of arthritis is usually pauciarticular (oligoarticular) and asymmetric, involving one to four joints.[27] The knee is the most commonly affected joint, followed by the ankle, wrist, and elbow (Table 4).[22] The small joints of the hand and foot are less frequently involved (20% and 10% respectively), whereas the shoulder and hip are affected in 10% of patients or less. Although any articulation can be affected, involvement of the cervical spine as well as the sternoclavicular, manubriosternal, and temporomandibular joints is rare in Behçet's syndrome. Occasionally, the pattern of involvement is polyarticular and symmetric with involvement of both large and small joints. When the small joints of the hands and/or feet are affected, the arthritis resembles rheumatoid arthritis.[22,30]

The duration of the initial or recurrent attacks of arthritis is

Table 4

Frequency of Joint Involvement in Behçet's Syndrome*

Affected Joints	Percentage
Knee	57
Ankle	47
Wrist	31
Elbow	29
Hands	20
Shoulder	11
Feet	10
Hip	6
Cervical spine	3
Sternoclavicular	2
Manubriosternal	0.5
Temporomandibular	0.5

*Adapted from Barnes, derived from seven published series of 265 patients.[22]

usually short, but may last from a few weeks to a few months.[27] Palindromic-like episodes of only a few days duration also are not unusual.[4,21] However, the arthritis may be chronic, especially with involvement of the knees, and effusions are common, particularly of the knees and other large joints. The arthritis of Behçet's syndrome is usually recurrent; however, occasionally, the synovitis is self-limiting with spontaneous and permanent remission even after many years of joint involvement.[6,22,23]

Pseudothrombophlebitis Syndrome

A fluid-filled synovial cyst may enlarge and rupture into the surrounding soft tissue. Sudden bending of the knee may precipitate rupture of a synovial cyst in the popliteal fossa behind the knee (Baker's cyst).[31,32] Thus, the patient complains of extreme tenderness and tightness in the calf, signs and symptoms that mimic acute thrombophlebitis, including a positive Homans' sign.[33-36] The synovial rupture can be confirmed by ultrasonography, arthrography, or radiographic examination with injection of contrast material into the knee, and needle aspiration of synovial fluid from the ruptured cyst.

Differentiation between rupture of a synovial cyst of the knee joint and thrombophlebitis is extremely important, since anticoagulants prescribed for a patient with a dissecting cyst may result in a massive hematoma with subsequent fibrosis and contracture of the calf muscles.[35] Consequently, any doubt regarding the occurrence of thrombophlebitis from Behçet's syndrome may require simultaneous ultrasonography and venography for diagnosis. The correct diagnosis is critical, especially in a disease with vascular manifestations such as Behçet's syndrome, since a ruptured synovial cyst and venous thrombosis may coexist in the same individual.[36] Since ruptured synovial cysts, either in the calf or elsewhere, respond dramatically to aspiration and corticosteroid injection, surgical intervention is rarely necessary.[33]

Synovial Fluid Characteristics

During active synovitis of Behçet's disease, aspiration of an affected joint will usually yield fluid that is inflammatory in character.[30] However, findings on synovial fluid analysis vary widely.[27] In fact, they may range from fluid that is noninflammatory or mildly inflammatory[37] to fluid that appears grossly purulent with a very high leukocyte count in the septic arthritis level.[38]

Generally, synovial fluid leukocyte counts less than 5,000 cells/mm³ or in excess of 50,000 cells/mm³ are uncommon in Behçet's syndrome.[27] The cells are predominantly polymorphonuclear leukocytes but may be primarily mononuclear when the arthritis is chronic rather than acute. The mucin clot test is usually good,[27] reflecting the mildly inflammatory nature of the synovitis, but may be fair or poor if the leukocyte count is high.[30] Synovial fluid glucose levels are usually normal, paralleling those found in simultaneously drawn serum. Occasionally, synovial fluid glucose values are reduced but rarely to the extremely low levels occurring in septic arthritis.[27,30] Synovial fluid complement levels are usually elevated, unlike the depressed levels noted in rheumatoid arthritis.[30,39]

Synovial Histology

On biopsy, the synovial histology in Behçet's syndrome is nonspecific, with an acute inflammatory reaction with polymorphonuclear infiltration. However, a wide spectrum of abnormalities may occur that are indistinguishable from those seen in either rheumatoid arthritis[40] or Reiter's syndrome.[30,38] Pannus formation and erosive changes of the articular surfaces may also evolve in Behçet's syndrome.[41] Electron microscopy also fails to reveal any distinctive features, although immunofluorescent studies reveal consistent deposition of IgG on the synovial lining surface.[40]

Other Laboratory Findings

Additional laboratory features are nonspecific, including the presence of acute-phase reactants such as C-reactive protein and elevation of the ESR,[42] a neutrophilic leukocytosis, low-grade anemia, and occasionally eosinophilia.[30] Serum protein electrophoresis may disclose an increase in gamma globulin, or less frequently, hypogammaglobulinemia.[30,37]

Unlike other forms of vasculitis, IgM rheumatoid factor (positive latex test) and antinuclear antibodies are not present in the sera of patients with Behçet's syndrome.[22] Serum complement levels may be either normal or elevated.[37]

Roentgenographic Features

Roentgenographic features are also nonspecific, consisting primarily of radiodensities from soft-tissue swelling and effusion. Periosteal reaction does not occur, even with florid arthritis. Erosions and joint-space narrowing of affected joints are rare manifestations of Behçet's syndrome.[21,22,27] In fact, erosive changes on x-ray examination occur in only 1% of patients.[22] In a study of 20 patients with Behçet's syndrome complicated by arthritis of the hands of more than five years' duration, roentgenographic features consisted of juxtaarticular demineralization, carpal bone rotation, and less commonly, bone destruction in the wrists and narrowing of the joint spaces.[43]

A Behçet's disease patient with atlantoaxial subluxation has been reported[44]; however, since a spur was also present at the anterior undersurface of the second cervical vertebra, the role of trauma in the pathogenesis of the subluxation remains unknown. Essentially, the sacroiliac and spinal articulations are not affected roentgenographically in Behçet's syndrome. Although uncommon, aseptic necrosis of the femoral head has also been observed in the triple symptom complex.[4]

Arthralgia, Myalgia, and Fibrositis

Joint discomfort without objective clinical synovitis may occur in Behçet's syndrome; these patients usually have arthralgia, myalgia, or secondary fibrositis.

Arthralgia

Joint pain and tenderness occur frequently in patients with Behçet's syndrome.[6,22,27] However, the frequency of arthralgia is uncertain because patients with only joint pain are not included in most reports of joint involvement.[22,27] Occasionally, arthralgia is an initial clinical manifestation, but most patients with this complaint develop joint swelling at a later date.[22]

Myalgia/Myositis

Myalgia may occur, either with or without arthralgia.[21] Moreover, subclinical muscle involvement, detectable only by electron microscopy, is common in Behçet's syndrome.[45] A necrotizing myositis that may be either localized or diffuse is a rare manifestation of Behçet's syndrome and may be associated with normal or elevated serum levels of muscle enzymes.[45–49] This myopathy is characterized clinically by severe leg pain, usually bilateral, that remits spontaneously. The most striking findings on muscle biopsy are inclusions within the muscle fiber that superficially resemble mitochondrial aggregates.[45] Histologically, vasculitis may also be present in tissue sections of skeletal muscle.[47,50]

In addition to myositis, two other types of myopathy may occur in Behçet's syndrome.[51,52] Afifi et al.[51] have reported seven patients, many of whom lacked neuromuscular symptoms and signs, whose gastrocnemius or deltoid muscle biopsies demonstrated on electron microscopy capillary basement membrane thickening; disorganization and disarray of the myofibrils; pleating of the sarcolemma; subsarcolemmal collection of mitochondria, glycogen, and lysosomes; central nucleation in areas lacking contractile material; and the presence of cytoplasmic inclusions. The latter varied from filamentous, cristae-like, and paracrystalline to concentrically laminated structures and were the most significant histologic finding.[51] The third form of myopathy, termed neurogenic muscular atrophy, has been described by Frayha et al.[52] in an 11-year-old boy with Behçet's syndrome complicated by nondeforming, relapsing polyarthritis of the elbows, wrists, knees, and ankles, erythema nodosum, and a brain-stem syndrome. Light microscopy of the gastrocnemius muscle biopsy showed small-size fibers, central nuclei, sparse necrotic fibers, and an increase in the number of nuclei, while electron microscopy demonstrated loss of myofilaments, swelling of the endothelial cells, multivesicular structures, and narrowing of the capillar lumina.[52]

Fibrositis (Fibromyalgia)

Fibrositis, also known as fibromyalgia or fibromyositis, is a common form of nonarticular rheumatism characterized by diffuse aches and stiffness and can be primary or secondary to other rheumatic or vasculitic diseases, including Behçet's syndrome.[53-55] In fact, it occurred in 6 of 30 patients with Behçet's syndrome in the Worcester series. Moreover, the unexplained episodic back complaints reported in 11 of 25 patients by Chamberlain,[17] and in 12 of 25 by Gow and associates,[24] could well have been examples of secondary fibrositis.

Patients with fibrositis complain of musculoskeletal pain and stiffness, usually worse in the morning.[53] Common tender sites include the neck, midback, and low back, as well as the elbows, shoulders, anterior chest wall, upper gluteal areas, and knees.[54] The presence of tender points at precisely predictable symmetrical sites confirms the diagnosis.[53,56]

Since fibrositis, in addition to arthritis, may occur in patients with Behçet's syndrome, the symptom complex may consist of back or other diffuse aches and pains with typical modulating factors in which symptoms are intensified by cold and damp weather, excessive physical activity, and emotional tension.[53] As a result, it would be inappropriate to alter the basic drug therapy of Behçet's syndrome, but instead, the primary-care physician must explain to the patient the benign nature of these additional complaints. Moreover, regular follow-up care is essential to assure continuous emotional support and implementation of other appropriate measures may be necessary.[57-59] Improvement often follows treatment with tricyclic agents such as low-dose cyclobenzaprine and amytriptyline, by physical measures, and by reduction of stress.[57]

Erythema Nodosum

As early as 1940, Behçet recognized that erythema nodosum, a form of hypersensitivity vasculitis, could occur in patients with the triple symptom complex.[60] However, this manifestation of the disease has not been adequately emphasized, particularly as a presenting feature.[23,25,61] Consequently, these patients pose difficulties in early diagnosis since most are believed to have sarcoidosis or idiopathic erythema nodosum.[61] The causes of erythema nodosum are multiple and variable (Table 5),[62,63] and currently, sarcoidosis, tuberculosis, and streptococcal infections are the three most common etiologies.[62]

The onset of erythema nodosum is often acute, accompanied by systemic manifestations such as fever and malaise. Myalgia and arthralgia are common, as is arthritis. Another feature is hilar adenopathy, which is often a clue to underlying sarcoidosis. However, the simultaneous occurrence of nodose skin lesions and hilar lymph node enlargement may have other etiologies.[62]

The skin eruption of erythema nodosum usually appears suddenly as crops of erythematous, painful, nonpruritic, slightly raised lesions on the anterior surfaces of both shins (Fig. 1). Occa-

Table 5

Major Causes of Erythema Nodosum*

Infectious causes:	Streptococcal disease†
	Tuberculosis†
	Psittacosis
	Yersinia infections
	Coccidioidomycosis
	Histoplasmosis
	Blastomycosis
	Leprosy
	Cat-scratch disease
	Lymphogranuloma venereum
	Trichophyton infections
Noninfectious causes:	Sarcoidosis†
	Behçet's syndrome
	Inflammatory bowel disease
	Ulcerative colitis
	Regional enteritis
	Neoplasms
	Leukemia
	Hodgkin's disease
	Pregnancy
	Drugs
	Vaccines

*From Calabro and Wolf.[62]
†Currently the three most common causes in the United States.

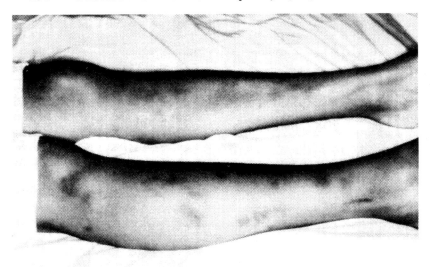

Figure 1-The nodules of erythema nodosum are exquisitely tender to palpation and the overlying skin is red, warm, and shiny. They have a predilection for the shins and a vivid play of colors, in which bright red spots gradually fade to dark red and blue and finally to purplish yellow "bruises."

sionally, a single lesion, unilateral crops, or involvement of the extensor surfaces of the forearms may characterize the erythema nodosum of Behçet's syndrome. Because lesions can occur wherever subcutaneous fat is present, they may appear almost anywhere, including the calves, thighs, buttocks, and even obscure areas such as the episclera of the eye.

The individual lesions of erythema nodosum vary in diameter from 0.5 to 5.0 cm. The skin over the nodules is red, smooth, shiny, and warm. Individual lesions may coalesce to form sizable indurations, which may then result in considerable edema of the affected limbs. Resolution without ulceration, scarring, or permanent pigmentary changes usually occurs within one to three weeks. During this time, the lesions progress from a bright red to a darker red or purple, along with intermediate color changes, including blue, green, and yellow.

Approximately two-thirds of patients with erythema nodosum have an associated arthropathy, which usually accompanies the febrile phase but occasionally may precede it by weeks. Some patients have only arthralgias, so that although the affected joints are tender to palpation, no joint swelling is present on examination. Early morning stiffness may also accompany erythema nodosum.

Approximately one-third of patients have objective evidence of arthritis, manifested as swelling, erythema, warmth, and effusion. The large peripheral joints (knees, ankles, wrists, and elbows) are usually involved, often symmetrically, but swelling may also occur in the small joints of the hands and feet.

The arthropathy of erythema nodosum usually resolves within a few weeks. Occasionally, it may become chronic, lasting for months, and only rarely for a year or longer. Deformity does not occur even when the duration of the arthritis is protracted.

Diagnosis of Behçet's Syndrome

Although most tissues and organs can be affected by Behçet's syndrome (Table 6),[4] generally, oral ulcers appear first, then

Table 6

Behçet's Syndrome: Major and Minor Clinical Features and Frequency*

Clinical Features	Frequency (%)
MAJOR	
Oral ulcers	99
Eye lesions: anterior uveitis (hypopyon-iritis), posterior uveitis, chorioretinitis, optic nerve atrophy	90
Skin lesions: erythema nodosum, thrombophlebitis, acneiform eruptions, hyperirritability ("needle reaction")	85
Genital ulcerations: primarily scrotum and vulva; also penis, perianal, and vaginal mucosa	67
MINOR	
Articular manifestations: arthralgia, arthritis (large joints), myalgia, fibrositis	50
Gastrointestinal complaints: abdominal pain, melena	50
Central nervous system manifestations: meningoencephalitis, sensory and motor involvement, psychologic changes	10
Vascular lesions: arterial occlusion, aneurysms, venous occlusion, varices	8
Epididymitis	8†

*Adapted from Schimizu et al.[4]
†Percentage of male patients.

cutaneous manifestations, followed by ocular, genital, and articular involvement. Nervous system or vascular lesions usually evolve later, although these may occasionally occur first.

Diagnostic Criteria

A number of diagnostic criteria have been proposed over the years. The one proposed by the 1977 International Symposium on Behçet's Syndrome held in Istanbul is practical and simple (Table 7).[64,65] The presence of three or more of seven criteria, provided one of these is recurrent oral ulcers, is sufficient for a definite diagnosis. Otherwise, the diagnosis of Behçet's syndrome is only tentative. Above all, the common and self-limiting entity of aphthous stomatitis and vulvitis in adolescent females should not be labeled Behçet's syndrome. Other clinical entities which one must consider include Crohn's disease, Herpes Simplex infections, and various causes of recurrent aseptic meningitis.

Differential Diagnosis

The patient who presents with the clinical impression of pauciarticular Behçet's syndrome may, if recently bitten by a tick, have Lyme disease.[66-68] However, oral and genital ulcerations do not occur in Lyme disease, and the test for serum antibodies to the spirochete *Borrelia burgdorferi* permits one to confirm the diagnosis of this tick-transmitted disorder.[69] If the skin rash, erythema chronicum migrans, is present, then early treatment with antibio-

Table 7

Behçet's Syndrome: Diagnostic Criteria*
(1) Recurrent aphthous stomatitis
(2) Recurrent genital ulcers
(3) Uveitis (anterior or posterior)
(4) Vasculitis (either cutaneous or of large vessels)
(5) Arthritis
(6) Meningoencephalitis
(7) Cutaneous hyperactivity to minor trauma

*The first criterion plus two others are required for a definite diagnosis.

tics may spare the patient with Lyme disease from chronic or prolonged recurrent bouts of arthritis.[70]

Confirming the arthritis of Behçet's syndrome is less difficult when two or more joints are swollen than when symptoms and signs affect only one joint. When a single joint is involved, arthrocentesis and synovial fluid analysis should be performed routinely to rule out infectious arthritis. Differentiating infectious from Behçet's arthritis must have the highest priority because infection can destroy a joint in only 7 to 10 days. The synovial fluid in septic arthritis is cloudy or purulent with a very high leukocyte count, usually 100,000/cm^3 or greater, and contains a preponderance of polymorphonuclear leukocytes. In infectious arthritis, the mucin clot is always poor, and the glucose level may be greatly reduced. Microorganisms can often be demonstrated on microscopic examination of gram-stained smears of synovial fluid, while bacterial cultures may result in the identification of the specific organism.

Infection can supervene in any joint affected by Behçet's syndrome. Septic arthritis is more likely to occur in patients with refractory arthritis treated by repeated joint aspiration plus intraarticular corticosteroid injections and/or by the systemic administration of immunosuppressive drugs including prednisone. Consequently, when there is unexplained persistent or progressive inflammation of a single joint, superimposed septic arthritis must be suspected, even in the absence of fever, leukocytosis, localized lymphadenopathy, or an obvious portal of infection. Septic arthritis is best treated with repeated aspiration of the affected joint and appropriate systemic antibiotic therapy. Occasionally, surgical drainage may be required for resolution of the infectious process.

When a patient is evaluated, especially a woman suspected of having polyarticular Behçet's syndrome, the most important disorders to consider in the differential diagnosis are systemic lupus erythematosus (SLE) and rheumatoid arthritis. The absence of antinuclear antibodies almost always excludes SLE, and thereby constitutes the single most helpful laboratory test in differentiating SLE from Behçet's syndrome. In rheumatoid arthritis, recurrent aphthous stomatitis and genital ulcers do not occur, whereas subcutaneous (rheumatoid) nodules and a positive latex fixation test for IgM rheumatoid factor, which are present in 20% and 85%, respectively, of adult patients with rheumatoid arthritis, are not characteristic of Behçet's syndrome.

Behçet's syndrome may be difficult to distinguish from relapsing polychondritis because of overlap in clinical manifestations. In fact, five patients have been reported with coexisting features of relapsing polychondritis and Behçet's syndrome.[71] The MAGIC syndrome, to emphasize the mouth and genital ulcers with inflamed cartilage complex, has been proposed for this overlap syndrome. A common immunological marker is likely, and elastin has been cited as a possible target antigen.[71]

The most difficult disorders to differentiate from Behçet's syndrome are Reiter's syndrome and psoriatic arthritis, since all three disorders are characterized by mucocutaneous manifestations and arthritis. Major differences among the three conditions are listed in Table 8. It is important to note that iridocyclitis probably in association with HLA-B27 and ulcerations of the oral mucosa rarely occur in psoriatic arthritis, whereas pitting of the nails is not characteristic of Reiter's syndrome. Neither onycholysis (nail discoloration and lifting of the nail bed) nor nail pitting is found in Behçet's syndrome.[9] Moreover, the oral ulcerations of Behçet's syndrome are painful, with sharply demarcated borders (Fig. 2), while those of Reiter's syndrome are not tender (Fig. 3).

Table 8

Differential Diagnostic Features of Reiter's Syndrome, Psoriatic Arthritis, and Behçet's Syndrome

Feature	Reiter's Syndrome	Psoriatic Arthritis	Behçet's Syndrome
Iridocyclitis	Yes	No	Yes
Nail pitting	No	Yes	No
Onycholysis of nails	Yes	Yes	No
Oral lesions	Yes	Rare	Yes
	Painless	Painless	Painful
Erythema nodosum	No	No	Yes
Sausage digits*	Yes	Yes	No
Enthesopathy	Yes	Yes	No
Sacroiliitis	Yes	Yes	No
Spondylitis	Yes†	Yes†	No
HLA-B27	Yes	Occasionally	No

*Sausage digits, or diffuse swelling of fingers or toes, result from acute synovitis of both distal and proximal interphalangeal joints.
†As Reiter's spondylitis and psoriatic spondylitis, respectively.

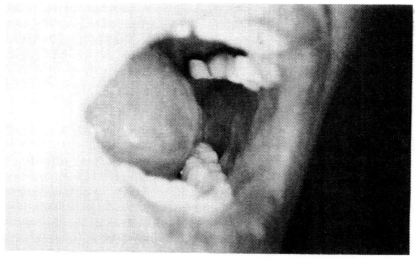

Figure 2—Oral ulceration of Behçet's syndrome. The outer border of the ulcer is sharply delineated and the lesion is usually exquisitely painful.

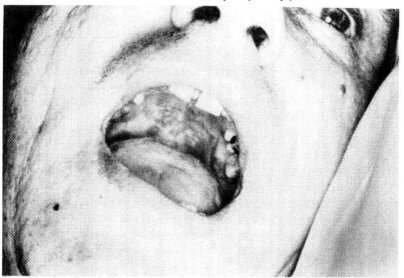

Figure 3—Patches of granular erythema and superficial ulcerations of the palate from Reiter's syndrome are painless and fleeting.

Erythema nodosum may be common in Behçet's syndrome but does not occur in either Reiter's syndrome or psoriatic arthritis.

The arthritis of all three disorders can be either pauciarticular or polyarticular.[9] However, sausage digits (Fig. 4), enthesopathy, sacroiliitis, and spondylitis, while prominent features of both Reiter's syndrome and psoriatic arthritis, do not occur in Behçet's syndrome (Table 8).

Management of Arthritis

The arthritis of Behçet's syndrome is usually responsive to drug therapy, unlike the ocular and neurological manifestations which are often refractory to antiinflammatory therapy but do respond to chlorambucil.[5] The comprehensive management of musculoskeletal manifestations includes both immediate and

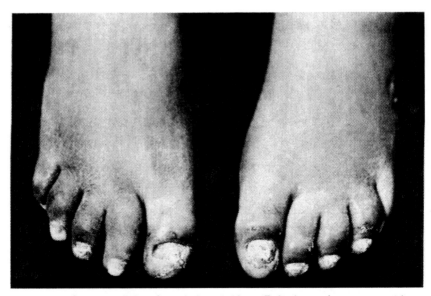

Figure 4—Sausage digits of psoriatic arthritis or Reiter's syndrome present in the second, third, and fourth toes bilaterally, result from acute synovitis of both distal and proximal interphalangeal joints.

long-term objectives. The immediate goal is to relieve joint discomfort with the use of nonsteroidal antiinflammatory drugs. Long-range plans are aimed at preventing, delaying, or correcting joint deformity. Thus, in patients with chronic or refractory arthritis, daily exercise and other physical modalities are vital to the maintenance of joint function.

Erythema Nodosum

Tender nodose lesions and associated arthropathy respond readily to nonsteroidal antiinflammatory drugs, usually prescribed for only a few weeks. If the skin lesions and arthropathy recur, another course of drug therapy can be administered with beneficial results. It is important to remember, however, that drugs are common causes of erythema nodosum.[62] These include salicylates and other nonsteroidal antiinflammatory drugs, as well as bromides, iodides, sulfonamides, antibiotics, vaccines or other biological preparations, and oral contraceptives.[63,72-74]

Behçet's Arthritis

A brief course of a nonsteroidal antiinflammatory drug will often control joint inflammation. Colchicine may also be beneficial. However, a double-blind controlled trial with colchicine disclosed that the drug improved arthralgia but not the arthritis of Behçet's syndrome.[75]

If the arthritis is monoarticular, a combination of joint aspiration and corticosteroid injection is an alternative to oral medication. Joint aspiration and steroid injection may also be beneficial if one or two joints are more seriously affected than others, especially when compromising ambulation and function. However, to minimize impairment of protective sensory mechanisms, no single joint should be injected more than three or four times in a given year. Moreover, the need for more frequent steroid injections should suggest reassessment of the basic drug therapy.

Of all the antirheumatic agents, corticosteroids appear to be most beneficial, especially in patients with polyarthritis. However, the response to steroids is inconsistent and variable.[23,30] Moreover, long-term use of steroids can be detrimental, predisposing the patient to steroid-induced compression fractures of the spine as well as to ischemic necrosis of the femoral head.[76] Thus, if prolonged corticosteroid therapy is unavoidable in Behçet's syndrome, every effort should be made to reduce the dosage to the lowest possible level.

Pseudotumor cerebri (benign intracranial hypertension), which causes headache, nausea, vomiting, and papilledema, can occur in untreated Behçet's disease secondary to intracranial venous sinus occlusion, but it is also an uncommon complication of corticosteroid therapy being caused either by an abrupt decrease in maintenance dosage or by a change from one corticosteroid compound to another. To correct this adverse effect, which may otherwise prove fatal, one must reinstitute the previous maintenance dosage or resume therapy with the original corticosteroid preparation.

Regardless of which medication is used, the physician must constantly monitor the patient for potential adverse reactions, particularly those that are common to all nonsteroidal antiinflammatory drugs (Table 9).[9,76] The combined use of two nonsteroidal drugs should be avoided because of enhanced toxicity. Gastric upset, the most common adverse reaction, can often be avoided if the drug is taken with meals or with milk or food at bedtime.

Table 9

Adverse Reactions Common to Nonsteroidal Antiinflammatory Drugs

- Gastrointestinal: upset, nausea, vomiting, dyspepsia, diarrhea, constipation, melena
- Major gastrointestinal bleeding, ulcer, or perforation
- Toxic hepatitis
- Mucocutaneous reactions. skin rash, pruritus, urticaria, alopecia, stomatitis
- Ocular toxicity: reversible blurring of vision
- Ototoxicity: reversible ringing in ears and difficulty with hearing
- CNS toxicity: headache, drowsiness, dizziness, confusion, lightheadedness, agitation, lethargy, malaise, depression
- Cardiopulmonary toxicity: palpitations, arrhythmias, pneumonitis, leg edema, and congestive heart failure from sodium and fluid retention
- Hematologic: alteration of platelet function, prolongation of bleeding time, aplastic anemia (rare)
- Nephrotoxicity, including the nephrotic syndrome

References

1. Behçet H. Über rezidivierende Aphthose, durch ein Virus verursachte Geschwüre am Mund, am Auge und an den Genitalien. *Derm Wschr* 1937; 105:1152–1157.
2. Behçet H, Gozcu N, Uc nahiyede nuksi tavazzular yapan ve hususi bir virus tesiriyle umumi intan hasil ettigine kanaatimiz artan (Entite morbide) hakkinda. *Deri Hastaliklari ve Frengi Arsivi* 1938; 5:1863–1873.
3. O'Duffy JD. Behçet's disease. In Kelly WN, Harris ED Jr, Ruddy S, Sledge CB, eds: *Textbook of Rheumatology.* Philadelphia, WB Saunders, 1985:1174–1178.
4. Shimizu T, Ehrlich GE, Inaba G, Hayashi K. Behçet disease (Behçet syndrome). *Semin Arthritis Rheum* 1979; 8:223–260.
5. Schiffman L, Giansiracusa D, Calabro JJ, et al. Behçet's syndrome. *Compr Ther* 1986; 12:62–66.
6. Chamberlain MA. Behçet's syndrome in 32 patients in Yorkshire. *Ann Rheum Dis* 1977; 36:491–499.
7. Decker JR. American Rheumatism Association nomenclature and classification of arthritis and rheumatism (1983). *Arthritis Rheum* 1983; 26:1029–1032.
8. Wright V. Seronegative polyarthritis: A united concept. *Arthritis Rheum* 1978; 21:619–633.
9. Calabro JJ. The seronegative spondyloarthropathies. A graduated approach to management. *Postgrad Med* 1986, Aug; 80:173–180, 185–188.
10. Wright V, Neumann V, Shinebaum R, Cooke EM. Pathogenesis of seronegative arthritis. *Br J Rheumatol* 1983; 22(suppl 2):29–32.
11. Calabro JJ. The spondylarthropathies: An overview. *Scand J Rheumatol* (Suppl) 1980; 9(suppl 32):21–24.
12. Wright V. Family studies implicating genetic factors in rheumatic diseases. *Ann Rheum Dis* 1975; 34(suppl 1):24–26.
13. Wright V. A unifying concept for the spondyloarthropathies. *Clin Orthop* 1979; 143:8–14.
14. Moll JMH. Pathogenetic mechanisms in B27 associated diseases. *Br J Rheumatol* 1983; 22(suppl 2):93–103.
15. Ball J. The enthesopathy of ankylosing spondylitis. *Br J Rheumatol* 1983; 22(suppl 2):25–28.
16. Calabro JJ. Clinical aspects of juvenile and adult ankylosing spondylitis. *Br J Rheumatol* 1983; 22(suppl 2):104–109.
17. Chamberlain MA. Epidemiologic features of Behçet's Syndrome. In Lehner T, Barnes CG, eds: *Behçet's Syndrome. Clinical and Immunologic Features. Proceedings of a Conference Sponsored by the Royal Society of Medicine, February 1979.* London, Academic Press, 1979:213–221.
18. Woodrow JC. Genetic aspects of the spondyloarthropathies. *Clin Rheum Dis* 1985; 11:1–24.

19. Yazici H, Tazlaci M, Yurdakul S. A controlled survey of sacroiliitis in Behçet's disease. *Ann Rheum Dis* 1981; 40:558–559.
20. Dilşen N, Koniçe M,. Aral O. Why Behçet's disease (BD) should be accepted as a seronegative arthritis (abstract 69)? Royal Society of Medicine international conference on Behçet's disease, September 5 and 6, 1985, London, England.
21. Ehrlich GE. Intermittent and periodic arthritic syndromes. In McCarty DJ, ed: *Arthritis and Allied Conditions. A Textbook of Rheumatology.* Philadelphia, Lea and Febiger, 1985:883–900.
22. Barnes CG. Behçet's syndrome—Joint manifestations and synovial pathology. In Lehner T, Barnes CG, eds: *Behçet's Syndrome. Clinical and Immunologic Features. Proceedings of a Conference Sponsored by the Royal Society of Medicine, February 1979.* London, Academic Press. 1979:199–212.
23. Mason RM, Barnes CG. Behçet's syndrome with arthritis. *Ann Rheum Dis* 1969; 28:95–103.
24. Gow P, Lehner T, Panayi GS. Joint manifestations in Behçet's syndrome and in recurrent oral ulcers. In Lehner T, Barnes CG, eds: *Behçet's Syndrome. Clinical and Immunologic Features. Proceedings of a Conference Sponsored by the Royal Society of Medicine, February 1979.* London, Academic Press, 1979:223–239.
25. Oshima Y, Shimizu T, Yokohari R, et al. Clinical studies on Behçet's syndrome. *Ann Rheum Dis* 1963; 22:36–45.
26. Dilşen N, Koniçe M, Övül C. Rheumatic patterns in Behçet's disease. In Dilşen N, Koniçe M. Övül C, eds: *Behçet's Disease. Proceedings of an International Symposium on Behçet's Disease, Istanbul, 29–30 September 1977.* Amsterdam-Oxford, Excerpta Medica, 1979:145–155.
27. Yurdakul S, Yazici H, Tüzün Y, et al. The arthritis of Behçet's disease: A prospective study. *Ann Rheum Dis* 1983; 42:505–515.
28. Chazek T, Fainaru M. Behçet's disease. Report of 41 cases and a review of the literature. *Medicine* 1975; 54:179–196.
29. Haim S. Contribution of ocular symptoms in the diagnosis of Behçet's disease. Study of 23 cases. *Arch Dermatol* 1968; 98:478–480.
30. Zizic TM, Stevens MB. The arthopathy of Behçet's disease. *Johns Hopkins Med J* 1975; 136:243–250.
31. Dawes PT, Raman D, Haslock I. Acute synovial rupture in Behçet's syndrome. *Ann Rheum Dis* 1983; 42:591–592.
32. Hanly JG, Molony J, Bresnihan B. Acute synovial rupture in Behçet's syndrome. *Ir J Med Sci* 1984; 153:286–287.
33. Hench PK, Reid RT, Reames PM. Dissecting popliteal cyst simulating thrombophlebitis. *Ann Intern Med* 1966; 64:1259–1264.
34. Dixon A St J, Grant C. Acute synovial rupture in rheumatoid arthritis. ·Clinical and experimental observations. *Lancet* 1964; 1:742–745.
35. Tait GBW, Bach F, Dixon A St J. Acute synovial rupture. Further observations. *Ann Rheum Dis* 1965; 24:273–277.
36. Simpson FG, Robinson PJ, Bark M, Losowsky MS. Prospective study of thrombophlebitis and "pseudothrombophlebitis." *Lancet* 1980; 1:331–333.

37. O'Duffy JD, Carney JA, Deodhar S. Behçet's disease. Report of 10 cases, 3 with new manifestations. *Ann Intern Med* 1971; 75:561–570.
38. France R, Buchanan RN, Wilson MW, Sheldon MB Jr. Relapsing iritis with recurrent ulcers of the mouth and genitalia (Behçet's syndrome). Review: With report of additional case. *Medicine* 1951; 30:335–355.
39. Hamza M'H, Ayed K, el Euch M, et al. Synovial fluid complement levels in Behçet's disease (letter). *Ann Rheum Dis* 1984; 43:767.
40. Gibson T, Laurent R, Highton J, et al. Synovial histopathology of Behçet's syndrome. *Ann Rheum Dis* 1981; 40:376–381.
41. Vernon-Roberts B, Barnes CG, Revell PA. Synovial pathology in Behçet's syndrome. *Ann Rheum Dis* 1978; 37:139–145.
42. Adinolfi M, Beck SE, Lehner T. Serum levels of acute phase proteins, C9, factor B and lysozyme in Behçet's syndrome and recurrent oral ulcers. In Lehner T, Barnes CG, eds: *Behçet's Syndrome. Clinical and Immunologic Features. Proceedings of a Conference Sponsored by the Royal Society of Medicine, February 1979.* London, Academic Press, 1979:107–125.
43. Takeuchi A, Mori M, Hashimoto A. Radiographic abnormalities in patients with Behçet's disease. *Clin Exp Rheumatol* 1984; 2:259–262.
44. Koss JC, Dalinka MK. Atlantoaxial subluxation in Behçet's syndrome. *AJR* 1980; 134:392–393.
45. Frayha R. Muscle involvement in Behçet's disease (letter). *Arthritis Rheum* 1981; 24:636–637.
46. Yazici M, Tüzüner N, Tüzün Y, Yurdakul S. Localized myositis in Behçet's disease (letter). *Arthritis Rheum* 1981; 24:636.
47. Di Giacomo V, Carmenini G, Meloni F, Valesini G. Myositis in Behçet's disease (letter). *Arthritis Rheum* 1982; 25:1025.
48. Arkin CR, Rothchild BN, Florendo NT, Popoff N. Behçet's syndrome with myositis. A case report with pathologic findings. *Arthritis Rheum* 1980; 23:600–604.
49. Finucane P, Doyle CT, Ferriss JB, et al. Behçet's syndrome with myositis and glomerulonephritis. *Br J Rheumatol* 1985; 24:372–375.
50. Lobo-Antunes J. Behçet's disease (letter). *Ann Intern Med* 1972; 76:332–333.
51. Afifi AK, Frayha RA, Bahuth NB, Tekian A. The myopathology of Behçet's disease. A histochemical, light-, and electron-microscopic study. *J Neurol Sci* 1980; 48:333–342.
52. Frayha RA, Afifi AK, Bergman RA, et al. Neurogenic muscular atrophy in Behçet's disease. *Clin Rheumatol* 1985; 4:202–211,
53. Yunus MB, Masi AT, Calabro JJ, et al. Primary fibromyalgia (fibrositis): Clinical study of 50 patients with matched normal controls. *Semin Arthritis Rheum* 1981; 11:151–171.
54. Smythe HA, Moldofsky H. Two contributions to understanding of the "fibrositis" syndrome. *Bull Rheum Dis* 1977; 28:928–931.
55. Wolfe F, Cathey MA. Prevalence of primary and secondary fibrositis. *J Rheumatol* 1983; 10:965–968.
56. Smythe H. Tender points: Evolution of concepts of the fibrositis/fibromyalgia syndrome. *Am J Med* 1986; 81(suppl 3A):2–6.

57. Wolfe F. The clinical syndrome of fibrositis. *Am J Med* 1986; 81(suppl 3A):7–14.
58. Bennett RM. Current issues concerning management of the fibrositis/fibromyalgia syndrome. *Am J Med* 1986; 81(suppl 3A):15–18.
59. Gatter RA. Pharmacotherapeutics in fibrositis. *Am J Med* 1986; 81(suppl 3A):63–66.
60. Behçet H. Some observations on the clinical picture of the so-called triple symptom complex. *Dermatologica* 1940; 81:73–83.
61. Frayha RA, Nasr FW. Erythema nodosum-arthropathy complex as an initial presentation of Behçet's disease. Report of five cases. *J Rheumatol* 1978; 5:224–228.
62. Calabro JJ, Wolf GL. Erythema nodosum. In Taylor RB, ed: *Difficult Diagnosis*. Philadelphia, WB Saunders, 1985:151–156.
63. Blomgren SE. Erythema nodosum. *Semin Arthritis Rheum* 1970; 4:1–24.
64. O'Duffy JD. Summary of international symposium on Behçet's disease, Istanbul, September 29–30, 1977. *J Rheumatol* 1978; 5:229–233.
65. Calabro JJ, Londino AV Jr, Wolf GL, et al. Behçet's disease (letter). *Clin Rheumatol Prac* 1984; 2:235.
66. Steere AC, Bartenhagen NH, Craft JE, et al. The early clinical manifestations of Lyme disease. *Ann Intern Med* 1983; 99:76–82.
67. Williamson PK, Calabro JJ. Lyme disease—A review of the literature. *Semin Arthritis Rheum* 1984; 13:229–234.
68. Shrestha M, Grodzicki RL, Steere AC. Diagnosing early Lyme disease. *Am J Med* 1985; 78:235–240.
69. Craft JE, Grodzicki RL, Steere AC. Antibody titers in Lyme disease: Evaluation of diagnostic tests. *J Infect Dis* 1984; 149:789–795.
70. Steere AC, Hutchinson GJ, Rahn DW, et al. Treatment of the early manifestations of Lyme disease. *Ann Intern Med* 1983; 99:22–26.
71. Firestein GS, Gruber HE, Weisman MH, et al. Mouth and genital ulcers with inflamed cartilage: MAGIC syndrome. Five patients with features of relapsing polychondritis and Behçet's disease. *Am J Med* 1985; 79:65–72.
72. Salvatore MA, Lynch PJ. Erythema nodosum, estrogens, and pregnancy. *Arch Dermatol* 1980; 116:557–558.
73. Merk H, Rusicka T. Oral contraceptives as a cause of erythema nodosum (letter). *Arch Dermatol* 1981; 117:454.
74. Darlington LG. Erythema nodosum and oral contraceptives. *Br J Dermatol* 1974; 90:209–212.
75. Aktulga E, Altaç M, Müftüoglu A, et al. A double blind study of colchicine in Behçet's disease. *Haematologica* (Pavia) 1980; 65:399–402.
76. Calabro JJ. Drug therapy of juvenile rheumatoid arthritis and the seronegative spondyloarthropathies. In Roth SH, ed: *Handbook of Drug Therapy in Rheumatology*. Littleton, MA, PSG/Wright Publishing, 1985:115–180.

11

MISCELLANEOUS CLINICAL MANIFESTATIONS, PART I: CARDIAC, VASCULAR, RENAL, and PULMONARY FEATURES

Gary R. Plotkin

TRADITIONALLY DESCRIBED AS A TRIAD consisting of recurrent aphthous stomatitis, genital ulcerations, and ocular inflammation, Behçet's disease is now recognized as a multisystem disorder whose clinical manifestations may be dominated by cardiac, vascular, pulmonary, renal, gastrointestinal, hepatic, rheumatologic, neuropsychiatric, and cutaneous complications.[1-18] Behçet's syndrome, which may be an intermittent disease characterized by symptom-free intervals, may not initially present with the classic triad of clinical findings.[7] The following four chapters focus on the diversity of those clinical features exclusive of the triple symptom complex.

Cardiac Manifestations

As mentioned in the previous chapter of this monograph, the Behçet's Disease Research Committee of Japan[19] established a set

From *Behcet's Disease: A Contemporary Synopsis*, edited by Gary R. Plotkin, M.D., John J. Calabro, M.D., and J. Desmond O'Duffy, M.B. © 1988, Futura Publishing Company, Inc., Mount Kisco, NY.

of criteria for the diagnosis of Behçet's disease. Included among these criteria, vascular lesions were considered a minor criterion[19]; however, these complications may indeed be associated with significant morbidity and mortality.[14,20-46] Cardiac involvement in Behçet's disease has been amply documented in the literature in the form of case reports, and it becomes evident that peripheral vascular involvement, especially venous, is much more common than cardiac or coronary artery disease in Behçet's syndrome. Most of the patients with Behçet's disease and cardiac manifestations have been less than 40 years of age, and these complications have been more frequent in men than in women. The cardiac complications may consist of coronary artery aneurysms, coronary artery occlusions, endocardial involvement, myocarditis, pericarditis, pericardial effusions with or without an associated mixed IgG and IgA cryoglobulinemia, congestive heart failure, arrhythmias including paroxysmal atrial fibrillation and ventricular ectopy, conduction system disturbances including heart block, myocardial infarction, endocardial and myocardial fibrosis, ruptured aneurysms of the sinus of Valsalva and right coronary artery, cardiomegaly, ventricular dilatation, congestive cardiomyopathy, ventricular aneurysms, intracardiac thrombi, and right ventricular mural thrombi with pulmonary emboli.[9,14,20-48] Valvular lesions may also occur in Behçet's disease and have included aortic and mitral insufficiency, tricuspid valve involvement, granulomatous endocarditis of the anterior mitral valve leaflet and chordae tendineae complicated by systemic emboli, endocarditis of the mitral and aortic valves, prolapse of the coronary cusp of the aortic valve associated with aortic incompetence, prolapse of the posterior mitral valve leaflet, and aortic insufficiency with sinus of Valsalva aneurysm.[24,27,33,34,39,40] In an accumulative autopsy series of 170 patients with Behçet's disease, 12 of 28 (43%) patients with cardiac involvement had cardiomegaly followed in order of decreasing frequency by endocarditis, pericardial effusion, myocardial fibrosis, aortic incompetence, mitral stenosis, tricuspid valve fibrosis, aortic sclerosis, and pancarditis.[9] It is not known if all of these autopsy findings were due to Behçet's disease or its treatment, or other unrelated conditions.

Since most patients with Behçet's disease and cardiac complications are below 40 years of age, coronary angiograms have often been normal[26,28,37]; nevertheless, several investigators have postulated coronary artery vasculitis as the initiating pathogenetic event.[22,28,29,43] Lakhanpal et al.[9] and Müftüoglu et al.[36] have reported respectively the occurrence of coronary arteritis and coronary artery occlusions in patients with Behçet's disease. Since coronary artery aneurysms and thrombotic coronary occlusions have been associated with other vasculitides including systemic lupus erythematosus and polyarteritis nodosa, Bowles et al.[22] have postulated that the coronary artery occlusions in patients with Behçet's syndrome may also be caused by an underlying vasculitis. Vasculitis may affect arteries of all sizes including the vasa vasorum.[14,29] However, accelerated atherosclerosis may occur in various syndromes characterized by vasculitis,[49] but coronary angiograms and pathological specimens obtained from patients with Behçet's disease have demonstrated a paucity of atherosclerotic changes involving the coronary vessels.[26,28,37] In light of the presence of pathergy or hyperreactivity in many patients with Behçet's disease, the trauma induced at the level of the arterial wall by arterial puncture, pressure of a cardiac catheter, or coronary artery bypass surgery itself may further propagate coronary artery pathology.[29,40] Additionally, abnormalities of coagulation and fibrinolysis, including the presence of platelet rosette formation around granulocytes,[50] enhanced platelet activity,[51] presence of anticardiolipin antibodies,[52] decreased levels of plasma prostacyclin (PGI$_2$)[53] and plasminogen activator activity,[54] defective release of tissue plasminogen activator,[55] increased plasma and tissue levels of prostaglandins E and F,[56] increased plasma viscosity and red cell rigidity,[57] endothelial cell dysfunction,[58] and neutrophil-induced oxidative damage of endothelial cells[59] which are characteristic of Behçet's disease may contribute to the pathogenesis of coronary artery thrombosis.[22,28] Therefore, a multitude of interrelated factors may influence the cardiovascular complications of Behçet's disease.

Wilkey et al.[46] reported a patient with Behçet's disease whose clinical course was complicated by myocarditis. Histologically, the myocardium showed extensive patchy and focal necrosis of both ventricles with the small intramural vessels revealing concentric intimal proliferation and fibrin thrombi.[46] In other postmortem examinations of patients with Behçet's disease and cardiac involvement, the heart demonstrated pathologically myocardial fiber degeneration; chronic inflammatory infiltrates in the endocardium; inflammatory cell infiltrates in the myocardium, endocardium, and within the interstitium around capillaries and small arterioles; and mononuclear infiltrates present within the myocardium, epicardium, and the intima of the aorta.[20,25,26,34,35]

Nojiri et al.[37] reported a patient with Behçet's disease with ruptured aneurysm of the sinus of Valsalva and conduction disturbance. The histology of the resected aortic wall demonstrated lamina elastica destruction, perivascular fibrosis, and cellular infiltrations in the tunica media. Histologically, the aneurysmal wall revealed fibrinoid degeneration with granuloma formation, and the aortic cusps showed fibrosis with inflammatory cell infiltrations. An associated conduction disturbance in this patient was presumably due to direct extension of the inflammatory process into the conduction tissues.[37]

Comess et al.[24] reported a patient with Behçet's disease and acute aortic regurgitation and sinus of Valsalva aneurysm. Histologically, the aortic valve showed extensive fibrosis, areas of vascularization and fibrin deposition, and foci of neutrophil, lymphocyte, and macrophage infiltration. The onset of the aortic insufficiency coincided with the other manifestations of acute disease activity, thus implicating an active vasculitis in the pathogenesis of the valvulitis and sinus of Valsalva aneurysm.[24] In two patients with Behçet's disease and prolapse of the posterior mitral valve leaflet, the diagnosis was established by echocardiographic tracings since there were no obvious physical findings.[33] The natural history of mitral valve prolapse in patients with Behçet's disease is not known, considering that arrhythmias, systemic emboli, and bacterial endocarditis are well-recognized complications of mitral valve prolapse in general.[33] Lu-Li et al.[33] also reported a patient with Behçet's disease and prolapse of the right coronary cusp of the aortic valve with associated aortic incompetence.

In the patient reported by Rae et al.[40] with aortic regurgitation and congestive heart failure, the resected aortic valve showed fibrotic changes without an inflammatory infiltrate; however, these pathological findings may have reflected the timing of the operative procedure. The postoperative course was complicated by the formation of a false aortic aneurysm of the ascending aorta which perhaps developed as a result of Behçet's disease itself. Histologically, the resected aneurysm showed fibrous tissue with focal calcification, proliferation of capillaries, and lymphatic infiltration.

These findings were similar to those reported in aneurysms in other patients with Behçet's syndrome.[40]

McDonald et al.[34] described two patients with Behçet's disease complicated by endocarditis of the mitral and aortic valves. Histologically, the valvular lesions showed a dense pleomorphic mononuclear inflammatory infiltrate. This inflammatory process extended along the cusps and into the elastica of the valve. These investigators postulated that endocarditis in Behçet's disease may represent valvulitis due to an underlying vasculitis.[34]

Huycek et al.[27] reported the occurrence of granulomatous endocarditis of the anterior mitral valve leaflet and chordae tendineae in a patient with Behçet's disease whose clinical course was complicated by systemic emboli. Histologically, the central portion of the vegetation contained granulomas, and its surface was lined by palisading histiocytes covered by polymorphonuclear leukocytes and an adherent superficial thrombus. Since the granulomatous nodules within the vegetation resembled rheumatoid nodules, these investigators postulated an underlying small-vessel vasculitis as the pathogenetic mechanism.[27]

Vascular Manifestations

Since the original description of Behçet's disease, the occurrence of both arterial and venous vascular disease in this syndrome has been reported by many authors.[9,14,29,31,34,40,46,60–90] Four types of vascular lesions are recognized in Behçet's disease; these consist of arterial and venous occlusions, aneurysms, and varices.[14,91] According to the Behçet's Disease Research Committee of Japan,[19] thrombophlebitis is listed as a major criterion while arterial occlusion and aneurysm are minor; however, like the cardiac ones, these complications may be associated with significant morbidity and mortality.[36,60,62,65–77,79–90]

Occlusive arterial lesions may involve vessels of various size including such arteries as the subclavian, pulmonary, common carotid, radial, femoral, tibial, brachial, ulnar, common iliac, external iliac, renal, popliteal, cerebral, aorta, coronary, arterioles, and vasa vasorum.[9,14,88] In one series of 31 patients with Behçet's disease and vascular complications, arterial occlusive disease more commonly affected the arteries of the upper and lower extremities.[88] Symptomatology is dependent upon the site of occlusion; for example, thrombosis of the subclavian artery may cause pulseless disease and syncope while occlusion of the renal artery may result in renovascular hypertension. Aseptic necrosis of the femoral head and hip pain have been associated with occlusion of the femoral artery, intermittent claudication may be due to thrombosis of the popliteal artery, and hemiplegia may result from involvement of the cerebral artery or its branches.[14] Takayasu's arteritis and thromboangiitis obliterans have been reported in four patients with Behçet's disease; however, the relationship between these two diseases and Behçet's disease is unknown.[9]

Aneurysmal dilatation has been reported in both small and large vessels including abdominal aorta; thoracic aorta; and femoral, common carotid, common iliac, external iliac, brachial, cerebral, subclavian, axillary, pulmonary, radial, ulnar, renal, splenic, superior mesenteric, and coronary arteries.[9,14,36,88] Aneurysms of the sinus of Valsalva and the left ventricle have also been reported in the literature.[21,36,37] Also, aneurysms may contain thrombi.[69,76]

Symptoms referable to aneurysms may mimic those due to vascular occlusive disease as described above[14]; however, aneurysms also have the propensity to rupture.[14,37,88] Gangrene of the feet and legs has been reported in patients with Behçet's disease due to aneurysms or occlusive arterial disease of both small and large vessels supplying the affected limbs.[68,81,84] In Behçet's disease there is a propensity for aneurysms to form following arterial puncture,[78] and trauma to arteries as produced by diagnostic angiography, cardiopulmonary bypass, or peripheral vascular surgery may also result in aneurysm formation.[29,76,78] Gruber et al.[71] reported a patient with Behçet's syndrome who developed acute paraparesis due to spinal cord ischemia secondary to thrombosis of the distal abdominal aorta which probably represented a complication of localized trauma induced at the time of sigmoidoscopy. Rae et al.[40] reported a patient with Behçet's disease and aortic regurgitation who developed a false aneurysm of the ascending aorta after aortic valve replacement.

Since ischemia due to thrombosed arteries and rupture of aneurysms in Behçet's disease are significant complications, surgical intervention to prevent these vascular catastrophies has been attempted by various individuals with variable results.[69,76,79,82,84, 88,92] Postoperatively, there has been a tendency for the bypass graft to dislodge, probably reflecting both the recurrent nature of Behçet's disease with aneurysm and thrombus formation and the failure to bypass inflammatory and endarteritic changes which may extend microscopically beyond the original aneurysm or occlusion.[69,76,83,86] Recurrent aneurysms and thrombi or formation of false aneurysms may occur at the sites of anastomoses following autogenous vein bypass procedures.[76,83,84] Jenkins et al.[76] have described two patients with Behçet's disease, one of whom underwent excision of an aneurysm of the common femoral artery with insertion of a prosthetic graft, while the second patient underwent an autogenous saphenous vein bypass graft for an aneurysm of the superficial femoral artery. In both patients recurrent aneurysms developed adjacent to the vascular anastomoses.[76] An autogenous vein bypass graft had been attempted in a patient with Behçet's disease and an aneurysm of the right femoral artery and an occlusion of the right popliteal artery; however, graft occlusion occurred during the postoperative period.[84] The postoperative clotting of a prosthetic axillary bifemoral bypass graft in a patient with Behçet's disease has also been reported.[79] Thus, these studies[69,76,79,82,84] have shown that vascular surgery in patients with Behçet's disease may be quite complicated and perhaps should be reserved for those patients with Behçet's disease who have potentially serious vascular compromise.[86] Nevertheless, Urayama et al.[88] reported four patients with Behçet's disease and aneurysms who improved with surgical intervention; however, the details of the surgical procedures were not described by the authors. Chavatzas[92] described a 29-year-old woman with Behçet's disease and a popliteal artery thrombosis who successfully underwent an autogenous saphenous vein bypass graft with postoperative restoration of the distal pulses. Aneurysms of the pulmonary artery will be discussed under the pulmonary complications of Behçet's disease in this chapter.

The histopathological findings of the arterial lesions in Behçet's disease have consisted of thickening of the intima and media, fragmentation and splitting of the elastic fibers of the media, perivascular lymphocytic cell infiltration of the vasa vasorum, thickening of the adventitia, and perivascular fibrosis.[14,93–95] Aneurysm formation results from rupture of the internal and external elastic laminae associated with thickening of the tunica intima and degeneration of the tunica media.[96] In one patient with Behçet's disease, a resected aneurysm of a popliteal artery histologically demonstrated a prominent and active inflammatory process with polymorphonuclear leukocytes, plasma cells, lymphocytes, and eosinophils. The arterial wall was completely destroyed and was replaced with fibrosis and granulation tissue. The adventitial blood vessels and vasa vasorum showed an obliterative endarteritis, and the lumen of the aneurysm also contained a thrombus.[69] The pathogenesis of the aneurysms in Behçet's disease thus probably reflects an obliterative endarteritis of the vasa vasorum resulting in either true aneurysm formation or arterial wall perforation with false aneurysm formation.[79] In addition, the occluded arteries in Behçet's disease, which are often friable with weakened walls, probably also result partly from an obliterative endarteritis of the vasa vasorum.[83] Defects in coagulation and fibrinolysis, as previously described in Chapter 6, which characterize Behçet's disease may contribute to thrombus formation.[14] Pathological examination of an excised thrombus from the abdominal aorta of a patient with Behçet's disease has revealed an acute inflammatory process with a predominance of polymorphonuclear leukocytes.[71] In a patient with Behçet's disease and an aneurysm of the ulnar artery reported by Oshima et al.,[38] the adjacent small arteries demonstrated pathologically obstruction of the lumen with fibrous tissue, swelling the lamina elastica interna, splitting of the elastic fibers of the media, and perivascular cell infiltration. Pathological examinations of resected arterial lesions in other patients with Behçet's disease have demonstrated false aneurysmal formation at the sites of previous bypass surgery, with destruction of the internal elastic membrane, lymphocytic infiltration in the arterial wall, and collagen deposition within the media, thus emphasizing underlying vasculitis as the predominant pathogenetic mechanism.[84]

Clausen et al.[63] described the pathological findings of the aorta of a 16-week-old fetus delivered from a patient with Behçet's disease. The fetal elastic artery demonstrated edema in the subendothelial space and the luminal side of the tunica media and sparse and disarranged smooth-muscle cells in the media. These changes were thought to be due to Behçet's disease itself and not secondary to the effects of corticosteroid treatment of the mother.[63]

In Behçet's syndrome, venous occlusions are more common than arterial thrombosis, may affect veins of all size, and may present as recurrent superficial or deep thrombophlebitis of the migratory type.[3,14,97] Depending upon the series, the frequency of thrombophlebitis in patients with Behçet's disease has ranged from 25 to 65%,[3,36,46,70,72,89] and according to the Behçet's Disease Research Committee of Japan,[19] thrombophlebitis of the cutaneous veins and obliterating thrombophlebitis are listed as major and minor criteria, respectively, in the diagnosis of Behçet's syndrome. Thus, thrombophlebitis is the most common vascular complication occurring in patients with Behçet's disease.[36] Thrombosis more commonly affects the superior and inferior venae cavae and those veins of the lower extremities; however, various thrombosed vieins have included the retinal, mesenteric, femoral, iliac, popliteal, saphenous, axillary, subclavian, brachiocephalic, portal, hepatic, splenic, and penile vessels,[3,14,36,77,88,89] and the brain-stem venous system.[98] Or et al.[48] have reported a 65-year-old man with Behçet's disease complicated by complete heart block and obstruction of the subclavian, innominate, and superior vena caval veins. Also, subcutaneous venules of the extremities may thrombose in Behçet's disease and on examination may be palpated as string-like hardening with reddening of the overlying skin.[14,19]

Clinically, peripheral superficial and deep vein thrombophlebitis may present as local signs of soft-tissue swelling, redness, and tenderness and may be accompanied by fever and prostration. Local sequelae may include postphlebitic edema of the extremities with prolonged leg ulcers (ulcus cruris).[3] Thrombophlebitis may follow minor trauma but spontaneous thrombosis may also occur in Behçet's disease.[69,99] Superficial thrombophlebitis also may result from venipunctures, intravenous injections of contrast material for phlebography, and intravenous infusions of heparin.[3,10,41,52,85,87] Thus, heparin therapy may not prevent recurrent thrombophlebitis or pulmonary emboli in Behçet's syndrome,[65,85] and clinical improvement of thrombophlebitis may be secondary to fibrosis and recanalization of the affected vessel or to formation and dilatation of collateral veins.[70,87]

Clinical syndromes of superior and/or inferior venae caval obstruction have been described in patients with Behçet's disease with the pathogenesis being either in-situ thrombus formation or propagation of a thrombus from a more distal vessel.[3,41,62,66,67,]

[72,77,85] Chajek and Fainaru[3] have mentioned that the occurrence of pulmonary emboli is rare in Behçet's syndrome. Nevertheless, pulmonary infarctions have been reported in patients with Behçet's disease; their pathogenesis, however, is not completely known. These infarctions may result from an intraatrial thrombus, right ventricular mural thrombus, emboli from the peripheral veins or venae cavae, in-situ thrombus formation within the pulmonary arteries, pulmonary arteritis or vasculitis, or rupture of pulmonary aneurysms.[10,25,65,74,77,85]

The Budd-Chiari syndrome due to occlusion of the hepatic veins has also occurred in patients with Behçet's syndrome.[9,14,34,36,46,75,100] In one patient with this complication, the liver on postmortem examination revealed centrilobular congestion and necrosis with reticulin collapse and infiltration of polymorphonuclear leukocytes. The hepatic veins and the intrahepatic venous structures were occluded by thrombi, and the wall of the hepatic vein contained lymphocytic infiltrations. Sections of the occluded veins revealed recanalized, organized thrombi consisting of collagenous tissue.[34] Similar hepatic pathology has been reported in another autopsied patient with Behçet's disease and the Budd-Chiari syndrome.[46]

With respect to the pathology of vascular structures in Behçet's disease, biopsy specimens have shown the underlying histologic process to consist of a vasculitis involving veins, venules, capillaries, and arterioles.[8,11,64,77,101-103] Sections of a scrotal ulcer from a patient with Behçet's disease revealed a venule with swelling of the endothelium, marked mural and periadventitial edema, and prominent infiltration of the wall with mononuclear cells.[70] The inflammatory process may affect postcapillary venules to a greater extent than arterioles.[64] Biopsy of a thrombosed vein from a patient with Behçet's disease has shown chronic inflammation of the wall with an organized adherent thrombus.[62]

The syndrome of benign intracranial hypertension or pseudotumor cerebri which is associated with an elevated cerebrospinal fluid pressure may complicate Behçet's disease and may present with headaches, vomiting, and papilledema.[60,61,73,90,104-106] This syndrome, which may be caused by thrombosis of the intracranial dural venous sinuses, had been in the past diagnosed by standard cerebral arteriography, but more recently has been detected by venous digital subtraction angiography.[61,73,90] The natural history of cerebral sinus thrombosis is unknown; however, the occluded sinuses may remain thrombosed with persistently increased intracranial pressure, recanalize, stimulate alternate drainage pathways, or develop into a dural arteriovenous malformation.[73,107] Imaizumi et al.[75] have reported a patient with Behçet's disease and both intracranial sigmoid sinus thrombosis and dural arteriovenous malformation.

The fourth and last type of vascular complication of Behçet's disease is the development of varices.[14] Chronic obliteration of the larger veins may result in enlargement and tortuosity of their collateral venous structures within the thoracic and abdominal walls, with resultant dilatation of the superficial veins of the chest wall and the formation of a caput medusae and hemothorax.[14,108,109] Esophageal varices have been described in Behçet's disease and have developed as a result of occlusion of the splenic and azygos veins, subclavian veins, superior and inferior venae cavae, and the cervical and internal mammary systems.[77,109] Additionally, rupture of the esophageal varices may complicate the Budd-Chiari syndrome.[95]

Renal Complications

Depending upon the series of patients with Behçet's syndrome, genitourinary involvement may be absent or detected in as many as one-third of patients upon random urinalyses.[3,38,110,111] Most commonly renal involvement is detected by the presence of microscopic hematuria and variable amounts of proteinura including amounts within the nephrotic syndrome range.[110-114] Associated leukocyturia and both red cell and white cell casts may also be present[46,101,112,115]; however, proteinuria and hematuria may not be pathognomonic of progressive deterioration of renal function in Behçet's syndrome.[110,111] In one study the renal biopsies of four patients with Behçet's disease were histopathologically normal, at least by light microscopy,[38] while other reported patients with normal urinalyses had abnormal renal biopsies.[112] The abnormal urinalyses in patients with Behçet's syndrome may be intermitent or persistent, and renal function may vary from normal or minimal impairment to renal failure requiring dialysis. Additionally, renal function may remain stable for years, deteriorate, or if impaired, improve with time.[30,110,111,113-115] Despite the presence of abnormal urinalyses or histopathology on renal biopsies in patients with Behçet's disease, intravenous pyelograms may be normal.[46,110-112,114]

In one large series of patients with Behçet's disease, symptoms referable to the genitourinary system were absent during periods in which the urinalyses were abnormal. Those patients with demonstrable renal disease were comparable to their counterparts without renal involvement with respect to the incidence, duration, and severity of the other nonrenal manifestations of Behçet's disease. Thus, there were no apparent precipitating factors to explain why certain patients with Behçet's disease developed renal abnormalities.[111]

Pathogenetically, renal involvement in Behçet's disease may consist of renal artery occlusion, renal artery aneurysm, renal artery stenosis and poststenotic aneurysmal dilation, renal vein thrombosis, glomerulonephritis, and amyloidosis.[3,9,14,30,38,46,83,86,101,110-129] Herreman et al.[112] have performed renal biopsies in 11 patients with Behçet's disease, 5 of whom had abnormal urinalyses consisting of proteinuria with or without associated leukocyturia. None of the 11 patients had symptoms referable to the genitourinary tract. In one patient glomerular lesions were focally and segmentally distributed and consisted of proliferation of mesangial cells with fibrinoid necrosis, crescent formation, an occasional capsular adhesion, and fibrinoid deposition on the epithelial side of the basement membrane.[112]

Interstitial and tubular lesions were present in two patients, and in one, areas of fibrosis, edema and round-cell infiltration with vacuolated tubular epithelial cells were present. All renal biopsies in this study contained arteriolar and interlobular arterial lesions with subendothelial or medial hyaline arteriolar deposits. The larger renal arteries showed variable intimal thickening and reduplication of the internal elastic lamina. There were no thromboses, vascular infiltrates, or fibrinoid necrosis within the renal biopsies. In essence three predominant forms of renal involvement were reported and consisted of focal glomerulonephritis with cellular epithelial crescent and fibrin, mesangial and extramembranous glomerular deposits of C3 complement and IgG and/or IgA immunoglobulin with a granular pattern of fluorescent staining, and subendothelial or medial hyaline deposits in the arterioles. Because of the presence of circulating immune complexes and the deposition of complement and immunoglobulins in the glomeruli, the pathogenesis of renal involvement in Behçet's disease was postulated to be immunologically mediated.[112]

Gamble et al.[101] extensively studied a patient with Behçet's disease with renal and pulmonary involvement. During the course of this patient's disease, the urinalysis showed proteinuria as high as 4.9 g/24 hr, microscopic hematuria, and the presence of red cell casts. Serum creatinine rose to 4.1 mg/dL before decreasing and stabilizing at 1.5 mg/dL with an associated creatinine clearance of 46 ml/min. Urinary sediment became benign and the proteinuria decreased to 38 mg/24 hr. The improvement in these parameters followed the initiation of corticosteroid therapy, beginning with 200 mg per day of intravenous methylprednisolone followed by tapering dosages of oral prednisone. This patient was of interest in that her chest roentgenogram abnormalities progressed as her renal function deteriorated. Chest roentgenograms showed a nodular noncalcified density in the anterior portion of the right lung followed by the development of interstitial infiltrates in the left lung and the superior segment of the right lower lobe. Histopathological and immunopathological studies of biopsies of the renal parenchyma demonstrated a focal segmental necrotizing glomerulonephritis with variable crescent formation characterized by the presence of many subendothelial and few intramembranous deposits containing IgG immunoglobulin, third and fourth components of complement, and fibrin(ogen); and therefore the finding of granular staining for IgG, C3, and C4 in the affected glomeruli strongly suggested that the glomerular lesions were due to circulating immune complex deposition with activation of the classic complement pathway. Similar immunological studies of biopsed right lung tissue showed an active venulitis and septal capillaritis, which on immunofluorescent microscopy, revealed granular staining of the walls of several small veins for C3, C4, and IgG. Immune complexes were also detected in the patient's serum.[101] Another patient with Behçet's disease and biopsy-proven acute focal necrotizing glomerulonephritis with early crescent formation had a creatinine clearance of 7 ml/min. Because of renal insufficiency, peritoneal dialysis was required temporarily; however, renal function improved after the initiation of corticosteroid therapy. In this case, the renal biopsy showed proliferative changes involving the glomeruli, focal fibrinoid necrosis, crescent formation, and interstitial inflammatory changes. Only by immunofluorescent staining was fibrinogen detected in the glomeruli, and no deposits of immune complexes were seen on electron microscopy. Despite the presence of glomerulonephritis, the urinalysis did not contain any red cell casts.[30] A similar patient with Behçet's disease and focal necrotizing glomerulonephritis has been reported by Mace and Jones.[122]

Wilkey et al.[46] reported a patient with Behçet's disease complicated by Budd-Chiari syndrome due to thrombotic occlusion of the hepatic veins and renal failure. On autopsy the kidneys showed a focal proliferative glomerulonephritis with occasional epithelial crescents. Some glomeruli revealed a mild increase in the endothelial and mesangial cellularity; however, many were also sclerosed. On electron microscopy electron-dense deposits were present subepithelially, and immunofluorescent studies of the glomeruli demonstrated 2+ linear and granular deposits of IgG within the capillary loops. According to the authors, the renal pathology was also compatible with end-stage focal necrotizing glomerulopathy.[46]

Williams and Lehner[114] reported one patient with Behçet's disease in whom a kidney biopsy consisting of 27 glomeruli showed a mild focal proliferative glomerulonephritis with segmental sclerosis and hyalinosis in one glomerulus. Immunofluorescent microscopy revealed diffuse granular mesangial deposits of IgA, IgG, and C3, while electron microscopy demonstrated electron-dense mesangial deposits. Since these microscopic findings have also been found in IgA mesangial nephropathy or Berger's disease, this patient's renal disease may not have been due to Behçet's disease.[114]

Beaufils et al.[116,117] performed renal biopsies in 11 patients with Behçet's syndrome. Five patients had proteinuria ranging from less than 500 mg/24 hr to 2 g/24 hr. At the time of renal biopsy microscopic hematuria was not detected in any of the 11 patients, and their creatinine clearances were normal. The renal biopsy specimen from one patient demonstrated on light microscopy focal and segmental glomerulonephritis with fibrinoid deposits. The segmental lesions were characterized by a proliferation of mesangial and epithelial cells, and some contained subepithelial deposits, capsular adhesions, and crescents. Immunofluorescent microscopy of biopsies from 10 patients revealed granular deposits of C3 in the mesangium and along the glomerular capillary basement membrane, and focal deposits containing IgA and/or IgG, and Clq were also present in the renal tissue obtained from four patients. Circulating immune complexes were detected in some patients. Electron microscopy demonstrated nonargyrophilic deposits scattered in the mesangial matrix associated with subepithelial hump-like glomerular deposits. These immunological data supported the role of immune complex deposition in the pathogenesis of certain types of renal disease in Behçet's syndrome.[116,117]

Olsson et al.[115] described a patient with Behçet's disease and diffuse proliferative glomerulonephritis with crescent formation. Histologic examination of the renal biopsy demonstrated focal and segmental mesangial sclerosis, tubular atrophy, and interstitial fibrosis, while immunofluorescent microscopy showed diffuse granular deposits of IgM and C3 and lesser amounts of granular deposits of IgG and fibrinogen in the capillary walls, and trace amounts of IgA, IgG, C3, and fibrinogen in the mesangium.[115] A patient with Behçet's disease complicated by myositis and diffuse proliferative glomerulonephritis with crescent formation has also been reported by Finucane et al.[130]

In a patient reported by Landwehr et al.[113] with Behçet's disease and rapidly progressive glomerulonephritis, renal pathology showed marked extracapillary proliferation with crescent formation, tubular loss associated with interstitial infiltration of lymphocytes and plasma cells, and granular deposition of mainly IgG with small amounts of IgA, IgM, and C3, in the capillary walls. Fibrinogen was present in a linear capillary pattern, and on electron microscopy a subepithelial deposit was present. A 24-hour urine collection revealed a proteinuria in the nephrotic syndrome range of 3.6 grams, and the evaluation for other causes of rapidly progressive glomerulonephritis was negative.[113] Thus, the spectrum of renal disease in patients with Behçet's disease varies from the asymptomatic patient with normal and stable renal function associated with a normal or abnormal urinalysis to the patient requiring maintenance dialysis because of the rapid deterioration of renal function.[110,111,113]

Mirua et al.[123] described a 35-year-old woman with Behçet's disease complicated by the nephrotic syndrome whose renal biopsy specimens revealed features of membranous glomerulonephritis. On histologic examination, light microscopy revealed diffuse thickening of the capillary walls with "spike" formation of the arygyrophilic glomerular basement membrane. Immunofluorescent studies demonstrated diffuse granular deposits of IgG, IgM, and C3 in the glomerular capillary walls, and electron microscopy revealed electron-dense deposits in the glomerular basement membrane.[123] Interstitial nephritis has additionally been reported in patients with Behçet's disease[131,132]; however, because of the rare occurrence of membranous glomerulopathy and interstitial nephritis in Behçet's disease, these disorders may represent independent processes.

Dilşen et al.[120,121] have reported three patients with Behçet's disease and biopsy-proven renal amyloidosis, all of whom had proteinuria ranging from 1 to 15 g/L. One patient with the nephrotic syndrome and renal insufficiency had a serum creatinine of 4.8 mg/dL. Electron microscopic examinations from two patients showed the deposition of amyloid fibrils in the glomerular basal lamina. According to this group of investigators, renal amyloidosis may be an intrinsic manifestation of Behçet's disease and may not be secondary to another disease entity. Since most patients with Behçet's disease and amyloidosis have resided in the Mediterranean countries where secondary amyloidosis is more commonly encountered, especially in patients with familial Mediterranean fever, genetic and environmental factors may be important in the pathogenesis of renal amyloidosis in Behçet's disease.[120,121] Based upon two autopsied patients with Behçet's disease, renal amyloidosis may occur in the absence of other associated disorders.[128]

Beroniade[118] reported three patients with Behçet's disease and renal amyloidosis, all of whom had massive proteinuria in the nephrotic syndrome range of 4–12 g/24 hr, and therefore it would appear that of the various renal lesions in Behçet's disease, amyloidosis probably accounts for the greatest quantity of proteinuria. Renal amyloidosis in Behçet's disease may result in uremia and death. Pathological findings of kidney tissue in two patients demonstrated amyloid deposition within the glomeruli, small arteries, and arterioles. Obliterating thrombi were also seen in the main renal veins plus the smaller intrarenal vessels. Thus renal vein thrombosis may contribute to the pathogenesis of the nephrotic syndrome in patients with Behçet's disease and renal amyloidosis[118]; however, not all patients with Behçet's disease and renal vein thrombosis will have detectable proteinuria.[126] Renal amyloidosis may also occur in association with generalized amyloidosis in Behçet's disease.[118,124] Necropsy of a patient with Behçet's syndrome complicated by the nephrotic syndrome revealed amyloid deposition within the spleen, kidneys, and adrenal glands and thromboses of the renal veins. Microscopically, the amyloid was demonstrated in the renal glomeruli and in the walls of the small arteries and arterioles within the myocardium, lungs, intestine, kidneys, and spleen.[124]

Penza et al.[133] have reported a 13-year-old Italian girl with Behçet's disease complicated by proteinuria of 350 mg/m²/hr and a chronic suppurative cutaneous condition. Renal biopsy revealed mesangial hypercellularity, several sclerosed glomeruli, nodular deposits of amyloid along the glomerular capillary loops and the small arterioles, and interstitial fibrosis with lymphocytic infiltration of the atrophic tubules. Peces et al.[127] have described a patient of Spanish descent with Behçet's disease and biopsy-proven renal amyloidosis who developed the nephrotic syndrome with chronic renal failure requiring maintenance hemodialysis. Histologically, the amyloid was of the AA protein type, and this was the second reported case of Behçet's disease with renal amyloidosis of this type.[129] In the review of the literature by Peces et al.,[127] renal amyloidosis was noted to occur 2 to 11 years after the diagnosis of Behçet's disease, with most of the patients residing in the Mediterranean countries. In essence, proteinuria of the nephrotic syndrome range has been associated in the vast majority of Behçet's disease patients with renal amyloidosis.[127,128]

In a collective autopsy review of patients with Behçet's syndrome, the pathological renal lesions consisted of pyelonephritis, nephrosclerosis, nephritis, urolithiasis, renal infarcts, and renal congestion.[9] However, these pathological findings may have been independent of Behçet's disease and have represented separate disease processes. In summary, the pathology of intrinsic renal disease in Behçet's disease has consisted of amyloidosis, diffuse proliferative glomerulonephritis with crescent formation, rapidly progressive (crescentic) glomerulonephritis, and focal necrotizing glomerulonephritis with variable crescents.[30,46,101,112,113,115–118, 120–122,127] The pathogenesis of the glomerulonephritides may represent a vasculitis, perhaps immune complex–mediated.[46,101,112,125]

Other renal complications reported in Behçet's disease have consisted of renal artery occlusion and aneurysm, stenosis and poststenotic aneurysmal dilatation of the renal artery, the renal vein thrombosis. These arterial abnormalities may be complicated by renovascular hypertension, while renal vein thrombosis may occur in association with the nephrotic syndrome and renal amyloidosis.[14,86,111,118,126] The reasons for the development of renal disease in certain patients with Behçet's syndrome is not known, and the optimal preventive and therapeutic regimens remain enigmas. Obviously, in order to better understand renal disease in patients with Behçet's syndrome, one must prospectively study a large number of affected individuals over a prolonged period of time.[114]

Pulmonary Involvement

The entire respiratory tract may be affected in Behçet's disease, from the nasal, palatal, pharyngeal, and laryngeal mucosae to the lungs.[3,9,14,20,25,38,46,102,134–153] Patients with upper respiratory tract involvement may present with rhinorrhea, recurrent sore throats, tonsillitis, hoarseness, dysphonia, odynophagia, dysphagia, and dyspnea.[46,102,136,152,154] Laryngoscopic examination has revealed ulcers of the pharynx, larynx, tonsils, palate, and epiglottis; fistulous tracts involving the oral and nasal pharynx, larynx, and esophagus; and strictures of the nasopharynx, uvula area, and mucous membranes of the mouth.[141,143,144,148,152,153] The oral ulcers may appear either as discrete aphthous ulcerations or as coalescent lesions with a gray-yellow eschar extending along the posterior pharyngeal wall and tonsillar fossae to the epiglottis.[148] As sequelae of the recurrent episodes of the oral ulcerations, there may be cicatricial contraction of the mouth with decreased range of motion, fusion of the base of the tongue with the soft palate, and pharyngeal stenosis at the junction of the oropharynx and hypopharynx.[136,141,149] Consequently, dysphagia, odynophagia, and dyspnea may ensue, and flow volume loop function tests may detect Behçet's disease patients with extrathoracic obstructive upper airway disease resulting from these anatomical complications.[136] Physical examination has occasionally revealed clubbing of the upper extremities in patients with Behçet's disease and obstructive upper airway disease, and surgical intervention may be necessary to improve this obstructive anatomy.[136,144]

Kobayashi et al.[114] reported two patients with Behçet's disease and ulcerative lesions of the hypopharynx, one of whom developed severe stenosis of the hypopharyngeal mucosa with resultant dyspnea. The epiglottis was also markedly deformed, and frontal tomography of the larynx revealed obliteration of the pyriform sinuses.[144] Another patient with Behçet's disease and oral ulcers who underwent otolaryngoscopy examination under anesthesia was observed to have a leukoplakia-like lesion of the piriform fossa.[145] Ulcerated lesions may also involve the arytenoid and aryepiglottic folds.[153] Difficulties in endotracheal intubation have been reported because of fusion of the base of the tongue with the palate and extensive scarring and adhesion formation in the pharynx. These structural abnormalities have occasionally necessitated tracheostomy.[149,151] Humaidan et al.[154] reported a patient with Behçet's disease who had repeated ulcerations of the hypopharynx with resultant scar formation and supraglottic constriction necessitating tracheostomy. Kenet[155] reported a patient with Behçet's disease and severe recurrent laryngeal ulcers who required repeated temporary tracheostomies for relief of respiratory embarrassment.

Pulmonary involvement in Behçet's disease has been amply described in the literature,[3,14,20,38,74,101,134,135,137-140,142,146,149,150] and its prevalence has been estimated to range from below 5% to 35%.[139,140] However, according to Efthimiou et al.,[140] pulmonary disease which is usually associated with active disease at other sites may be the presenting and most important clinical manifestation of Behçet's disease. The most common clinical symptom referable to the respiratory tract is hemoptysis, which is often massive in character, may be associated with significant morbidity and mortality, and often is accompanied by clinical exacerbations of extrapulmonary disease activity including peripheral deep and superficial thrombophlebitis and ocular, oral, genital, cutaneous, and rheumatologic manifestations.[137,140] As many as one-third of patients with Behçet's disease and pulmonary complications may have accompanying inferior and/or superior venae caval thrombosis.[137,140] Other signs and symptoms include fever, cough, dyspnea, thoracic pain which may be pleuritic, clubbing, bronchial aphthae, superior vena caval syndrome, and right heart failure due to cor pulmonale.[25,140,142]

In one series[139] of Behçet's disease, patients with and without pulmonary manifestations were comparable with respect to age and duration of disease. Patients with pulmonary involvement tended to be male, and a higher percentage of these patients had cutaneous lesions, thrombophlebitis of small and large veins, and amyloidosis; a lower percentage had ocular and articular manifestations. In contradistinction to other studies, many patients with pulmonary involvement were asymptomatic or had minimal hemoptysis, and the course of the pulmonary manifestations which persisted for a few weeks to a few months was benign.[139] Petty et al.[146] described a patient with Behçet's disease who experienced recurrent pulmonary infiltrates during a 13-year period unassociated with severe hemoptysis and respiratory failure. The pulmonary function tests did not reveal any evidence of obstructive or restrictive lung disease, thus reemphasizing the potentially benign course of lung involvement in Behçet's syndrome.[146]

The pathogenesis of hemoptysis in Behçet's disease may be multifactorial, including superimposed infections, pulmonary infarctions, vasculitis, rupture of aneurysms, pulmonary and bronchial arterial occlusions, erosion of a newly formed vessel located within an arterial thrombus, erosion of a pulmonary aneurysm into an adjacent bronchus, spread of inflammation from a destroyed artery into the wall of an adjacent bronchus, inflammatory disruption of alveolar capillaries, and rupture of bronchial veins.[25,77,134-153] Pulmonary arteritis may precede aneurysm formation with hemoptysis resulting from rupture either of the aneurysm wall or anastomotic vessels in the bronchial wall.[25] Since obstruction of the superior vena cava may be commonly encountered in patients with Behçet's disease and pulmonary complications, hemoptysis may result from rupture of the bronchial veins.[77,137] In Behçet's disease, prominent intercostal and bronchial venous channels under increased pressure may result from blockage in the azygos vein which can be secondary to obstruction in the superior vena cava.[77]

An association between Behçet's disease and obstructive lung disease, including emphysema, has been raised in the literature.[9,101,134,139,156-358] Ahonen et al.[156] reported two patients, aged 30 and 41 years, with Behçet's disease who developed objective evidence of irreversible obstructive airway disease based upon pulmonary function tests with bronchodilating medications. The patient reported by Gibson et al.[158] with Behçet's disease had severe and irreversible airway obstruction. However, Evans and Jenkins[157] questioned the association of airway obstruction and Behçet's syndrome. They described one 44-year-old patient with Behçet's disease and reversible airway obstruction whose sputum showed eosinophils and laminar plug formation. This patient, who smoked cigarettes heavily for 28 years, had a past history of extensive pulmonary tuberculosis and the chest roentgenograms showed right upper lobe fibrosis and calcification with decreased vascular markings at the lung bases. They postulated that the pulmonary disease may have been associated with asthma, the smoking habits, and/or previous pulmonary tuberculosis.[157] A restrictive ventilatory defect has also been reported in Behçet's disease.[140]

In the series reported by Dilşen et al.,[139] the chest radiographic findings in patients with Behçet's disease consisted of pleural effusions or adhesions, hilar enlargement, apical cavitary lesions, apical or subapical fibrous or fibrocalcific changes, apical opacification, and bilateral fibroproductive infiltrates. The hilar enlargement may represent aneurysms of the pulmonary arterial vessels.[140,142] Most of the roentgenographic abnormalities were unilateral, nonprogressive, small to medium in size, and transient.[139]

In another series of Behçet's syndrome and pulmonary disease reported by Akkaynak et al.,[134] the main roentgenographic findings were single or bilateral recurrent lung infiltrates, evanescent round lesions, basal linear atelectasis, hilar enlargement, pleural effusions, and diaphragmatic elevation. Roentgenographically, one may also observe transient alveolar infiltrates, lobar consolidations, diffuse interstitial process, pulmonary fibrosis, mediastinal lymphaenopathy, subpleural opacities, peripheral or central rounded or nodular densities, cavitation of the rounded opacities, and hydropneumothorax secondary to rupture of a subpleural nodule.[84,137,139,140,142,147] The opacities may correspond to hemorrhage, tissue necrosis, infarction, or aneurysms.[20,142] However, since these various roentgenographic findings are not pathognomonic of Behçet's disease, one should always consider other superimposed disease processes that may account for these abnormalities. The pleural effusions may be bilateral, and upon analysis are often nonbloody transudates. However, if pulmonary emboli with infarcts are present, the effusions may become hemorrhagic exudates.[77] A hemothorax may also result from variceal rupture of the subclavian vein.[95,108] Additionally, Hannun and Frayha[159] have reported the occurrence of a pseudochylothorax in Behçet's disease with the fluid analysis demonstrating type IV lipoprotein phenotype, elevated triglyceride level, low cholesterol level, and negative Sudan III stain.

Pulmonary angiography in patients with Behçet's disease and abnormal chest roentgenograms may reveal widespread occlusions of the pulmonary arteries and aneurysms of the lobar or segmental pulmonary arteries.[140,142] These aneurysms, which may be situated proximal to an occluded artery and which may account for the founded opacities, may be reversible[140,142]; however, rupture of a pulmonary artery aneurysm may result in massive hemoptysis and death.[140,160] Additionally, the thrombosed pulmonary arteries may undergo partial recanalization.[142] Gibson et al.[160] described a patient with Behçet's disease who was evaluated for several episodes of large hemoptysis which required transfusions. A ventilation perfusion radionuclide lung scan revealed multiple bilateral perfusion defects, and the pulmonary angiogram demonstrated multiple occluded segmental branches of the pulmonary arteries. A chest roentgenogram demonstrated a rounded opacity adjacent to a prominent main pulmonary artery, and computed tomographic scans with contrast material of this nodule revealed a partially thrombosed saccular aneurysm. Because of massive hemoptysis this patient expired and necropsy revealed intrapulmonary hemorrhage with a communication between an aneurysm of the left lower lobe pulmonary artery and its related bronchus. This aneurysm corresponded anatomically to the roentgenographic pulmonary nodule. Pulmonary aneurysms in Behçet's disease may be either segmental or lobar and may be located proximal to an occluded artery.[160]

As previously mentioned, pulmonary infarction has been reported in patients with Behçet's disease with various prevalence rates; however, their pathogenesis is unknown. These infarctions may result from emboli from the peripheral veins or venae cavae, intraatrial thrombus, right ventricular mural thrombus, concomitant thromboses of pulmonary arteries and veins, in-situ thrombus formation within the pulmonary arteries, pulmonary arteritis or vasculitis, or rupture of pulmonary aneurysms.[10,25,65,75,77,85,128,137,140,150] In one study consisting of 14 patients with Behçet's disease and occlusion of the superior vena cava, pulmonary emboli or infarction were not mentioned as complicating events.[14] The role of heparin therapy in the treatment of pulmonary emboli or infarction complicating Behçet's disease is controversial since its use has been associated with therapeutic failures including its inability to prevent recurrent thrombophlebitis, hemoptysis, and pulmonary emboli and infarction.[20,65,85,140] In addition, intravenous heparin therapy may actually induce local thrombophlebitis.[3] Corticosteroids and immunosuppressive agents including cyclophosphamide and methotrexate have been used in the treatment of pulmonary vasculitis in Behçet's disease with variable results.[20,101,137,140,142] Lacombe et al.[161] reported the use of selective transcatheter arterial embolization with nonresorbable occlusive agents in a patient with Behçet's disease complicated by pulmonary aneurysms. In this patient, pulmonary infarction occurred in the distribution of one of the occluded vessels 72 hours after embolization. Since some of the pulmonary complications associated with Behçet's disease may be benign, self-limited, and even reversible, it may be difficult to assess the value of these various therapeutic modalities accurately.[139,140,142]

Pulmonary Pathology

Histologically, lung tissue from patients with Behçet's disease may show an active vasculitis,[14,135,140,150,162] and in one patient in whom the chest roentgenograms revealed a nodular, noncalcified density in the right upper lobe and interstitial infiltrates in the right lower lobe and the left lung, the lung biopsy specimen from the right middle lobe showed an acute venulitis and septal capillaritis which on immunofluorescent microscopy revealed granular deposits containing IgG, C3, C4, and fibrin(ogen) within the walls of the small pulmonary veins and alveolar septal capillaries, thus implying an immune complex–mediated inflammatory process. Light microscopy revealed mild fibrosis of the pleural surfaces, infiltration of the small veins by polymorphonuclear leukocytes and mononuclear cells, and infiltration of the interalveolar septa by neutrophils. This patient also had evidence of a focal segmental necrotizing glomerulonephritis.[101] Biopsy of the pulmonary opacities may also reveal diffuse fibrosis with neovascularization, thrombosis, hemorrhage, and periarterial infiltrations with lymphocytes and plasma cells.[138] The fluctuating roentgenographic abnormalities may reflect reversible aneurysm formation, organization of the arterial occlusions, or resolution of the small intrapulmonary hemorrhages.[25]

In one autopsied patient reported by Davies,[25] the larger elastic pulmonary arteries revealed medial mucoid degeneration and intimal thickening, and the muscular arteries showed medial hyperplasia and intimal fibroplasia. The pulmonary arteries demonstrated focal thrombosis with transmural inflammatory infiltrates consisting predominantly of polymorphonuclear or mononuclear cells. Some of the walls of the pulmonary arteries were destroyed by these inflammatory infiltrates. There also were thrombosed pulmonary aneurysms, some of which were recanalized. The bronchial arterial walls were normal; however, perivascular mononuclear infiltration and endothelial proliferation characterized the capillaries and small veins of the pulmonary septa. Similar lesions affected the alveolar capillaries.[25] In the patient with Behçet's disease reported by Bank,[135] the bronchial arteries were also markedly abnormal; however, the histology was not described in extensive detail. According to Davies,[25] patients with Behçet's disease and pulmonary complications may have histologic evidence of pulmonary hypertension, right ventricular hypertrophy, aneurysms and recanalized thrombi of the pulmonary arteries, periarterial and peribronchial vascularization, and intrapulmonary hemorrhage.[25] Pulmonary hypertension, which may result from vasculitis or arterial thromboses, may cause right heart failure and other manifestations of cor pulmonale.[25,140,142,150,160] The pulmonary vasculitis of Behçet's disease may affect pulmonary arteries of all sizes, capillaries, and the small pulmonary veins.[25,140]

According to Slavin and de Groot,[150] the basic pulmonary lesion in Behçet's disease is histologically a lymphocytic necrotizing vasculitis involving arteries and veins of all sizes and septal capillaries. This vasculitic process may result in the formation of aneurysms of the elastic pulmonary arteries, arterial and venous thromboses, pulmonary infarcts, bronchial erosions by the pulmonary artery aneurysms, and periadventitial fibrosis. A resected right lower lobe from a patient with Behçet's disease and hemoptysis revealed the vasculitis to involve the elastic and muscular arteries, veins, arterioles, and the septal capillaries. The inflammatory infiltrate was predominantly lymphocytic; however, plasma cells, eosinophils, macrophages, and polymorphonuclear leukocytes were also present in the walls of the vessels. In some elastic and muscular pulmonary arteries, the elastica and the media were replaced by fibrous and granulation tissue. Aneurysms, some with recanalized and neovascularized thrombi, were also present in tissue sections. Extension of inflammation and necrosis from an elastic pulmonary artery aneurysm into an adjacent bronchus resulted in the formation of a pulmonary artery-bronchial fistula. Bronchial hemorrhage resulted from the erosion of a newly formed vessel located within an intraarterial thrombus situated in the lumen of the pulmonary artery-bronchial fistula. Alveolar capillaries revealed chronic and acute inflammatory cells infiltrates, and some pulmonary veins which were located in the lobular septa and which surrounded a pulmonary infarct revealed transmural inflammation and organizing thrombi.[150] According to Efthimiou et al.,[140] histologic examination of postmortem lung tissue from a Behçet's disease patient with massive and lethal hemoptysis also revealed a necrotizing vasculitis affecting the elastic and muscular pulmonary arteries. Fibrinoid necrosis was absent, and the inflammatory infiltrate consisted mainly of mononuclear cells.[140]

In summary the pulmonary complications in Behçet's disease may result from repeated episodes of vasculitis which may affect vessels of all sizes, including elastic and muscular pulmonary arteries, arterioles, capillaries, venules, and small and large veins. Complications of this pulmonary angiitis include arterial and venous thrombosis, pulmonary artery aneurysms, pulmonary infarction, and pulmonary arterial hypertension. In addition, pulmonary vasculitis may be responsible for the development of periadventitial arterial and intrapulmonary fibrosis.[150]

According to other authors,[20,146] an active vasculitis may not always be demonstrated pathologically. The open-lung biopsy from the patient reported by Petty et al.[146] histologically showed organized pneumonitis, sparse eosinophils, round-cell infiltration, and thickening of the pleural and parenchymal arteries without evidence of active vasculitis. Similarly, the pulmonary nodules from the patient reported by Arkin et al.[20] histologically did not show a vasculitis but revealed areas of infarction with organized thrombi within the vasculature. However, the demonstration of a vasculitic process may be dependent upon obtaining the biopsy specimen at a specific time in the patient's clinical course. Amyloid deposition may also affect the lungs of patients with Behçet's disease, and these deposits may be present predominantly in the walls of the small arteries and arterioles.[118,128]

Hughes-Stovin Syndrome

In 1959, J. P. Hughes and P.G.I. Stovin[163] described a syndrome which now bears their names as consisting of segmental pulmonary artery aneurysms, and peripheral venous thrombosis which may be accompanied by elevated intracranial pressure or pseudotumor cerebri due to thrombosis of the dural sinuses or jugular veins. Additional cases of this syndrome have been reported[164-168]; however, the Hughes-Stovin syndrome may not be a distinct clinical or pathological entity but may represent a variant of Behçet's disease.[150,162,164] Some of these patients have had other manifestations of Behçet's disease, including oral ulcerations, peripheral arterial aneurysms, and epididymitis; and thus there is an overlap of these two disorders. There is also evidence of vasculitis that is histologically similar to the type traditionally described in patients with Behçet's disease.[150,163-168] Recently, magnetic resonance imaging has been shown to be useful in detecting pulmonary artery aneurysms and thus offers a noninvasive means of diagnosing these vascular abnormalities.[169]

References

1. Barnes CG. Behçet's syndrome. *J Roy Soc Med* 1984; 77:816–819.
2. Berlin C. Behçet's disease as a multiple symptom complex. Report of ten cases. *Arch Dermatol* 1960; 82:73–79.
3. Chajek T, Fainaru M. Behçet's disease. Report of 41 cases and a review of the literature. *Medicine* 1975; 54:179–196.
4. Ehrlich GE. Intermittent and periodic arthritic syndromes. In McCarty DJ, ed: *Arthritis and Allied Conditions. A Textbook of Rheumatology*. Philadelphia, Lea and Febiger, 1985:883–900.
5. Feagin OT. Behçet's disease: The Ochsner experience, 1979 to 1982. *South Med J* 1984; 77:442–446.

6. Fife RS. Behçet's disease. *Clin Rheumatol Prac* 1983; 1:249–254.
7. Gilliland BC, Mannik M. Reiter's syndrome, psoriatic arthritis, arthritis associated with gastrointestinal disease, and Behçet's syndrome. In Petersdorf RG, Adams RD, Braunwald E, et al, eds: *Harrison's Principles of Internal Medicine.* New York, McGraw-Hill, 1983:1989–1994.
8. Jorizzo JL. Behçet's syndrome: Pathogenesis, diagnosis, and treatment. *Cutis* 1983; 32:441–442, 444–445, 448.
9. Lakhanpal S, Tani K, Lie JT, et al. Pathologic features of Behçet's syndrome: A review of Japanese autopsy registry data. *Hum Pathol* 1985; 16:790–795.
10. Michelson JB, Chisari FV. Behçet's disease. *Surv Ophthalmol* 1982; 26:190–203.
11. O'Duffy JD. Behçet's disease. In Kelley WN, Harris ED Jr, Ruddy S, Sledge CB, eds: *Textbook of Rheumatology.* Philadelphia, WB Saunders, 1985:1174–1178.
12. O'Duffy JD. Summary of international symposium of Behçet's disease, Istanbul, September 29–30, 1977. *J Rheumatol* 1978; 5:229–233.
13. O'Duffy JD, Lehner T, Barnes CG. Summary of the third international conference on Behçet's disease, Tokyo, Japan, October 23–24, 1981. *J Rheumatol* 1983; 10:154–158.
14. Shimizu T, Ehrlich GE, Inaba G, Hayashi K. Behçet disease (Behçet syndrome). *Semin Arthritis Rheum* 1979; 8:223–260.
15. Snyderman R. Behçet's disease. In Wyngaarden JB, Smith LH Jr, eds: *Cecil Textbook of Medicine.* Philadelphia, WB Saunders, 1985:1960–1962.
16. Tokoro Y, Seto T, Abe Y, et al. Skin lesions in Behçet's disease. *Int J Dermatol* 1977; 16:227–244.
17. Venkatasubramaniam KV, Swinehart DR. Behçet's syndrome: Case report and literature review. *Henry Ford Hosp Med J* 1981; 29:153–159.
18. Wong RC, Ellis CN, Diaz LA. Behçet's disease. *Int J Dermatol* 1984; 23:25–32.
19. Behçet's Disease Research Committee of Japan. Behçet's disease: Guide to diagnosis of Behçet's disease. *Jpn J Ophthalmol* 1974; 18:291–294.
20. Arkin CR, Rothschild BM, Florendo NT, Popoff N. Behçet's syndrome with myositis. A case report with pathologic findings. *Arthritis Rheum* 1980; 23:600–604.
21. Binak K, Ucak D, Yalcin B, et al. Left ventricular aneurysm and acute pericarditis in a case of Behçet's disease (letter). *J Rheumatol* 1980; 7:578–580.
22. Bowles CA, Nelson AM, Hammill SC, O'Duffy JD. Cardiac involvement in Behçet's disease. *Arthritis Rheum* 1985; 28:345–348.
23. Buge A, Escourelle R, Chomette G, et al. La maladie de Behçet avec manifestations neurologiques et fibrose endocardique du coeur droit. Etude anatomoclinique d'une observation. *Ann Med Interne* (Paris) 1977; 128:411–419.

24. Comess KA, Zibelli LR, Gordon D, Fredrickson SR. Acute, severe, aortic regurgitation in Behçet's syndrome. *Ann Intern Med* 1983; 99:639–640.
25. Davies JD. Behçet's syndrome with haemoptysis and pulmonary lesions. *J Pathol* 1973; 109:351–356.
26. Higashihara M, Mori M, Takeuchi A, et al. Myocarditis in Behçet's disease—A case report and review of the literature. *J Rheumatol* 1982; 9:630–633.
27. Huycke EC, Robinowitz M, Cohen IS, et ai. Granulomatous endocarditis with systemic embolism in Behçet's disease. *Ann Intern Med* 1985; 102:791–793.
28. Hutchison SJ, Belch JJF. Behçet's syndrome presenting as myocardial infarction with impaired blood fibrinolysis. *Br Heart J* 1984; 52:686–687.
29. James DG, Thomson A. Recognition of the diverse cardiovascular manifestations in Behçet's disease. *Am Heart J* 1982; 103:457–458.
30. Kansu E, Deglin S, Cantor RI, et al. The expanding spectrum of Behçet's syndrome. A case with renal involvement. *JAMA* 1977; 237:1855–1856.
31. Kaseda S, Koiwaya Y, Tajimi T, et al. High false aneurysm due to rupture of the right coronary artery in Behçet's syndrome. *Am Heart J* 1982; 103:569–571.
32. Lewis PD. Behçet's disease and carditis. *Br Med J* 1964; 1:1026–1027.
33. Lu-Li S, Guang-Gen C, Ru-Lian L. Valve prolapse in Behçet's disease. *Br Heart J* 1985; 54:100–101.
34. McDonald GSA, Gad-Al-Rab J. Behçet's disease with endocarditis and the Budd-Chiari syndrome. *J Clin Pathol* 1980; 33:660–669.
35. McMenemey WH, Lawrence BJ. Encephalomyelopathy in Behçet's disease. Report of necropsy findings in two cases. *Lancet* 1957; 2:353–358.
36. Müftüoglu AÜ, Yurdakul S, Yazaci H, et al. Vascular involvement in Behçet's disease (abstract 63). Royal Society of Medicine international conference on Behçet's disease, September 5 and 6, 1985, London, England.
37. Nojiri C, Endo M, Koyanagi H. Conduction disturbance in Behçet's disease. Association with ruptured aneurysm of the sinus of valsalva into the left ventricular cavity. *Chest* 1984; 86:636–638.
38. Oshima Y, Shimizu T, Yokohari R, et al. Clinical studies on Behçet's syndrome. *Ann Rheum Dis* 1963; 22:36–45.
39. Peña JM, Garcia-Alegria J, Garcia-Fernandez F, et al: Mitral and aortic regurgitation in Behçet's syndrome. *Ann Rheum Dis* 1985; 44:637–639.
40. Rae S, Vandenburg M. Scholtz CL. Aortic regurgitation and false aortic aneurysm formation in Behçet's disease. *Postgrad Med J* 1980; 56:438–439.
41. Roguin N, Haim S, Reshef R, et al. Cardiac involvement and superior vena caval obstruction in Behçet's disease. *Thorax* 1978; 33:375–377.
42. Scarlett JA, Kistner ML, Yang LC. Behçet's syndrome. Report of a

case associated with pericardial effusion and cryoglobulinemia treated with indomethacin. *Am J Med* 1979; 66:146–148.

43. Schiff S. Moffatt R, Mandel WJ, Rubin SA. Acute myocardial infarction and recurrent ventricular arrhythmias in Behçet's syndrome. *Am Heart J* 1982; 103:438–440.

44. Sigel N, Larson R. Behçet's syndrome. A case with benign pericarditis and recurrent neurologic involvement treated with adrenal steroids. *Arch Intern Med* 1965; 115:203–207.

45. Stucchi C, Vollenweider A. Maladie de Behçet et manifestations atypiques. *Ophthalmologica* 1958; 135:573–578.

46. Wilkey D. Yocum DE, Oberley TD, et al. Budd-Chiari syndrome and renal failure in Behçet disease. Report of a case and review of the literature. *Am J Med* 1983; 75:541–550.

47. Hyman NM, Sagar HJ. Behçet's syndrome: Unusual multisystem involvement and immune complexes. *Postgrad Med J* 1980; 56:182–184.

48. Or I, Roguin N, Yahalom M, et al. Pacemaker implantation in a patient with a Behçet's disease associated with superior vena cava obstruction. *Cardiovasc Intervent Radiol* 1986; 9:13–14.

49. Parrillo JE, Fauci AS. Coronary vasculitis. *Cardiovasc Rev Rep* 1985; 6:322, 328–334, 339–340, 343–344.

50. Ehrlich GE, Kajani M. Schwartz IR, McAlack RF. Further studies of platelet rosettes around granulocytes in Behçet's syndrome. *Inflammation* 1975–76; 1:223–229.

51. Matsuda T, Kaneko K, Hoshi K, Mizushima Y. Platelet function in Behçet's disease (abstract 34). Royal Society of Medicine international conference on Behçet's disease, September 5 and 6, 1985, London, England.

52. Hull RG, Harris EN, Gharavi AE, et al. Anticardiolipin antibodies: Occurrence in Behçet's syndrome. *Ann Rheum Dis* 1984; 43:746–748.

53. Hizli N, Sahin G, Sahin F, et al. Plasma prostacyclin levels in Behçet's disease (letter). *Lancet* 1985; 1:1454.

54. Mishima H, Masuda K, Shimada S, et al. Plasminogen activator activity levels in patients with Behçet's syndrome. *Arch Ophthalmol* 1985; 103:935–936.

55. Jordan JM, Allen NB, Pizzo SV. Defective release of tissue plasminogen activator in systemic and cutaneous vasculitis. *Am J Med* 1987; 82:397–400.

56. Hizli N, Sahin G, Duru S, et al. Plasma and tissue prostaglandin E and $F_2\alpha$ levels in Behçet's disease (abstract 39). Royal Society of Medicine international conference on Behçet's disease, September 5 and 6, 1985, London, England.

57. Souza-Ramalho P, Freitas JP, Martins R, et al. Blood viscosity changes in Behçet's disease (abstract 40). Royal Society of Medicine international conference on Behçet's disease, September 5 and 6, 1985, London, England.

58. Schmitz-Huebner U, Knop J. Evidence for an endothelial cell dysfunction in association with Behçet's disease. *Thromb Res* 1984; 34:277–285.

59. Niwa Y, Miyake S, Sakane T, et al. Auto-oxidative damage in Behçet's disease endothelial cell damage following the elevated oxygen radicals generated by stimulated neutrophils. *Clin Exp Immunol* 1982; 49:247–255.

60. Bank I, Weart C. Dural sinus thrombosis in Behçet's disease. *Arthritis Rheum* 1984; 27:816–818.

61. Brissaud P, Laroche L, de Gramont A, Krulik M. Digital angiography for the diagnosis of dural sinus thrombosis in Behçet's disease (letter). *Arthritis Rheum* 1985; 28:359–360.

62. Chajek T, Fainaru M. Behçet's disease with decreased fibrinolysis and superior vena caval occlusion. *Br Med J* 1973; 1:782–783.

63. Clausen J, Bierring F. Fetal arterial involvement in Behçet's disease: An electron microscope study. *Acta Pathol Microbiol Immunol Scand [A]* 1983; 91:133–136.

64. Clausen J, Bierring F. Involvement of post-capillary venules in Behçet's disease: an electronmicroscopic study. *Acta Derm Venereol (Stockh)* 1983; 63:191–197.

65. Cunliffe WJ, Menon IS. Treatment of Behçet's syndrome with phenformin and ethyloestrenol. *Lancet* 1969; 1:1239–1240.

66. Dündar S, Yazici H. Superior vena cava syndrome (letter). *Mayo Clin Proc* 1982; 57:785.

67. Dündar-Kaldirimci SV, Ates KA, Akpolat T, Nazli N. Iliac artery aneurysm in Behçet's disease: A case report. *Angiology* 1985; 36:549–551.

68. Enoch BA. Gangrene in Behçet's syndrome (letter). *Br Med J* 1969; 3:54.

69. Enoch BA, Castillo-Olivares JL, Khoo TCL, et al. Major vascular complications in Behçet's syndrome. *Postgrad Med J* 1968; 44:453–459.

70. France R, Buchanan RN, Wilson MW, Sheldon MB Jr. Relapsing iritis with recurrent ulcers of the mouth and genitalia (Behçet's syndrome). Review: With report of additional case. *Medicine* 1951; 30:335–355.

71. Gruber HE, Weisman MH. Aortic thrombosis during sigmoidoscopy in Behçet's syndrome. *Arch Intern Med* 1983; 143:343–345.

72. Haim S, Barzilai D, Hazani E. Involvement of veins in Behçet's syndrome. *Br J Dermatol* 1971; 84:238–241.

73. Harper CM Jr, O'Neill BP, O'Duffy JD, Forbes GS. Intracranial hypertension in Behçet's disease: Demonstration of sinus occlusion with use of digital subtraction angiography. *Mayo Clin Proc* 1985; 60:419–422.

74. Hills EA. Behçet's syndrome with aortic aneurysms. *Br Med J* 1967; 4:152–154.

75. Imaizumi M, Nukada T, Yoneda S, Abe H. Behçet's disease with sinus thrombosis and arteriovenous malformation in brain. *J Neurol* 1980; 222:215–218.

76. Jenkins AM, Macpherson AI, Nolan B, Housley E. Peripheral aneurysms in Behçet's disease. *Br J Surg* 1976; 63:199–202.

77. Kansu E, Özer FL, Akalin E, et al. Behçet's syndrome with obstruction of the venae cavae. A report of seven cases. *Q J Med* 1972; 41:151–168.
78. Kingston M, Ratcliffe JR, Alltree M, Merendino KA. Aneurysm after arterial puncture in Behçet's disease. *Br Med J* 1979; 1:1766–1767.
79. Little AG, Zarins CK. Abdominal aortic aneurysm and Behçet's disease. *Surgery* 1982; 91:359–362.
80. Mamo JG, Baghidassarian A. Behçet's disease. A report of 28 cases. *Arch Ophthalmol* 1964; 71:4–14.
81. Mowat AG, Hothersall TE. Gangrene in Behçet's syndrome (letter). *Br Med J* 1969; 2:636.
82. Park JH, Han MC, Bettman MA. Arterial manifestations of Behçet disease. *AJR* 1984; 143:821–825.
83. Piers A. Behçet's disease with arterial and renal manifestations. *Proc R Soc Med* 1977; 70:540–544.
84. Reza MJ, Demanes DJ. Behçet's disease: A case with hemoptysis, pseudotumor cerebri, and arteritis. *J Rheumatol* 1978; 5:320–326.
85. Rosenthal T, Halkin H, Shani M, Deutch V. Occlusion of the great veins in the Behçet syndrome. *Angiology* 1972; 23:600–605.
86. Rosenthal T, Rubenstein Z, Adar R, Gafni J. Major vessel arteritis with aortic aneurysm in Behçet's disease. *Vasa* 1982; 11:124–127.
87. Tibbutt DA, Durack DT, MacFarlane JT, Teddy PJ. Behçet's disease and venous thrombosis (letter). *Br Med J* 1973; 3:236.
88. Urayama A, Sakuragi S, Sakai F, et al. Angio-Behçet syndrome. In Inaba G, ed: *Behçet's Disease. Pathogenetic Mechanism and Clinical Future. Proceedings of the International Conference on Behçet's Disease, Tokyo, October 23–24, 1981.* Tokyo, University of Tokyo Press, 1982:171–176.
89. Vella MA, James DG. Vascular and neurological involvement in 25 patients with Behçet's disease (abstract 67). Royal Society of Medicine international conference on Behçet's disease, September 5 and 6, 1985, London, England.
90. Wechsler B, Bousser MG, Huong Du LT, et al. Central venous sinus thrombosis in Behçet's disease (letter). *Mayo Clin Proc* 1985; 60:891–892.
91. Shimizu T, Inaba G. Epidemiology of Behçet's disease: Status of Behçet's disease in Japan. *Ryumachi* 1976; 16:224–233.
92. Chavatzas D. Popliteal artery thrombosis in Behçet's syndrome. A new manifestation of a very little known condition (letter). *Angiology* 1974; 25:773–776.
93. Fukuda Y, Sakuma Y, Sumita M. Pathological studies of vascular changes in Behçet's disease. In Shiokawa Y, ed: *Vascular Lesions of Collagen Diseases and Related Conditions. Proceedings of the International Workshop of Vascular Lesions of Collagen Diseases and Related Conditions, February 6–7, 1976, Tokyo.* Tokyo, University Park Press, 1977:212–225.
94. Murakami T. Pathological changes in the large blood vessels caused by Behçet's disease, especially by neuro-Behçet's disease. In

Shiokawa Y, ed: *Vascular Lesions of Collagen Diseases and Related Conditions. Proceedings of the International Workshop on Vascular Lesions of Collagen Diseases and Related Conditions, February 6–7, 1976, Tokyo.* Tokyo, University Park Press, 1977:229–235.

95. Shimizu T. Behçet's disease: A systemic inflammatory disease. In Shiokawa Y, ed: *Vascular Lesions of Collagen Diseases and Related Conditions. Proceedings of the International Workshop on Vascular Lesions of Collagen Diseases and Related Conditions, February 6–7, 1976, Tokyo.* Tokyo, University Park Press, 1977:201–211.

96. Katoh K, Matsunaga K, Ishigatsubo Y, et al. Pathologically defined neuro-, vasculo-, entero-Behçet's disease. *J Rheumatol* 1985; 12:1186–1190.

97. Haim S, Sobel JD, Friedman-Birnbaum R. Thrombophlebitis. A cardinal symptom of Behçet's syndrome. *Acta Derm Venereol* (Stockh) 1974; 54:299–301.

98. Mavioğlu H. Behçet's recurrent disease. Analytical review of the literature. *Mo Med* 1958; 55:1209–1222.

99. Carr AR. Cellulitis and thrombophlebitis in Behçet's syndrome. *Lancet* 1957; 2:358–359.

100. Nakayama S, Sakata J, Kusumoto S. Ultrasonic appearance of the liver in hepatic venous outflow obstruction (Budd-Chiari syndrome): A case of pseudohepatic infarct associated with Behçet's disease. *JCU* 1986; 14:300–303.

101. Gamble CN, Wiesner KB, Shapiro F, Boyer WJ. The immune complex pathogenesis of glomerulonephritis and pulmonary vasculitis in Behçet's disease. *Am J Med* 1979; 66:1031–1039.

102. O'Duffy JD, Carney JA, Deodhar S. Behçet's disease. Report of 10 cases, 3 with new manifestations. *Ann Intern Med* 1971; 75:561–570.

103. White JW Jr. Hypersensitivity and miscellaneous inflammatory disorders. In Moschella SL, Hurley HJ, eds: *Dermatology.* Philadelphia, WB Saunders, 1985:464–498.

104. Ben-Itzhak J, Keren S, Simon J. Intracranial venous thrombosis in Behçet's syndrome. *Neuroradiology* 1985; 27:450.

105. Kalbian VV, Challis MT. Behçet's disease. Report of twelve cases with three manifesting as papilledema. *Am J Med* 1970; 49:823–829.

106. Masheter HC. Behçet's syndrome complicated by intracranial thrombophlebitis. *Proc R Soc Med* 1959; 52:1039–1040.

107. Houser OW, Campbell JK, Campbell RJ, Sundt TM Jr. Arteriovenous malformation affecting the transverse dural venous sinus—An acquired lesion. *Mayo Clin Proc* 1979; 54:651–661.

108. Özer ZG, Çetin M, Kahraman C. Thrombophlebitis in Behçet's disease. *Vasa* 1985; 14:379–382.

109. Yashiro K, Nagasako K, Hasegawa K, et al. Esophageal lesions in intestinal Behçet's disease. *Endoscopy* 1986; 18:57–60.

110. Rosenthal T, Weiss P, Gafni J. Evidence of a benign renal lesion in Behçet's disease. In Dilşen N, Koniçe M, Övül C, eds: *Behçet's Disease. Proceedings of an International Symposium on Behçet's Disease, Istanbul, 29–30 September 1977.* Amsterdam-Oxford, Excerpta Medica, 1979:157–159.

111. Rosenthal T, Weiss P, Gafni J. Renal involvement in Behçet's syndrome. *Arch Intern Med* 1978; 138:1122–1124.
112. Herreman G, Beaufils H, Godeau P, et al. Behçet's syndrome and renal involvement: A histological and immunofluorescent study of eleven renal biopsies. *Am J Med Sci* 1982; 284:10–17.
113. Landwehr DM, Cooke CL, Rodriguez GE. Rapidly progressive glomerulonephritis in Behçet's syndrome. *JAMA* 1980; 244:1709–1711.
114. Williams DG, Lehner T. Renal manifestations of Behçet's syndrome. In Lehner T, Barnes CG, eds: *Behçet's Syndrome. Clinical and Immunological Features. Proceedings of a Conference Sponsored by the Royal Society of Medicine, February 1979.* London, Academic Press, 1979:259–264.
115. Olsson PJ, Gaffney E, Alexander RW, et al. Proliferative glomerulonephritis with crescent formation in Behçet's syndrome. *Arch Intern Med* 1980; 140:713–714.
116. Beaufils H, Cassou B, Auriol M. et al. Kidney involvement in Behçet's syndrome. A report of 11 cases studied by optic, ultrastructural and immunopathological techniques. *Virchows Arch [A]* 1980; 388:187–198.
117. Beaufils H, Cassou B, Roujeau JC, et al. Renal pathological and immunofluorescent findings in Behçet's disease: A report of 11 cases (abstract). *Kidney Int* 1978; 14:541–542.
118. Beroniade V. Amyloidosis and Behçet's disease (letter). *Ann Intern Med* 1975; 83:904–905.
119. Carswell GF. A case of Behçet's disease involving the bladder. *Br J Urol* 1976; 48:199–202.
120. Dilşen N, Koniçe M, Erbengi T, et al. Amyloidosis in two cases of Behçet's disease. In Dilşen N, Koniçe M, Övül C, eds: *Behçet's Disease. Proceedings of an International Symposium on Behçet's Disease, Istanbul, 29–30 September 1977.* Amsterdam-Oxford, Excerpta Medica, 1979:171–177.
121. Dilşen H, Koniçe M, Övül C, et al. Three cases of Behçet's disease with amyloidosis. In Inaba G, ed: *Behçet's Disease. Pathogenetic Mechanism and Clinical Future. Proceedings of the International Conference on Behçet's disease, Tokyo, October 23–24, 1981.* Tokyo, University of Tokyo Press, 1982:449–457.
122. Mace BEW, Jones JG. Renal involvement in Behçet's disease. *J R Soc Med* 1978; 71:74.
123. Miura M, Tomino Y, Suga T, et al. A case of Behçet's disease associated with membranous nephropathy. *Tokai J Exp Clin Med* 1984; 9:231–235.
124. Nestor G, Beroniade V, Cârnaru S, Badea I. Behçet's disease with renal involvement (with reference to three anatomico-clinical cases). *Rom Med Rev* 1970; 14:27–32.
125. Olsson PJ. Glomerulonephritis in Behçet's syndrome (letter). *JAMA* 1981; 246:1087.
126. Oro-genital ulceration with phlebothrombosis (? Behçet's syndrome) complicated by osteomyelitis of lumbar spine and ruptured aorta.

Demonstrated at the Postgraduate Medical School of London. *Br Med J* 1965; 5431:357–361.

127. Peces R, Riesgo I, Ortega F, et al. Amyloidosis in Behçet's disease. *Nephron* 1984; 36:114–117.
128. Rosenthal T, Bank H, Aladjem M, et al. Systemic amyloidosis in Behçet's disease. *Ann Intern Med* 1975; 83:220–223.
129. Case records of the Massachusetts General Hospital. Weekly clinicopathological exercises. Case 19-1982. Recent onset of proteinuria in a young woman with a chronic multisystem disease. *N Engl J Med* 1982; 306:1162–1167.
130. Finucane P, Doyle CT, Ferriss JB, et al. Behçet's syndrome with myositis and glomerulonephritis. *Br J Rheumatol* 1985; 24:372–375.
131. Nagata K. Recurrent intracranial hemorrhage in Behçet disease (letter). *J Neurol Neurosurg Psychiatry* 1985; 48:190–192.
132. Yudis M. Nephropathy with Behçet's syndrome (letter). *Arch Intern Med* 1979; 139:602–603.
133. Penza R, Brunetti L, Francioso G, et al. Renal amyloidosis in a child with Behçet's syndrome. *Int J Pediatr Nephrol* 1983; 4:35–37.
134. Akkaynak S, Enacar N, Cobanli B, et al. Behçet's disease and lungs. In Dilşen N, Koniçe M, Övül C, eds: *Behçet's Disease. Proceedings of an International Symposium on Behçet's Disease, Istanbul, 29–30 September 1977*. Amsterdam-Oxford, Excerpta Medica, 1979:160–162.
135. Bank H. Thrombotic pulmonary manifestations in Behçet's syndrome. *Is J Med Sci* 1973; 9:955.
136. Brookes GB. Pharyngeal stenosis in Behçet's syndrome. The first reported case. *Arch Otolaryngol* 1983; 109:338–340.
137. Cadman EC, Lundberg B, Mitchell MS. Pulmonary manifestations in Behçet syndrome. Case report and review of the literature. *Arch Intern Med* 1976; 136:944–947.
138. Decroix AG. Thoracic manifestations of Behçet's syndrome. *Thorax* 1969; 24:380.
139. Dilşen N, Koniçe M, Gazioğlu K, et al. Pleuropulmonary manifestations in Behçet's disease. In Dilşen N, Koniçe M, Övül C, eds: *Behçet's Disease. Proceedings of an International Symposium on Behçet's Disease, Istanbul, 29–30 September 1977*. Amsterdam-Oxford, Excerpta Medica, 1979:163–170.
140. Efthimiou J, Johnston C, Spiro SG, Turner-Warwick M. Pulmonary disease in Behçet's syndrome. *Q J Med* 1986; 58:259–280.
141. Fromer JL. Behçet's syndrome. *Arch Dermatol* 1970; 102:116–117.
142. Grenier P, Bletry O, Cornud F, et al. Pulmonary involvement in Behçet disease. *AJR* 1981; 137:565–569.
143. James DG. Behçet's syndrome. *N Engl J Med* 1979; 301:431–432.
144. Kokayashi T, Kikaweda T, Shima K, Fukuda O. Ulceration and stenosis of the hypopharynx and its surgical management. *Head Neck Surg* 1982 Sept–Oct; 5:65–69.
145. Morrison AW. Behçet's syndrome. *J Laryngol Otol* 1959; 23:833–837.
146. Petty TL, Scoggin CH, Good JT. Recurrent pneumonia in Behçet's syndrome. Roentgenographic documentation during 13 years. *JAMA* 1977; 238:2529–2530.

147. Prakash UBS, Divertie MB. Neuromuscular, skeletal, and dermatologic disease. In Baum GL, Wolinsky E, eds: *Textbook of pulmonary diseases*. Boston: Little, Brown, 1983:1179–1195.
148. Rapport P, Duckert LG, Boies LR Jr. Behçet's disease. *Ear Nose Throat J* 1979; 58:45–52.
149. Screech G. An unusual cause of respiratory obstruction during anaesthesia. A case report. *Br J Anaesth* 1965; 37:978–979.
150. Slavin RE, de Groot WJ. Pathology of the lung in Behçet's disease. Case report and review of the literature. *Am J Surg Pathol* 1981; 5:779–788.
151. Turner ME. Anaesthetic difficulties associated with Behçet's syndrome. A case report. *Br J Anaesth* 1972; 44:100–102.
152. Wright MI. Behçet's disease in the mouth, pharynx, and larynx: An under-diagnosed disease? (abstract 56). Royal Society of Medicine international conference on Behçet's disease, September 5 and 6, 1985, London, England.
153. Yassin A, Girgis IH. Behçet's disease. *J Laryngol Otol* 1966; 80:481–494.
154. Humaidan P, Manthorpe R, Rasmussen N, Velander B. Behçet's disease (a severe case from Greenland). *J Laryngol Otol* 1986; 100:367–370.
155. Kenet DS. Cortisone in Behçet's syndrome. Report on a patient with lesions of the genitalia, mouth, pharynx, and larynx necessitating repeated tracheostomies. *Arch Otolaryngol* 1951; 54:505–509.
156. Ahonen AV, Stenius-Aarniala BSM, Viljanen BC, et al. Obstructive lung disease in Behçet's syndrome. *Scand J Resp Dis* 1978; 59:44–50.
157. Evans WV, Jenkins RM. Pulmonary function in Behçet's syndrome. *Scand J Resp Dis* 1979; 60:314–316.
158. Gibson JM, O'Hara MD, Beare JM, Stanford CF. Bronchial obstruction in a patient with Behçet's disease. *Eur J Resp Dis* 1982; 63:356–360.
159. Hannum Y, Frayha R. Behçet's disease with pseudochylothorax (letter). *J Rheumatol* 1985; 12:817–818.
160. Gibson RN, Morgan SH, Krausz T, Hughes GRV. Pulmonary artery aneurysms in Behçet's disease. *Br J Radiol* 1985; 58:79–82.
161. Lacombe P, Frija G, Parlier H, et al. Transcatheter embolization of multiple pulmonary artery aneurysms in Behçet's syndrome. Report of case. *Acta Radiol [Diagn]* (Stockh) 1985; 26:251–253.
162. Leavitt RY, Fauci AS. Pulmonary vasculitis. *Am Rev Respir Dis* 1986; 134:149–166.
163. Hughes JP, Stovin PGI. Segmental pulmonary artery aneurysms with peripheral venous thrombosis. *Br J Dis Chest* 1959; 53:19–27.
164. Durieux P, Bletry O, Huchon G, et al. Multiple pulmonary arterial aneurysms in Behçet's disease and Hughes-Stovin syndrome. *Am J Med* 1981; 71:736–741.
165. Kopp WL, Green RA. Pulmonary artery aneurysms with recurrent thrombophlebitis. The "Hughes-Stovin syndrome." *Ann Intern Med* 1952; 56:105–114.
166. Meireles A, Sobrinho-Simões A, Capucho R, Brandão A. Hughes-

Stovin with pulmonary angiitis and focal glomerulonephritis. A case report with necropsy study. *Chest* 1981; 79:598–600.
167. Teplick JG, Haskin ME, Nedwich A. The Hughes-Stovin syndrome. Case report. *Radiology* 1974; 113:607–608.
168. Wolpert SM, Kahn PC, Farbman K. The radiology of the Hughes-Stovin syndrome. *AJR* 1971; 112:383–388.
169. Jeang MK, Adyanthaya A, Kuo L, et al. Multiple pulmonary artery aneurysms. New use for magnetic resonance imaging. *Am J Med* 1986; 81:1001–1004.

12

MISCELLANEOUS CLINICAL MANIFESTATIONS, PART II: GASTROINTESTINAL, HEPATIC, SPLENIC, PANCREATIC, GENITOURINARY, AND DERMATOLOGIC FEATURES

Gary R. Plotkin

Gastrointestinal Features

ACCORDING TO THE BEHÇET'S DISEASE Research Committee of Japan,[1] recurrent aphthous ulcerations of the oral mucous membranes and intestinal ulcers in the ileocecal region constitute major and minor criteria, respectively, in the diagnosis of Behçet's disease. However, gastrointestinal involvement may affect all areas from the lips to the anus with complications that include hematemesis; melena; hematochezia; toxic megacolon; fissures; strictures; intraabdominal, enterocutaneous, and perianal fistulas; perirectal abscesses; bowel perforation; and peritonitis. Gastrointestinal symptoms, which may be present, depending upon the series, in as

From *Behcet's Disease: A Contemporary Synopsis*, edited by Gary R. Plotkin, M.D., John J. Calabro, M.D., and J. Desmond O'Duffy, M.B. © 1988, Futura Publishing Company, Inc., Mount Kisco, NY.

many as 60% of patients with Behçet's disease, include recurrent sore throats, oral fetor, referred otalgia, odynophagia, dysphagia, oropharyngeal pain, anorexia, vomiting, flatulence, dyspepsia, regurgitation, eructation, retrosternal and abdominal pain, abdominal distention, diarrhea which may be accompanied by mucus and/or blood, constipation, tenesmus, pain on defecation, and anal pain.[2-81] These various gastrointestinal manifestations are more frequent during the acute exacerbations of disease activity but definitely may also occur during periods of remission or recovery.[60,68] However, there may be discordance between the symptoms of Behçet's colitis and the extraintestinal complications; that is, the gastrointestinal symptoms may predominate when the other manifestations of disease activity are quiescent. In addition, rectal biopsies may show inflammatory changes in asymptomatic patients with Behçet's disease.[2,65]

The salivary glands may be involved in Behçet's disease and may be swollen and slightly painful[46,49,82]; in one postmortem examination of a patient with Behçet's syndrome, the parotid gland was enlarged and revealed histologically dilated acini, focal necrosis, and a nonspecific chronic inflammatory infiltrate.[83] The presence of Sjögren's syndrome in a patient with Behçet's disease has also been reported by Ramírez-Peredo et al.[84]; however, these two diseases may have been independent processes. As discussed in previous chapters, recurrent aphthous ulcerations may affect the upper respiratory and digestive tracts including the labial and buccal mucosae, gingivae, alveolar ridges, tongue, tonsils, palate, pharynx, larynx, and epiglottis.[29,30,81] Many patients with Behçet's disease experience a prodromal phase of oral soreness or burning sensation one to two days prior to ulcer formation.[30] The oral ulcers are often multiple, ranging from 2 to 18 mm in diameter, may be surrounded by a small erythematous areola, and may persist for several days to weeks only to recur days to months later.[13,81] These ulcerations also may produce pain and heal with scarring, and consequently there may be difficulties in speaking, chewing, and swallowing liquids and solids, resulting in dehydration and weight loss.[30,47,64,81]

The lingual ulcers may be well demarcated with gray or yellow membranes on their bases, and biopsy specimens have revealed acute and chronic inflammation in the epithelium and numerous polymorphonuclear leukocytes and lymphocytes within the submucosa. The blood vessels were lined by hyperplastic endothelium, and the walls of the vessels contained inflammatory infiltrates. Thus, vasculitis may be the underlying pathogenetic mechanism in oral ulcer formation.[30] The tongue ulcers may also heal with scar formation.[16] Other features of the oral lesions of Behçet's disease have been extensively reviewed in Chapter 9.

Other less common oral physical findings in patients with Behçet's syndrome include leukoplakia or plaque-like lesions, furred tongue, absent or sparse lingual fungiform papillae as determined by ocular slit lamp examination, and soft-palate perforation.[17,43,54,62,73] Absent lingual fungiform papillae is not pathognomonic for Behçet's disease since this physical finding may occur in Riley-Day syndrome (familial dysautonomia) and various other medical conditions. Also, patients with either isolated aphthous stomatitis or uveitis but without other evidence of Behçet's disease have normal distribution of the lingual fungiform papillae.[17]

Shuttleworth et al.[69] reported a patient with neuro-Behçet's disease with palatal myoclonus secondary to brain-stem disease with involvement of the dentatoolivary system. On examination there were rhythmic contractions of the muscles of the soft palate. Other structures derived from the branchial arches including the pharynx, larynx, tongue, mouth, face, orbicularis oculi, diaphragm, and extraocular and neck muscles may also undergo synchronous contractions due to brain-stem lesions of various origins.[69]

The most common cause of swallowing problems in Behçet's disease is odynophagia from oral ulcerations; however, dysphagia may result from pharyngeal obstruction or esophageal abnormalities including ulcerations and strictures.[11,12,78] Brookes[12] reported a patient with dysphagia due to severe pharyngeal stenosis resulting from recurrent episodes of multiple ulcerations of the mouth and pharynx; indirect laryngoscopy showed a scarred pharynx at the junction of the oropharynx and hypopharynx. This patient required endoscopic dilatation for control of his gastrointestinal symptoms.[12] Kobayashi et al.[41] also described a patient with Behçet's disease and dysphagia due to a stenotic hypopharynx resulting from an ulcerating mucosal lesion of the hypopharyngeal walls. Although most aphthous ulcers resolve without scarring, the fusion of several ulcers may result in a larger one that can heal into a stenotic lesion.[41] Scarring with adhesion formation in the pharynx and fusion of the soft palate to the base of the tongue with scar tissue have been reported in patients with Behçet's disease, and these anatomical abnormalities have resulted in difficulties in nasotracheal and oropharyngeal intubation.[66,76] Recurrent ulcerations of the mouth and throat may result in fistulas among the oral and nasal pharynx, larynx, and esophagus; strictures of the nasopharynx, uvula area, and mucous membranes of the mouth; and decreased range of motion of the mouth due to cicatricial changes.[25,79] More commonly, the oral ulcers in Behçet's disease may be minute, less invasive, and heal without sequelae.[14,68] Arma et al.[5] have postulated that dysphagia in Behçet's disease may also result from focal degenerative changes in the brain stem affecting the vagus supply of the esophageal wall with resultant absent ganglion cells of Auerbach's plexus.

Esophagus

Excluding the oral mucosa, the most common sites of gastrointestinal involvement in Behçet's disease are the terminal ileum, cecum, and ascending colon[53]; however, esophageal involvement has been amply described in the literature and may manifest itself by substernal pain, bleeding, dysphagia, and mediastinal abscess formation secondary to esophageal perforation.[5,11,28,35,40,45,46,53,61,67,78,79] Hemorrhagic ulcerative esophagitis has also been reported.[40] Various studies have shown that esophageal ulcers in Behçet's disease may be single, multiple, painless, painful, small, large, discrete, diffuse, shallow, penetrating, hemorrhagic, perforating, self-limited, located throughout the esophagus, and independent of corticosteroid administration.[35,40,46,53,67] In a comprehensive analysis of esophageal involvement in Behçet's disease, Mori et al.[53] concluded that the entire esophagus may be affected; however, the midportion was the most common site of disease activity with lesions consisting of erosions, ulcers, perforations, diffuse esophagitis, stenosis, strictures, and esophagobronchial fistulas. Esophageal stenosis may be extensive with rigidity and irregularity extending over 15 centimeters.[53] The posterior wall of the lower esophagus may also be involved frequently.[40] According to Mori et al.,[53] the ulcers histologically may reveal nonspecific lymphocytic or neutrophilic infiltrations with or without vasculitis. In one autopsy specimen, the esophageal erosions demonstrated vasculitis with lamillar proliferative exudative arteriolitis.[53] Some esophageal ulcers may have heaped-up inflamed margins, and some may heal with scarring.[40,67] Anticytoplasmic antibodies to human cadaver esophagus cells may be present in the sera of patients with Behçet's disease; however, their role in the pathogenesis of esophageal ulcerations is unknown.[59]

Kaplinsky et al.[35] described one patient with hematemesis, and on upper endoscopy the distal five centimeters of the esophagus revealed multiple, discrete, apparently superficial ulcers with normal intervening mucosa. Radiographic examination did not reveal these ulcerations, and the hematemesis was self-limited.[35] In the patient reported by Kikuchi et al.,[40] the barium swallow examination revealed multiple kissing-type gastric ulcers on the anterior and posterior walls of the body; however, esophagoscopy was necessary to visualize the four oval shallow esophageal ulcerations. The shape and motility of the esophagus at least by roentgenographic studies were normal; however, an esophageal mamometric study performed two weeks later revealed normal pressure of the lower esophageal sphincter, normal relaxation of the lower esophageal sphincter after swallowing, and normal acid clearance. The pressure at the level of the esophageal ulcer scars was slightly higher than normal. Biopsies of the active esophageal ulcers revealed nonspecific changes of the squamous epithelium underlined with infiltrates of acute and chronic inflammatory cells. There was no evidence of active vasculitis.[40] Similar histology was reported by Lockhart et al.[46]; however, biopsies of esophageal ulcers may also show suppurative esophagitis.[67] According to Kikuchi et al.,[40] the gastric ulcers in their patient responded to antacid therapy while the esophageal ulcers healed with scarring two weeks after beginning corticosteroid therapy.

In the patient with Behçet's disease and esophageal ulceration reported by Lockhart et al.,[46] esophageal motility was normal and there was no evidence of reflux esophagitis. Since the patient also had not received corticosteroid therapy prior to the diagnosis of her esophageal ulcer, the authors postulated that ulcer formation in Behçet's syndrome is part of the primary disease process. Repeat endoscopy six weeks later revealed an apparently normal esophageal mucosa without scar formation.[46] However, distal esophageal dilatation, gastroesophageal reflux, and disordered esophageal motility with spasm have been reported in Behçet's disease.[11,78]

Levack and Hanson[45] reported a patient with Behçet's disease who had a tracheoesophageal fistula involving the area of esophageal ulceration. Barium swallow revealed a distorted upper esophagus with a filling defect below the larynx, and at surgery a fistulous communication was seen in the tracheoesophageal septum. This was amenable to surgical intervention.[45] Wright[79] reported another patient with a fistula involving the pharynx, larynx, and esophagus.

In summary, esophageal ulcers in Behçet's disease may not be visualized roentgenographically, and thus esophagoscopy should be considered in those patients with hematemesis, substernal pain, and dysphagia for liquids or solid foods.[40] Since esophageal ulcers may be self-limited, it is difficult to accurately assess the therapeutic efficacy of various modalities, including antacids and corticosteroid therapy. Nevertheless, these medications have been used with apparently favorable experiences.[35,40,46,53,67]

According to Yashiro et al.,[85] three types of esophageal lesions can be identified in Behçet's syndrome; these consist of ulcers, varices, and dissection of the esophageal mucosa. As stated in the previous chapter, esophageal varices have developed as a result of occlusion of the splenic and azygos veins, subclavian veins, superior and inferior venae cavae, and the cervical and internal mammary systems.[85,86] In addition, the Budd-Chiari syndrome may be complicated by rupture of the esophageal varices.[87]

Stomach and Small Intestine

Patients with Behçet's disease may also have ulcerations of the stomach, duodenum, ampulla of Vater, ileum, and jejunum.[7,8,27,36,40,48,53,61] Clinically, these ulcers may produce symptoms mimicking those due to gastritis, peptic ulcer disease, inflammatory bowel disease, or appendicitis.[7,21,28,36,60,68,71] These gastrointestinal ulcers may be single or multiple, shallow or deep, circumscribed or diffuse, and may penetrate or perforate with resultant peritonitis.[61,88] Ulcerative hemorrhagic lesions may also involve the stomach and small bowel,[40] and the terminal ileum may become stenotic or form fistulous tracts with other portions of the intestinal tract, including the cecum.[78] However, if gastrointestinal fistulae are present, one must also consider Crohn's disease as the underlying disease process.

In a patient with Behçet's disease and gastric involvement, a barium roentgenographic examination revealed a ragged antral mucosa, and prepyloric ulcerated and elevated areas were demonstrated by endoscopy. Biopsy of an ulcerated lesion showed moderate inflammatory infiltration in the lamina propria, and the surface was covered by a single layer of cuboidal epithelial cells infiltrated by neutrophils. Also, beneath the epithelium, a fibrous reaction with associated lymphocytic cells was observed. The patient improved clinically after the initiation of prednisolone therapy.[89]

In one large series of 136 patients with Behçet's disease and intestinal ulcers requiring surgical intervention, the ulcers were most frequently found in the terminal ileum and the cecum. The patients' ages ranged from 10 to 66 years with a mean age of 35; 60% were males, 35% females, and 5% were of unspecified gender.[36] However, Behçet's syndrome with gastrointestinal tract involvement has also been reported during childhood even under the age of five years.[90] The interval between the initial diagnosis of Behçet's disease and laparotomy ranged from one month to 30 years with a mean of 6.6 years. The common sites of ulcer formation were the terminal ileum, ileocecal region, and the cecum, while the less frequent areas included the stomach, duodenum, jejunum, ileum, and the ascending and transverse colon. The indications for surgery were abdominal pain (92%), abdominal mass (21%), and/or melena (17%). Ulcer perforation occurred in 28 (41%) of 68 patients treated with corticosteroids and 5 of 15 (33%) of untreated patients.[36] However, according to Baba et al.,[7] steroids may not influence the incidence of perforation. The surgical specimens revealed the ulcers to be either localized or diffuse with undermining of the tissue and edema formation. Multiple perforations were also observed; however, the intestinal wall between the ulcers may be normal. Postoperatively, complications occurred in 44% and included reperforation, wound dehiscence, wound infection, hematemesis, melena, or loosening of the sutures. Ulcers recurred in 22 of 34 patients (65%) within six months; the significant incidence of these complications may reflect the recurrent nature of Behçet's disease.[36]

In another study[8] of 131 patients with Behçet's disease and intestinal involvement, the ulcers in the ileum were usually small, deep, and perforated readily, while those in the cecum were larger and seldom perforated. Histopathologically, the ulcers showed fissuring and nonspecific inflammatory reactions. The smaller arteries revealed intimal thickening and perivascular cellular infiltration, while the larger vessels were thrombosed. The venous structures demonstrated intimal proliferation and thrombus formation, and these changes were more prominent than those involving the arteries. Lymphatic dilatation and edema may be observed in both the submucosa surrounding the ulcers and the nonulcerative regions. Since microangiograms revealed avascular areas at the ulcer sites, thromboses of both arteries and veins may contribute to gastrointestinal ulcer formation in Behçet's disease. Additional pathogenetic factors postulated included the hypercoagulability state, ischemia, and vasculitis, which are characteristic features in Behçet's disease.[8]

The intestinal ulcers in Behçet's disease may be characterized by penetration to the serous membrane or fascia, tendency to irregular undermining of the tissue, and by edematous swelling and crater-shape formation. Histologically, the inflammation is transmural with lymphocytic infiltration and edema present in the submucosal layer. Also, intimal thickening, thrombi in vessels, and pericapillary and perivenular mononuclear infiltration may be observed in the vessels surrounding the ulcers. These histologic changes represent nonspecific inflammation.[36] In a pathological study by Fukuda and Watanabe,[91] the intestinal ulcers in patients with Behçet's disease histologically revealed nonspecific changes with inflammation of the venules, lymph vessel dilatation, and arterial intimal fibrous thickening. The microscopic changes of the venous structures were more prominent than those affecting the arterial vessels.[91] Besides nonspecific acute and chronic inflammation, the walls of the arteries and veins of the small bowel ulcers may reveal acute inflammatory changes with nuclear dust and fibrinoid necrosis affecting the arterioles.[61] The capillaries may also contain thrombi; these changes were compatible with vasculitis, including the leukocytoclastic type.[7,61,68] In an autopsy examination of a patient with Behçet's disease, the intestinal ulcerations were characterized by vasculitis of the small arteries, thrombophlebitis, and diffuse lymphocytic infiltration, especially prominent in the submucosa.[92] According to Katoh et al.,[92] an underlying systemic vasculitis is critical in the pathogenesis of the gastrointestinal complications in Behçet's disease. Also, as mentioned in Chapter 11, the vascular complications of Behçet's syndrome may result in aneurysms and occlusions of all sizes of intraabdominal arteries, including the abdominal aorta and mesenteric vessels.[68,93,94]

According to Asakura et al.,[6] 4 of 15 biopsy specimens of jejunal mucosa from patients with Behçet's disease revealed lymphangiectasia in the lamina propria, and electron microscopy showed precipitated lipoprotein-like substances in the extracellular spaces of the lamina propria and in the basal portions of the epithelium. Those villi with dilated lymphatic vessels and edema in the lamina propria were clubbed, finger-shaped, and roentgenographically, there was thickening of the intestinal folds with fragmentation or stippling of barium. Although the entity primary lymphangiectasia is characteristic of a protein-losing enteropathy, the serum levels of albumin and immunoglobulins were not decreased in patients with Behçet's disease and lymphangiectasia of the small intestine.[6,95]

According to McLean et al.,[58] one may demonstrate roentgenographically multiple discrete nodular lesions 8 to 12 mm in diameter with central ring-like collections of barium in the terminal ileum in Behçet's disease, and this sign may be pathognomonic of intestinal involvement in Behçet's syndrome. Oshima et al.[60] performed 141 gastrointestinal radiological examinations in 70 patients with Behçet's disease and observed abnormalities especially involving the small intestine. These abnormalities, which were more prominent during periods of disease activity as compared to periods of remission, consisted of localized or extensive dilatation, gas retention, hypotonia, fluid retention, flocculation, segmentation, and loss of the normal mucosal pattern.[60] Similarly, Shimizu et al.[68] have reported findings of the small intestine in Behçet's disease to include roughened folds, incomplete mixing of barium, "moulage sign," dilatation, distention, and gas retention. In light of these observations, malabsorption and abnormal digestion may be frequently present in those patients with Behçet's disease who have small-bowel involvement, especially during the acute phases of disease activity.[60,68] Decreased fat absorption has been reported in patients with Behçet's disease who had abnormal barium studies of the small intestine, and was most marked during the acute phases of gastrointestinal disease.[60]

Indium-111 granulocyte scanning of the gastrointestinal tract, which would identify areas of neutrophil infiltration, was studied in three patients with Behçet's disease including one with right-sided colitis associated with diarrhea and abdominal pain. All three patients had positive scans detected by gamma camera views, thus suggesting that white blood cell scans may offer a noninvasive means of identifying areas of intestinal abnormalities.[38]

Large Intestine

In Behçet's disease both hemorrhagic and nonhemorrhagic ulcerations may be detected in all portions of the large intestine including the cecum, ascending, transverse, and descending colon, sigmoid, rectum, and anus.[7,8,21,22,31,40,55,68] In one series of 60 cases of intestinal ulcers, the most common site was the ileum (75%), followed by the cecum (42%), ascending colon (13%), transverse colon (13%), descending colon (7%), sigmoid (5%), and rectum (3%). Many patients had multiple sites of involvement.[68] Large-bowel ulcers may be complicated by perforation, peritonitis, and hematochezia, and barium enema and colonoscopy may reveal large discrete deep ulcers with normal intervening mucosa and haustral markings.[21,22,39,55,90] Symptoms mimicking inflammatory bowel disease and acute appendicitis may occur in Behçet's syndrome.[7,28,36,57–59,71] The resected appendix from one Behçet's disease patient revealed three separate, sealed perforations with small abscesses at its base,[28] and in another patient, generalized purulent peritonitis due to a perforated ulcer at the base of the appendix was observed at laparotomy.[21] Histologically, lymphocytic vasculitis primarily involved the small veins and venules of the colonic ulcers of Behçet's disease.[32]

As suggested in this discussion, the relationships between inflammatory bowel disease and Behçet's disease are complex and somewhat controversial.[58,71] Difficulties may be encountered in distinguishing between Behçet's colitis with Crohn's disease and ulcerative colitis since all three illnesses may be associated with mucocutaneous, ocular, musculoskeletal, and vasculature complications.[56] In Behçet's disease the terminal ileum may become stenotic and ulcerated, with resultant fistula formation with the cecum,[78] and rectovaginal fistulas have been reported as complications of intestinal disease.[7,26,32,39,56,59,71] Nevertheless, the presence of intestinal fistulae is usually more indicative of Crohn's disease.

The distribution of ulcers in Behçet's disease may differ from those due to ulcerative colitis. In the latter condition the ulcers usually start in the rectum, whereas in Behçet's disease, the ileocecal area may be the most frequent site. In addition, the ulcers in Behçet's disease may be localized, deeper, multiple, scattered, and undermined; bowel involvement may be discontinuous; and the haustral markings may be intact. However, pseudopolypoid change and bridging formation have been reported in Behçet's colitis.[7] In one patient with presumed Behçet's disease and lower intestinal bleeding, superior mesenteric angiography did not reveal tortuous arteries, mucosal hyperemia or early venous filling, which are common radiographic findings in inflammatory bowel disease. Thus, angiography may assist in distinguishing between Behçet's colitis and ulcerative colitis.[72]

Rectal biopsies were performed in eight patients with Behçet's disease, and these were compared histologically with biopsies from normal controls and patients with ulcerative colitis. The biopsies from 50% of the patients with Behçet's disease showed mononuclear cell infiltration with eosinophils and mast cells. Additionally, IgM producing plasma cells and a few OKT4 (helper-inducer) positive cells were seen; however, there were no OKT8 (cytotoxic-suppressor) positive cells. In contrast the OKT8 positive cells were increased in rectal biopsies from patients with ulcerative colitis. Capillary deposits of immunoglobulins and complement components were not detected within the rectal specimens in Behçet's disease; however, they were positive in ulcerative colitis. Focal colitis as documented by rectal biopsy was demonstrable even in patients with Behçet's disease who lacked gastrointestinal symptoms.[2] In a surgical intestinal specimen from a patient with intestinal Behçet's disease, collections of lymphocytes as defined by anti-Leu series monoclonal antibodies surrounded the edges of the ulcers. Sixty percent of the T cells were Leu-3a positive (helper-inducer), and 30% were Leu-2a positive (cytotoxic-suppressor) T cells. The Leu-llb reactive cells or NK subsets were not detected.[96]

In comparison with Crohn's disease, there may be less of an inflammatory process surrounding the ulcer in Behçet's disease, that is, less thickening of the intestinal wall and less stenosis. Granulomas are infrequently observed in Behçet's disease, but the ulcers can be complicated by fistula formation. In Behçet's syndrome the intestinal ulcers are often multiple, distributed over a wider area, and perforate more readily.[7] However, Behçet's colitis and Crohn's disease have certain similar features, in that both disorders can affect the terminal ileum, have discrete ulcerations and skip areas of inflammation, are transmural in character, may involve the proximal colon with rectal sparing, and are characterized by aphthoid ulcerations.[25,56] In the report by O'Connell et al.,[56] one patient with Behçet's colitis had pancolitis with transmural inflammation, aphthoid ulcerations, and noncaseating granuloma formation, while a second patient had endoscopically aphthous colitis of the proximal colon and inflammatory changes in the distal ileum. Transmural lymphoid aggregates and submucosal fibrosis are more common in Crohn's colitis.[32]

According to various authors, patients with both Behçet's disease and inflammatory bowel disease have been reported in the literature.[52,58,59,62,97] Dr. O'Duffy[58] reported the histologic findings of chronic granulomatous colitis and granulomatous ileocolitis in patients meeting the diagnostic criteria of Behçet's disease. A subset of patients with Behçet's disease including those with central nervous system involvement may develop Crohn's disease at a later date.[37,52,57-59] Ramsay[63] reported a patient with Behçet's disease and acute ulcerative colitis, and Mir-Madjlessi and Farmer[52] described the occurrence of toxic megacolon plus Crohn's disease in a patient with Behçet's syndrome. Yim and White[97] reported three members of a family in whom the propositus had features of Behçet's disease plus Crohn's ileocolitis, a daughter without Behçet's disease who underwent a colectomy for ulcerative colitis, and a second daughter who had classic Behçet's disease including recurrent episodes of colitis with colonic aphthous ulcerations. In essence, Behçet's colitis is generally characterized by penetration of the ulcers to the serosa, often with perforation, clustering of discrete ulcers in the ileocecal area, and by the absence of granulomatous lesions histologically. Thus, the findings of this family suggested that inflammatory bowel disease and Behçet's syndrome may be interrelated and represent a disease continuum rather than distinct entities.[97]

Compounding the difficulties in distinguishing· between inflammatory bowel disease and Behçet's colitis, patients with Behçet's disease and either ischemic colitis or celiac disease have been reported.[65,70] The patient with celiac disease did improve with a gluten-free diet.[70] In addition, patients with Behçet's disease and renal involvement, especially those with the nephrotic syndrome, may have amyloidosis of the AA type detected on rectal biopsies. The amyloid may also be deposited within the walls of the small arteries and arterioles of various portions of the intestinal tract.[98–101] As mentioned in Chapter 9, patients with features of coexistent relapsing polychondritis and Behçet's disease have been reported by Firestein et al.[102] These patients had cartilage inflammation, gastrointestinal manifestations, oral and genital ulcers, arthritis, ocular inflammation, thrombosis, audiovestibular dysfunction, and vasculitis in various combinations. This constellation of findings was named the "mouth and genital ulcers with inflamed cartilage (MAGIC) syndrome," and the authors postulated that there may be a common mechanism of pathogenesis. Specifically, autoimmunity to components of cartilage, including proteoglycans or elastic tissue (elastin) but not type II collagen may be responsible for this disorder.[102]

Liver, Spleen, and Pancreas

Other intraabdominal organs including the liver, spleen, and pancreas may be affected in Behçet's disease.[13,27,68] Hepatomegaly and abnormal liver function tests have been occasionally reported in Behçet's disease.[23,27,60,103] In one series,[13] transient elevations in alkaline phosphatase with other normal liver function tests were detected during periods of disease activity; however, liver biopsies performed in five patients were normal. Elevations in liver function tests may not be accompanied by symptoms indicative of hepatic dysfunction.[13]

Good et al.[27] described a patient with Behçet's disease with massive hemobilia and multiple hepatic abscesses secondary to a penetrating ulcer at the ampulla of Vater. When initially evaluated, the patient had mild elevations in his liver function tests; however, the liver biopsy was normal. Subsequently, the patient developed hepatosplenomegaly with persistent mild to moderate elevations in the liver function tests. His clinical course was eventually complicated by gastrointestinal bleeding, necessitating an exploratory laparotomy which disclosed a penetrating bleeding duodenal ulcer at the ampulla of Vater. The gallbladder and common bile duct were distended with blood. The patient did not survive the operative procedure, and at autopsy the pancreas was hemorrhagic and edematous, and the liver revealed multiple abscesses. Histologically, the gallbladder showed acute and chronic inflammation, and the bile ducts revealed diffuse cholangitis with purulent exudates in the ductal structures. Other findings included an enlarged congested spleen, and fibrosis, edema, and fat necrosis of the pancreas. The authors maintained that the precipitating event in this patient was the penetrating duodenal ulcer which involved the ampulla of Vater and obstructed the biliary tract.[27]

In patients with Behçet's disease, one may encounter thrombophlebitis affecting the portal and hepatic veins with the latter presenting as the Budd-Chiari syndrome.[42,68,83,86,104-108] Kansu et al.[86] have reported a patient with Behçet's disease and probable Budd-Chiari syndrome who on physical examination had hepatomegaly, marked ascites, and rapidly developing hepatic coma. The abdomen was moderately distened with free fluid, and there were numerous collateral vessels on its wall. Except for a minimal elevation in the alanine aminotransferase, the liver function tests were normal; however, the liver spleen scan revealed hepatomegaly with small scattered defects. Histologically, the liver biopsy demonstrated congestion of the sinusoids, marked cholestasis, and focal necrosis of the parenchymal cells. These changes were compatible with the Budd-Chiari syndrome; however, the patient did not survive his acute illness.[86]

McDonald and Gad-Al-Rab[83] reported another patient with Behçet's disease complicated by the Budd-Chiari syndrome. Physical findings consisted of hepatomegaly, distended abdomen, prominent collateral veins on the abdominal wall, and jaundice. Ascites was not present; however, the patient developed hepatic coma. Tests of liver function including bilirubin, alkaline phosphatase, and asparate aminotransferase were moderately elevated. The liver on postmortem examination revealed centrilobular congestion and necrosis with reticulin collapse and infiltration by polymorphonuclear leukocytes. The hepatic veins and the intrahepatic venous structures were occluded by thrombi, and the walls of the hepatic veins contained lymphocytic infiltrations. Sections of the veins revealed recanalized organized thrombi consisting of collagenous tissue. In other areas of the liver, cholestasis and hemosiderin deposits were detected, and the spleen, which weighed 280 grams, was congested.[83]

Ferraris et al.[105] reported a 16-year-old Italian boy with Behçet's disease and the Budd-Chiari syndrome who developed ascites and suprahepatic portal hypertension. Tests of liver function including bilirubin, alkaline phosphatase, gamma-glutamyltransferase, alanine aminotransferase, and asparate aminotransferase were elevated, and selective celiac arteriography revealed delayed emptying of the portal venous system and the presence of a collateral venous circulation which drained the liver through the superior vena cava and the inferior mesenteric vein. There was no evidence of cirrhosis at least by peritoneoscopy.[105]

The simultaneous occurrence of focal proliferative glomerulonephritis with occasional crescent formation, ascites, and the Budd-Chiari syndrome in a patient with Behçet's disease has been described by Wilkey et al.[108] The alkaline phosphatase and gamma-glutamyltransferase were moderately elevated; however, aspartate aminotransferase was normal. Analysis of the ascitic fluid was compatible with an exudate. The liver tissue obtained at premortem and postmortem was congested and showed multiple large venous channels with organizing thrombi. The larger hepatic veins contained adherent thrombi, and the hepatic architecture revealed extensive centrilobular necrosis.[108] The Budd-Chiari syndrome in Behçet's disease is thus very similar to the Budd-Chiari syndrome due to various other causes with respect to clinical findings, laboratory data, hepatic congestion, histopathology, and generally poor prognosis.[109,110] The patient reported by Ferraris et al.,[105] however, had resolution of his ascites and hepatic enlargement concomitantly with the institution of furosemide, spironolactone, prednisone, and azathioprine.

Anti et al.[3] have reported fatty metamorphoresis of the liver and chronic active hepatitis in patients with Behçet's disease, but these disorders may have represented complications of therapy or the presence of other unrelated illnesses. Manna et al.[111] described the occurrence of chronic active hepatitis in a patient with Behçet's disease. Histologically, the needle biopsy specimen of the liver demonstrated piecemeal necrosis and portal lymphomonocytic infiltration with extension into the lobule. Additionally, the degree of elevation in liver function tests paralleled the manifestations of extrahepatic disease activity.[111]

Various investigators have focused on the incidence, of hepatitis B virus antigenemia in patients with Behçet's disease.[112-115] Although a significant proportion of patients with Behçet's disease may possess hepatitis B virus antigenemia especially if they reside in countries with a high frequency of infection with this agent, the specific role of this virus in the pathogenesis of Behçet's syndrome is unknown.[112-115] Patients with either Behçet's disease or hepatitis B virus infection may indeed manifest clinical signs and symptoms due to an immune complex–mediated vasculitis affecting the small, medium, and large arteries.[68,116-121] Anecdotal case reports of patients with Behçet's disease and hepatitis B antigenemia manifesting unusual features of their illnesses have appeared in the literature.[122-124]

Cadman et al.[122] have reported a patient with Behçet's disease complicated by diffuse bilateral pulmonary infiltrates and hemoptysis whose peripheral blood tested positive for hepatitis B antigen by radioimmunoassay. Despite normal liver function tests and a liver spleen scan, the liver biopsy specimen showed nonspecific portal and parenchymal focal inflammation with vasculitis. The patient's pulmonary symptoms were controlled with prednisone and cyclophosphamide.[122] In one report a patient with Behçet's syndrome who was a chronic carrier of hepatitis surface antigen experienced recurrent leg ulcerations which histologically demonstrated leukocytoclastic vasculitis. Many of these ulcerations were covered by eschar, and the leg ulcers responded to prednisone and chlorambucil therapy. A liver biopsy was not performed.[123] Schiff et al.[124] described a 31-year-old patient with Behçet's disease who years after the onset of his illness developed hepatitis B viral infection and recurrent episodes of ventricular tachyarrhythmias. Cardiac catheterization showed total occlusion of the left anterior descending coronary artery, and the patient subsequently died from an acute myocardial infarction complicated by refractory ventricular tachycardia. On autopsy the left anterior descending vessel was completely occluded; however, the histology of the liver was not mentioned.[124] The role of hepatitis B virus antigenemia in the clinical manifestations of these patients remains an enigma.

Splenomegaly, which may be secondary to portal hypertension, has been described in patients with Behçet's disease,[16,27,105,125-127] and in the patient reported by Good et al.[27] with duodenal ulcer, hepatic abscesses, and fatal hemobilia, the spleen at postmortem examination revealed congestive changes. Kiernan et al.[127] described the clinical courses of two patients with Behçet's disease and splenomegaly. One patient with hepatomegaly had a spleen 15 cm below the costal margin, and splenoportography showed normal splenic and portal veins with no varices. The liver biopsy specimen demonstrated inflammatory cells around the portal tracts, and at the time of a diagnostic laparotomy the resected spleen weighed 1,330 grams but did not reveal any specific histologic abnormalities. The second patient's spleen at one time was palpable at the umbilicus, but this rapidly decreased in size to 3 cm below the costal margin within 24 hours after initiating prednisone therapy. The patient expired two years later, and at necropsy the spleen, which weighed 560 grams, had normal histology.[127] Kansu et al.[106] reported esophageal varices in a patient with Behçet's disease which were probably secondary to thrombosis of the splenic vein. Also, amyloidosis may involve the spleen in patients with Behçet's disease,[98,128] and the necropsy of one patient revealed systemic amyloidosis and a "sago" spleen.[128]

The occurrence of pancreatitis and diabetes mellitus has been reported by Lakhanpal et al.[42] and Fishof[129] in patients with Behçet's disease. In a cumulative review of the Japanese autopsy registry data, pathological findings have included fatty liver, hepatic congestion, hepatomegaly, cirrhosis, acute hepatitis, chronic hepatitis, toxic hepatitis, liver abscess, cholelithiasis, acute cholecystitis, splenitis, splenic congestion, splenomegaly, hemosiderosis, splenic infarction, autosplenectomy, pancreatitis, and diabetes mellitus. It is not known, however, if these conditions were secondary to Behçet's disease and/or its therapy or represented other unrelated disease processes.[42]

Genitourinary Involvement

This discussion of the lower genitourinary tract will not include genital ulcerations since these have been reviewed in another chapter as part of the triple symptom complex. Several distinct clinical entities may affect the lower genitourinary tract in Behçet's disease, including thrombophlebitis of the penile veins, urine retention, and transient or recurrent urethritis, epididymitis, and orchitis.[9,13,33,47,49,68,73,130-133] According to the Behçet's Disease Research Committee of Japan,[1] epididymitis, which is listed as a minor criterion, presents as a transient swelling with haphalgesia. Epididymitis may occur with variable frequency, can present as spontaneous painless or painful swelling lasting for one to two weeks, and may be recurrent.[13,49,68] Urethroscopic examination in a patient with Behçet's disease and recurrent epididymitis associated with a urethral discharge disclosed aphthous ulcerations of the urethral mucous membrane.[131] Orchitis may be painful, affect both testes, and may be accompanied by fever.[49]

Bladder involvement may also occur in Behçet's disease,[134,135] and one patient reported by Carswell[134] presented with profuse hematuria. Intravenous urography revealed right-sided hydroureter and hydronephrosis, and biopsy of a bladder lesion showed acute inflammation with mucosal ulceration. Since several of the blood vessels were surrounded by inflammatory infiltrates and contained thrombi, it was suggested that vascular occlusion accounted for the bladder necrosis. Repeat investigations at a later date showed resolution of the hematuria and a normal pyelogram.[134] Thus, bladder ulcers may also occur in patients with Behçet's disease.[134,135]

In a venereological practice in London, Dunlop[136] evaluated 45 patients with Behçet's disease and reported such genitourinary disorders as candidosis, herpes progenitalis, "nonspecific urethritis," trichomoniasis, gonorrhea, and syphilis. Thus, patients with Behçet's syndrome and symptoms referable to the lower genitourinary tract must be evaluated for various diseases that are probably unrelated to their primary illness. Other genitourinary complications reported in Behçet's disease have included hydrocele, varicocele, neurogenic bladder from nervous system involvement, trigonal ulcerations, cystitis, ruptured urinary bladder, prostatic enlargement, pyogenic prostatitis, ovarian cysts, and rectovesical and rectovaginal fistulae.[7,42,47,49,68,71] However, some of these conditions may represent disorders occurring independently of Behçet's disease.[42] In an autopsy of a patient with Behçet's syndrome, the arteries and veins in the parovarian region revealed thrombi and there was extensive inflammation in the surrounding adipose and muscle tissues.[83]

Dermatologic Manifestations

Of the various cutaneous manifestations occurring in Behçet's disease, erythema nodosum-like lesions, subcutaneous thrombophlebitis, folliculitis or acne-like lesions, and cutaneous hypersensitivity or pathergy are listed as one major criterion.[1] The erythema nodosum-like lesions were described by the Behçet's Disease Research Committee of Japan[1] as consisting of tender, raised red nodes that appear more commonly on the anterior surfaces of the legs and slowly resolve within a few weeks without scar formation. These lesions can also occur at other sites, including the face, neck, and buttocks, may be recurrent, and may heal with cutaneous hyperpigmentation.[59,68] According to several investigators, the erythema nodosum-like lesions may also be small, sparse or multiple, grouped together, tender, and colorless, red, or blue.[47,137] Systemic symptoms including malaise and fever may accompany erythema nodosum in Behçet's disease.[49] Histologically, one may observe perivascular cell infiltration, fibrin deposition in the vessel walls, and perivascular connective tissue within the dermis and subcutaneous tissues. This inflammatory process affects venules to a greater extent than the arterioles.[68] According to Nazarro,[138] the erythema nodosum-like lesions in Behçet's disease differ histologically from classic erythema nodosum since they lack giant cells and histiocytic granulomas; however, this differential point may be controversial.[57,139] In one study, biopsy specimens from the early-appearing erythema nodosum-like lesions revealed predominately lymphocytes, while the cellular infiltrates in the chronic ones consisted mainly of polymorphonuclear leukocytes; using monoclonal antibodies in an immunoperoxidase technique, Yamana et al.[140] have shown that of the infiltrating T lymphocytes, 60 to 80% possessed the helper-inducer phenotype, 20 to 40% were cytotoxic-suppressor cells, and 5% of the infiltrating lymphocytes in four of seven patients were NK cells. According to Marufi et al.,[141] apparently normal skin in patients with Behçet's disease may also demonstrate histologic abnormalities. In this study there were endothelial proliferation and perivascular lymphocytic infiltrates affecting the blood vessel walls in skin biopsies obtained from the deltoid region in 12 of 15 patients with Behçet's disease.[141]

The subcutaneous venules in Behçet's disease may develop thrombosis leading to sclerosis, and on examination the venous structures can be palpated as painful subcutaneous nodules or string-like hardenings with reddening of the overlying skin.[1,68] These palpable subcutaneous strands may occur after injection or venipuncture, may resemble migrating obliterative thrombophlebitis, and may resolve spontaneously.[1,13,68] Superficial thrombophlebitis may be migrating, may occur spontaneously or following venipuncture and intravenous infusions including heparin and radiographic contrast material, may be accompanied by fever, prostration, local pain, swelling, and tenderness, may persist for several weeks, may spontaneous resolve only to recur, and may be complicated by local sequelae including postphlebitic edema of the extremities and prolonged leg ulcers (ulcus cruris).[13]

The acneiform skin eruptions probably represent a folliculitis resembling acne vulgaris and may appear as numerous papules and postules on the face, breast, thorax, neck, and extremities. However, pruritus and comedone formation are unusual manifestations.[1,9,68,138] In one study of 297 patients with Behçet's disease, folliculitis and thrombophlebitis were more common among males, while erythema nodosum was more prominent among female patients.[142] Other cutaneous lesions occurring in Behçet's disease include nodules, vesicles, ulcerations with or without eschar, furuncles, abscesses, pyodermas, impetigo, cellulitis, erythema multiforme-like lesions, psoriasis, purpura, dermatographism, urticaria, eczema, paronychia, hidradenitis suppurativa, and subungual flame-shaped hemorrhagic lesions or infarcts.[13, 14,23,48,49,59,68,73,80,123,126,137–139,143–145] Some of these, as for example purpura, dermatographism, urticaria, eczema, and hidradenitis suppurativa, may represent unrelated diseases, and the relationship of sepsis to the cutaneous manifestations of Behçet's disease remains unknown.[14,48,80] Many patients with Behçet's disease may have several different cutaneous lesions concurrently, with the lesions spontaneously remitting within 7 to 14 days only to recur days to months later. These various lesions may be painful, may heal with scar formation, and because of cutaneous hyperirritability or hyperreactivity (pathergy), may be initiated by local trauma. [13,48,68,138,143,144] According to Nazarro,[138] the papulopustular skin lesions are the most characteristic of Behçet's disease. These lesions commence as minute, erythematous, slightly tender papules and may either regress within a few days or evolve into pustules with occasional ulcer formation. Pathogenetically, Jorizzo et al.[146] have described pustular vasculitis of Behçet's disease as arising from an interaction between circulating immune complex–mediated vessel damage and enhancement of polymorphonuclear leukocyte migration by a heat-stable serum factor. The papulonodular manifestations of Behçet's syndrome are larger than the papulopustular lesions, are typically painful and transient, resolve within a few days without scar formation, and do not evolve into ulcers or pustules.[138] Dermo-hypodermitis may be the most frequent cutaneous manifestation of Behçet's syndrome, may resemble circular dermo-hypodermic nodules, and may appear as erythematous, tender, and slightly painful nodules. Spontaneous regression may occur within 10 to 15 days and without ulceration or residuum. Occasionally, however, minute sclerotic areas remain after the regression of the lesions. These nodules generally appear with recrudescence of the other manifestations of Behçet's disease and may be accompanied by a systemic febrile response.[138]

Gangrene, which may affect either small or large areas, as for example fingertips or feet, has also been reported in patients with Behçet's disease, and histologic studies of the amputated tissues have shown thrombotic occlusion of the arteries and veins accompanied by an acute inflammatory process involving the walls of these vessels. Thus, the underlying pathogenetic mechanism accounting for gangrene in Behçet's disease may be a vasculitis affecting different-sized vessels.[73,147,148]

Similarly, the underlying histopathological feature in many of the cutaneous manifestations in Behçet's syndrome is an inflammatory vasculitis, probably immune complex–mediated, involving veins, venules, capillaries, arterioles, and arteries with vascular and perivascular infiltration by varying proportions of polymorphonuclear leukocytes, mononuclear cells, and plasma cells.[13, 41,57,59,68,116,118,138,149,150] However, vasculitis may not always be demonstrable; rather, one may observe microscopically perivascular infiltrates with predominantly polymorphonuclear or mononuclear cells.[138,149,151,152] Mast cells may also be present in the cutaneous lesions in patients with Behçet's disease, and these were quantified in spontaneous and localized trauma-induced (reactive) skin lesions and in apparently normal skin. Based upon the histologic studies of biopsy specimens, there was a significant increase in the number of mast cells in the reactive and spontaneous skin lesions as compared with the apparently uninvolved skin of patients during the active stage of Behçet's disease. The "uninvolved skin" revealed either normal or a slightly elevated number of mast cells. The mast cell counts were also increased in the erythema nodosum-like lesions in Behçet's disease as compared to the erythema nodosum lesions associated with other conditions. The histamine content was increased twofold in the reactive or pathergic lesions, and the percentage of degranulating mast cells was markedly increased in both the pathergic and spontaneously occurring skin lesions, thus implying an active role for the mast cell in the pathogenesis of the cutaneous lesions in Behçet's disease. Mechanisms similar to cutaneous basophil hypersensitivity may enable the mast cell to contribute to the production of skin lesions in Behçet's disease.[151–154] Many patients with Behçet's disease will also have elevated serum IgE levels.[151]

Langerhans cells are normally located in the midepidermis of the skin, as well as in lymph nodes, spleen, tonsils, thymus, dermis, and the epithelia of the oral and genital mucous membranes.[155–158] These cells originate from the bone marrow mesenchymal precursors and, like marcophages, have cell surface Ia antigens and membrane receptors for the C3b complement component and the Fc portion of IgG. These markers participate in the recognition of antigens and in the interactions with T lymphocytes, thus enabling the Langerhans cells to participate in cell-mediated reactions.[157] The Langerhans cells probably process foreign antigen for presentation to the T lymphocytes possessing identical Ia antigens, and as a result, these activated T lymphocytes react with foreign antigen-bearing Ia antigen compatible Langerhans cells in the epidermis, causing the Langerhans cells to produce an interleukin-1-like molecule named epidermal cell-derived thymocyte-activation factor (ETAF), and to release lysosomal enzymes which may contribute to the production of inflammation, especially T-cell-dependent immune responses including syngeneic and allogeneic T-cell activation and epidermal cell-induced cytotoxic T-cell responses.[156-159] Skin biopsies from erythema nodosum-like lesions in patients with Behçet's disease were compared with biopsies obtained from normal controls. The Langerhans cells in biopsies in Behçet's disease were mainly situated in the midepidermis (89%), but some were just beneath the stratum granulosum (11%), as compared to controls in which these cells were distributed unevenly throughout the epidermis. In addition, the Langerhans cells in Behçet's disease had more prominent rough endoplasmic reticulum and granules than in controls. Thus, the Langerhans cells in Behçet's disease are in a more active metabolic state; however, the role of these cells in the cutaneous expressions of Behçet's disease is unknown.[160]

Pathergy

A peculiar characteristic of patients with Behçet's disease is the phenomenon of skin pathergy or hyperirritability (hyperreactivity) occurring at the site of minor trauma.[13,68] This phenomenon was initially mentioned by Blobner[161] (Blobner phenomenon) and Jensen,[162] and was further reviewed by Katzenellenbogen.[82] Pathergy is manifested clinically by erythematous induration, a papule or an aseptic pustule at the site of a needle stick or trauma; may be maximally visible by 48 hours; and may evolve into a sterile ulcer.[13,68,138,144,151-154,163] The pustule usually resolves in four to five days.[138] The presence of only erythema without induration is considered a negative test.[164] Injection of such substances as physiological saline, isoosmotic phosphate buffer, phosphate-buffered saline, distilled water, heat-aggregated human gamma globulin, saliva, autogenous plasma, or an aseptic extract of a genital ulcer can induce grossly similar reactions.[13,68,132,138,144,151-154,]

[163,165-167] The pathergic lesion produced by the latter antigen was named the Behçetin reaction.[47,68,144,166,168] Depending upon the study, the intracutaneous injection of physiological saline and sterile needle prick might elicit the more pronounced reactions,[163,167] and according to Dilsen et al.,[169] the subcutaneous application of a needle stick may be the most sensitive means of eliciting pathergy. The topical application of hydrocortisone and ointments containing gentamicin, bacitracin and fradiomycin, and tetracycline may impair or prevent pathergy; and of these antibiotics, the latter had the greatest effect in suppressing cutaneous hyperreactivity.[138,164,167]

Pathergy may be demonstrated experimentally on the skin, including the integument of the genitalia and the oral mucosa; and aphthous ulcers and cutaneous lesions including edematous induration, papules, pustules, and folliculitis have been reported to follow natural trauma. Needle stick or injection of physiological saline may produce oral and genital ulcers whose clinical courses are similar to spontaneously appearing lesions, and systemic symptoms including headache, weakness, and fever may accompany the pathergic lesions.[138,144] Generally, pathergy is not invariably present in untreated Behçet's disease; pathergy is not consistently reproduced in the same individual; variations in the interpretation of the pathergy test exist among different observers and the same observer; the presence of pathergy may be demonstrable only microscopically; and pathergy may not predictably correlate with the presence of clinical symptoms, including aphthae, ocular manifestations, erythema nodosum, folliculitis, and thrombophlebitis or the results of laboratory tests including leukocytosis and sedimentation rate.[68,167,170-174] Thus, there may exist discordance between the presence or strength of the pathergy reaction and the clinical severity of Behçet's disease[132,167,173-176]; however, the degree of positivity of the cutaneous hyperirritability reaction may occasionally correlate with disease activity.[138,177,178] According to Aksungur et al.,[175] the presence and not the absolute degree of pathergy might be a better indicator of disease activity in Behçet's syndrome.

Since not all needle sticks or injections applied concurrently in the same individual to different areas of apparently normal skin will demonstrate pathergy, one visibly negative test does not negate the presence of cutaneous hyperirritability.[167,169] According to

Dilşen et al.,[169] the intensity of the cutaneous reactions at four different sites of concurrent injections in the same individual revealed homogeneous or heterogeneous reactions. The highest number of positive reactors was detected by subcutaneous needle pricks using four different cutaneous areas. In another study, the false-negative reaction rate was reduced from 48% to 16% in Behçet's disease by applying 10 intradermal injections of physiological saline.[167]

Male patients with Behçet's disease may have a higher prevalence of pathergy positivity and stronger pathergy reactions as compared to females.[176] Aral et al.[179] have observed positive skin pathergy reactions in healthy family members of patients with Behçet's disease and negative results in 122 healthy controls and 240 patients with diseases other than Behçet's syndrome. Thus, Aral et al.[179] have postulated that skin pathergy may represent a specific genetic marker of Behçet's disease. Also, Turkish patients with Behçet's disease have a higher prevalence of pathergy and the HLA-B5 (Bw 51 split) antigen as compared to North American and British patients with Behçet's disease, and at least in Turkish patients the absence of these two markers virtually excluded the diagnosis of Behçet's disease. These observations were not observed in British patients with Behçet's disease since the possession of the HLA-B5 (Bw 51 split) histocompatibility antigen was not increased as compared to normal controls. Also, normal British subjects carrying the HLA-Bw 51 antigen had negative pathergy tests. In summary, there was no correlation between pathergy and either the possession of the HLA-B5 (Bw 51 split) antigen or types of clinical manifestations in British patients with Behçet's syndrome. The high prevalence of this allele is also observed in Japan, South France, and Israel but not in the United States.[171,180-185]

Pathergy is not pathognomonic for Behçet's disease since it may occur in patients with recurrent idiopathic aphthous ulcerations, iridocyclitis, idiopathic erythema nodosum, continuous elevated erythema syndrome, pyoderma gangrenosum, herpes genitalis, rheumatoid arthritis, and healthy family members of patients with Behçet's disease.[68,132,152,164,171,179,186] Although patients with isolated aphthous ulcerations, iridocyclitis, or erythema nodosum and pathergy have been reported, it is not known if any of these patients evolved into classic Behçet's disease.[152,164,171,181] Both pyoderma gangrenosum and pathergy have been reported by Powell et al.[186] in patients lacking the complete triad of Behçet's disease; that is, some of these patients had recurrent aphthous stomatitis. Therefore, long-term follow-up is needed to determine if any of these patients will evolve into classic Behçet's disease. According to Powell et al.[186] and Domonkos et al.,[187] pyoderma gangrenosum has been reported in patients with Behçet's disease. Nevertheless, since the incidence of pathergy in patients with pyoderma gangrenosum was 25% of 86 patients in the series by Powell et al.,[186] one would predict that not all of these patients would develop Behçet's disease. Patients with sarcoidosis may demonstrate the formation of scar tissue at the sites of trauma, including the tuberculin skin test site, and these areas may later reveal inflammatory changes histologically similar to spontaneously occurring skin lesions.[188]

In patients with Behçet's disease, false-positive or hyperreactive cutaneous reactions have been widely reported to such antigens as tuberculin, lepromin, *Canadida albicans*, trichophytin, histoplasmin, coccidioidin, streptococcus toxoid, streptokinase-streptodornase, Staphylococcus vaccine, Hemophilus Ducrey vaccine, dmelcos (Hemophilus ducreyi), Frei and leishmanin.[16,49,73,82,130,138,144,175,189,190] According to Aksungur et al.,[175] patients with Behçet's disease may show hyperreaction to the PPD skin test with the center of the induration forming a bullous lesion within a short time. Biopsies obtained from a spontaneous skin lesion, positive skin reactivity test, and the positive PPD test site all showed similar histology which resembled the Arthus reaction. The positive tuberculin skin site revealed vasculitis with nuclear dust comparable to leukocytoclastic vasculitis and thus is different from the pathology observed in patients with a true positive PPD skin test which demonstrates changes histologically indicative of cell-mediated immunity.[175] According to Lee et al.,[191] the positive rate of tuberculin reactivity in Behçet's disease was not dependent upon the types of clinical manifestations. False-positive cutaneous reactions have not usually been reported following routine allergy skin testing, perhaps since such reactions represent a Type I hypersensitivity response.[166,172] Despite these various inadequacies, skin pathergy may serve as a useful marker for the internist or rheumatologist confronted with a patient not manifesting the classic triple symptom complex.[192]

Various studies have been performed in attempts to correlate the diminution in the degree of positivity of pathergy skin testing with the suppression of clinical disease activity by immunosuppressive and antiinflammatory agents including prednisone, thalidomide, cyclophosphamide, dapsone, and colchicine. Despite the many variables in pathergy skin testing, several investigators have observed a correlation between the suppression of the clinical symptoms and negative or diminished skin pathergy; however, this has definitely not been a universal observation.[123,138,146,165,173–177,178,193] Also, immunosuppressive agents may not alter either the gross appearance or the histology of the pathergy test,[164] and there may exist disordance between skin hyperreactivity and clinical disease activity.[123]

The histopathological findings of cutaneous pathergy lesions are dependent on methodology of induction and time of biopsy.[137,138,144,146,152,163,164,173,174] Cutaneous biopsies obtained at four hours following the intradermal injection of histamine phosphate (modified Braverman's "histamine trap test") may reveal by immunofluorescent microscopy deposition of immunoreactants (IgM, IgG, Clq, C3) or fibrin in the walls of the dermal blood vessels.[146,173,174] At six hours following the application of a needle prick, there may be an inflammatory infiltrate composed mainly of polymorphonuclear leukocytes which may be immune complex and complement–mediated.[164] At 24 hours one may observe findings consistent with either leukocytoclastic vasculitis or Sweet's-like vasculitis (neutrophilic vascular reaction). Pathological findings in leukocytoclastic vasculitis consist of endothelial swelling of dermal blood vessels; perivascular neutrophilic infiltration with degeneration of the leukocytes (leukocytoclasis); invasion of the walls of arterioles, capillaries, and venules by neutrophils; fibrinoid necrosis; and extravasation of erythrocytes. Histologically, the neutrophilic vascular reaction is characterized by minimal or absent fibrinoid necrosis, and leukocytoclasia and extravasation of erythrocytes are not prominent features.[146,174] Direct immunofluorescence of 24-hour-old cutaneous hyperreactivity lesions may reveal IgG or IgM, Clq, C3, C4, and fibrin in the dermal vessel walls.[194] Alternatively, one may observe at 24 hours endothelial swelling of blood vessel walls and perivascular accumulation of polymorphonuclear leukocytes or an inflammatory infiltrate consisting of neutrophils, mononuclear cells, and a significant mast cell infiltration.[164,173] In a study of pathergy conducted by Haim et al.,[152] vasculitis was not observed, but rather perivascular lymphocytic infiltrates were demonstrable by light microscopy. Small clusters of polymorphonuclear leukocytes were observed in a few specimens; however, these were thought to result directly from tissue damage induced by the injections. Immunofluorescent microscopy did not reveal any evidence of immunoglobulins or complement.[152]

According to Yazaki,[195] light microscopy of skin lesions induced by the intracutaneous injection of physiological saline revealed edema, fibrin deposition, polymorphonuclear infiltration, and microabscesses surrounded by perivascular infiltration with mononuclear cells, histiocytes, and neutrophils. The reaction peaked at 24 hours and persisted for 48 hours. Based upon electron microscopic studies, the infiltrating neutrophils contained phagocytic vacuoles and phagocytized erythrocytes. Also, the neutrophil granules were present more commonly adjacent to or within the phagocytic vacuoles, and degranulation of polymorphonuclear leukocytes with degeneration of cytoplasm and nuclei were present.[195] In another study, skin biopsies obtained after 24 hours showed a predominance of mononuclear cells.[164]

Based upon histologic studies of skin biopsies obtained from patients with Behçet's disease, Lichtig et al.[153,154] and Haim et al.[151,152] have shown the presence of an increased number of mast cells in the reactive or pathergic lesions induced by either needle prick or the intracutaneous injection of normal saline. In addition, the histamine content of the reactive lesions showed a twofold increase in comparison to apparently normal skin in patients with active Behçet's disease, and there was a marked increase in the percentage of degranulating mast cells in the pathergic lesions.[153,154] Thus, the mast cell is metabolically active in the hyperreactive lesion, and it may contribute to the pathogenesis of this phenomenon. The number of mast cells was either normal or slightly increased in apparently normal skin from patients with active Behçet's disease.[152]

Biopsies of needle-prick-induced skin lesions in Behçet's disease have revealed histologically an increased number of Langerhans cells in the prickle cell layer. These Langerhans cells contained lattice-shaped granules in their mitochondria and were in contact with lymphocytes.[196] Thus in patients with Behçet's disease, the Langerhans cells may be just as important in the pathogenesis of pathergy as they are in the development of spontaneous lesions.[160,196]

Sobel et al.[163] studied the specific cutaneous responses to needle prick and to the intradermal injections of autologous plasma and normal saline. At the sites of needle prick or saline injection, various degrees of perivascular mononuclear cell infiltration were demonstrated histologically, and the skin biopsy at the site of the needle prick from one patient also revealed an acute inflammatory response with necrosis. In contradistinction, the intradermal injection of autologous plasma produced more frequently acute inflammation with perivascular granulocytic infiltration and necrosis within the dermis.[163] In another study of four patients with Behçet's disease, the pathergic lesions produced by the intradermal injection of sterile heparinized autologous plasma histologically showed an acute inflammatory reaction in the dermis with endothelial swelling and infiltrates of neutrophils and eosinophils. Leukocytoclastic vasculitis was observed in one biopsy specimen, and the pathological findings were postulated to represent an Arthus reaction.[165] Djawari et al.[197] studied the Rebuck skin window examination in patients with active Behçet's disease and positive pathergy tests. This study revealed a more rapid acceleration of an influx of polymorphonuclear leukocytes compared to normal controls followed by a rapid depletion of these cells and an influx of mononuclear cells, some of which phagocytized erythrocytes. There was a paucity of polymorphonuclear leukocytes observed in 8- to 16-hour-old skin puncture lesions, and after 24 hours mononuclear cells predominated.[197]

In summary, pathergy may reflect a mucocutaneous reaction of hyperirritability or hyperreactivity induced by trauma with resultant papules or aseptic pustules that are similar both macro- and microscopically to those appearing spontaneously in patients with Behçet's disease. Since the inflammatory cells in the early and late lesions are the polymorphonuclear leukocyte and lymphocyte, respectively, immune complex-Arthus-type reactions and delayed hypersensitivity may explain the pathogenesis of these early and late reactions, respectively.[151,152,163,165,175] Not only do the neutrophils from patients with Behçet's syndrome show enhanced chemotaxis, but similar data have been obtained from studies of mononuclear cells.[123,198] Thus, the mononuclear cell may be of primary immunopathogenic importance[199] in the cutaneous manifestations of Behçet's syndrome, including the phenomenon of pathergy.

References

1. Behçet's Disease Research Committee of Japan. Behçet's disease: Guide to diagnosis of Behçet's disease. *Jpn J Ophthalmol* 1974; 18:291–294.
2. Akoğlu T, Tuncer I, Sandicki M, et al. Focal colitis in Behçet's disease (abstract 72). Royal Society of Medicine international conference on Behçet's disease, September 5 and 6, 1985, London, England.
3. Anti M, Marra G, Bochicchio GB, et al. Gut problems in Behçet's syndrome (abstract 73). Royal Society of Medicine international conference on Behçet's disease, September 5 and 6, 1985, London, England.
4. Anti M, Marra G, Rapaccini GL, Fedeli G. Ulcerative esophagitis in Behçet's syndrome (letter). *Gastrointest Endosc* 1985; 31:389.
5. Arma S. Habibulla KS, Price JJ, Collis JL. Dysphagia in Behçet's syndrome. *Thorax* 1971; 26:155–158.
6. Asakura H, Morita A, Morishita T, et al. Histopathological and electron microscopic studies of lymphangiectasia of the small intestine in Behçet's disease. *Gut* 1973; 14:196–203.
7. Baba S, Maruta M, Ando K, et al. Intestinal Behçet's disease: Report of five cases. *Dis Colon Rectum* 1976; 19:428–440.
8. Baba S, Morioka S. Treatment of intestinal Behçet's disease. In Inaba G, ed: *Behçet's Disease. Pathogenetic Mechanism and Clinical Future. Proceedings of the International Conference on Behçet's Disease, October 23–24, 1981, Tokyo.* Tokyo, University of Tokyo Press, 1982:559–570.
9. Berlin C. Behçet's disease as a multiple symptom complex. Report of ten cases. *Arch Dermatol* 1960; 82:73–79.
10. Bøe J, Dalgaard JB, Scott D. Mucocutaneous-ocular syndrome with intestinal involvement. A clinical and pathological study of four fatal cases. *Am J Med* 1958; 25:857–867.
11. Brodie TE, Ochsner JL. Behçet's syndrome with ulcerative oesophagitis: Report of the first case. *Thorax* 1973; 28:637–640.
12. Brookes GB. Pharyngeal stenosis in Behçet's syndrome. The first reported case. *Arch Ophthalmol* 1983; 109:338–340.
13. Chajek T, Fainaru M. Behçet's disease. Report of 41 cases and a review of the literature. *Medicine* 1975; 54:179–196.
14. Chamberlain MA. Behçet's syndrome in 32 patients in Yorkshire. *Ann Rheum Dis* 1977; 36:491–499.
15. Chong SKF, Wright VM, Raafat F, et al. Neonatal chronic inflam-

matory bowel disease (abstract 74). Royal Society of Medicine international conference on Behçet's disease, September 5 and 6, 1985, London, England.

16. Curth HO. Recurrent genito-oral aphthosis and uveitis with hypopyon (Behçet's syndrome). Report of two cases. *Arch Dermatol Syphilol* 1946; 54:179–196.

17. Davies E, Melzer E. A new sign in Behçet's syndrome. Scanty fungiform papillae in tongue. *Arch Intern Med* 1969; 124:720–721.

18. Ehrlich GE. Intermittent and periodic arthritic syndromes. In McCarty DJ, ed: *Arthritis and Allied Conditions. A Textbook of Rheumatology.* Philadelphia, Lea and Febiger, 1985:883–900.

19. Empey DW. Rectal and colonic ulceration in Behçet's disease. *Br J Surg* 1972; 59:173–175.

20. Empey DW, Hale JE. Rectal and colonic ulceration in Behçet's disease. *Proc R Soc Med* 1972; 65:163–164.

21. Eng K, Ruoff M, Bystryn J-C. Behçet's syndrome. An unusual cause of colonic ulceration and perforation. *Am J Gastroenterol* 1981; 75:57–59.

22. Fallingborg J, Laustsen J. Colitis of Behçet's syndrome. *Acta Med Scand* 1984; 215:397–399.

23. Feagin OT. Behçet's disease: The Ochsner experience, 1979–1982. *South Med J* 1984; 77:442–446.

24. Fife RS. Behçet's disease. *Clin Rheumatol Prac* 1983; 1:249–254.

25. Fromer JL. Behçet's syndrome. *Arch Dermatol* 1970; 102:116–117.

26. Goldstein SJ, Crooks DJM. Colitis in Behçet's syndrome. Two new cases. *Radiology* 1978; 128:321–323.

27. Good AE, Mutchnick MG, Weatherbee L. Duodenal ulcer, hepatic abscesses, and fatal hemobilia with Behçet's syndrome: a case report. *Am J Gastroenterol* 1982; 77:905–909.

28. Griffin JW Jr, Harrison HB, Tedesco FJ, Mills LR IV. Behçet's disease with multiple sites of gastrointestinal involvement. *South Med J* 1982; 75:1405–1408.

29. Gustafson RO, McDonald TJ, O'Duffy JD, Goellner JR. Upper aerodigestive tract manifestations of Behçet's disease: Review of 30 cases. *Otolaryngol Head Neck Surg* 1981; 89:409–413.

30. Hersh SP, Grimes CD JR, Harrison W, Nonkin P. Behçet's syndrome. An overlooked entity in otolaryngology. *Arch Otolaryngol* 1982; 108:250–252.

31. Iwana T, Utzunomiya J. Anal complication in Behçet's syndrome. *Jpn J Surg* 1977; 7:114–117.

32. Lee RG. The colitis of Behçet's syndrome. *Am J Surg Pathol* 1986; 19:888–893.

33. Kalbian VV, Challis MT. Behçet's disease. Report of twelve cases with three manifesting as papilledema. *Am J Med* 1970; 49:823–829.

34. Kaneko H, Nakajima H. Okamura A, et al. Histopathology of Behçet disease. Review of the literature with a case report. *Acta Pathol Jpn* 1976; 26:765–769.

35. Kaplinsky N, Neumann G, Harzahav Y, Frankl O. Esophageal ulceration in Behçet's syndrome. *Gastrointest Endosc* 1973; 23:160.
36. Kasahara Y, Tanaka S, Nishino M, et al. Intestinal involvement in Behçet's disease: Review of 136 surgical cases in the Japanese literature. *Dis Colon Rectum* 1981; 24:103–106.
37. Kaunitz JD, Sleisenger MH. Effects of systemic and extraintestinal disease on the gut. In Sleisenger MH, Fordtran JS, eds: *Gastrointestinal Disease. Pathophysiology Diagnosis Management.* Philadelphia, WB Saunders, 1983:369–404.
38. Keshavarzian A, Saverymuttu SH, Chadwick VS, et al. Noninvasive investigation of the gastrointestinal tract in collagen-vascular disease. *Am J Gastroenterol* 1984; 79:873–877.
39. Ketch LL, Buerk CA, Liechty D. Surgical implications of Behçet's disease. *Arch Surg* 1980; 115:759–760.
40. Kikuchi K, Suga T, Senoue I, et al. Esophageal ulceration in a patient with Behçet's syndrome. *Tokai J Exp Clin Med* 1982; 7:135–143.
41. Kobayashi T, Kikawada T, Shima K, Fukuda O. Ulceration and stenosis of the hypopharynx and its surgical management. *Head Neck Surg* 1982; 5:65–69.
42. Lakhanpal S, Tani K, Lie JT, et al. Pathologic features of Behçet's syndrome: A review of Japanese autopsy registry data. *Hum Pathol* 1985; 16:790–795.
43. Lavalle C, Gudiña J, Reinoso SR, et al. Behçet's syndrome and palate perforation (letter). *Arthritis Rheum* 1979; 22:308.
44. Lebwohl O, Forde KA, Berdon WE, et al. Ulcerative esophagitis and colitis in a pediatric patient with Behçet's syndrome. Response to steroid therapy. *Am J Gastroenterol* 1977; 68:550–555.
45. Levack B, Hanson D. Behçet's disease of the oesophagus. *J Laryngol Otol* 1979; 93:99–101.
46. Lockhart JM, McIntyre W, Caperton EM Jr. Esophageal ulceration in Behçet's syndrome. *Ann Intern Med* 1976; 84:572–573.
47. Mamo J, Baghdassarian A. Behçet's disease. A report of 28 cases. *Arch Ophthalmol* 1964; 71:38–48.
48. Mason RM, Barnes CG. Behçet's syndrome with arthritis. *Ann Rheum Dis* 1969; 28:95–103.
49. Mavioǧlu H. Behçet's recurrent disease. Analytical review of the literature. *Mo Med* 1958; 55:1209–1222.
50. McLean AM, Simms DM, Homer MJ. Ileal ring ulcers in Behçet syndrome. *AJR* 1983; 140:947–948.
51. Michelson JB, Chisari FV. Behçet's disease. *Surv Ophthalmol* 1982; 26:190–203.
52. Mir-Madjlessi SH, Farmer RG. Behçet's syndrome, Crohn's disease and toxic megacolon. *Cleve Clin Q* 1972; 39:49–55.
53. Mori S, Yoshihira A, Kawamura H, et al. Esophageal involvement in Behçet's disease. *Am J Gastroenterol* 1983; 78:548–553.
54. Morrison AW. Behçet's syndrome. *J Laryngol Otol* 1959; 73:833–837.
55. Nilsen KH, Jones SM, Shorey BA. Behçet's syndrome with perfora-

tions of the colon. *Postgrad Med J* 1977; 53:108–110.
56. O'Connell DJ, Courtney JV, Riddell RH. Colitis of Behçet's syndrome—Radiologic and pathologic features. *Gastrointest Radiol* 1980; 5:173–179.
57. O'Duffy JD. Behçet's disease. In Kelley WN, Harris ED Jr, Ruddy S, Sledge CB, eds: *Textbook of Rheumatology*. Philadelphia, WB Saunders, 1985:1174–1178.
58. O'Duffy JD. Behçet's disease. Comments. *Bull Rheum Dis* 1978–79; 29:977–979.
59. O'Duffy JD, Carney JA, Deodhar S. Behçet's disease. Report of 10 cases, 3 with new manifestations. *Ann Intern Med* 1971; 75:561–570.
60. Oshima Y, Shimizu T, Yokhari R, et al. Clinical studies on Behçet's syndrome. *Ann Rheum Dis* 1963; 22:36–45.
61. Parkin JV, Wight DGD. Behçet's disease of the alimentary tract. *Postgrad Med J* 1975; 51:260–264.
62. Pope CE II. Involvement of the esophagus by infections, systemic illnesses, and physical agents. In Sleisenger MH, Fordtran JS, eds: *Gastrointestinal Disease. Pathophysiology Diagnosis Management*. Philadelphia, WB Saunders, 1983:495–504.
63. Ramsay CA. Behçet's syndrome with large bowel involvement. *Proc R Soc Med* 1967; 60:185–187.
64. Rapport PN, Duckert LG, Boies LR Jr. Behçet's disease. *Ear Nose Throat J* 1979; 158:45–52.
65. Reuben A, Jones RR, Lovell D. Behçet's syndrome with colonic involvement and arterial thrombosis. *J R Soc Med* 1980; 73:520–524.
66. Screech G. An unusual cause of respiratory obstruction during anaesthesia. A case report. *Br J Anaesth* 1965; 37:978–979.
67. Shapiro LS, Notis WM, Romanoff NR. Self-limited esophageal ulcerations in Behçet's syndrome (letter). *Arthritis Rheum* 1983; 26:690–691.
68. Shimizu T, Ehrlich GE, Inaba G, Hayashi K. Behçet disease (Behçet syndrome). *Semin Arthritis Rheum* 1979; 8:223–260.
69. Shuttleworth EC, Voto S, Sahar D. Palatal myoclonus in Behçet's disease. *Arch Intern Med* 1985; 145:949–950.
70. Sladen GE, Lehner T. Gastro-intestinal disorders in Behçet's syndrome and a comparison with recurrent oral ulcers. In Lehner T, Barnes CG, eds: *Behçet's Syndrome. Clinical and Immunological Features. Proceedings of a Conference Sponsored by the Royal Society of Medicine, February 1979*. London, Academic Press, 1979: 151–158.
71. Smith GE, Kime LR, Pitcher JL. The colitis of Behçet's disease: a separate entity? Colonoscopic findings and literature review. *Am J Dig Dis* 1973; 18:987–1000.
72. Stanley RJ, Tedesco FJ, Melson GL, et al. The colitis of Behçet's disease: A clinical-radiographic correlation. *Radiology* 1975; 114:603–604.
73. Strachan RW, Wigzell FW. Polyarthritis in Behçet's multiple symptom complex. *Ann Rheum Dis* 1963; 22:26–35.

74. Sulheim O, Dalgaard JB, Andersen SR. Behçet's syndrome. Report of case with complete autopsy performed. *Acta Pathol Microbiol Scand* 1959; 45:145–158.
75. Thach BT, Cummings NA. Behçet syndrome with "aphthous colitis." *Arch Intern Med* 1976; 136:705–709.
76. Turner ME. Anaesthetic difficulties associated with Behçet's syndrome. Case report. *Br J Anaesth* 1972; 44:100–102.
77. Venkatasurbramaniam KV, Swinehart DR. Behçet's syndrome: Case report and literature review. *Henry Ford Hosp Med J* 1981; 29:153–159.
78. Vlymen WJ, Moskowitz PS. Roentenographic manifestations of esophageal and intestinal involvement in Behçet's disease in children. *Pediatr Radiol* 1981; 10:193–196.
79. Wright MI. Behçet's disease in the mouth, pharynx, and larynx: An underdiagnosed disease? (abstract 56). Royal Society of Medicine international conference on Behçet's disease, September 5 and 6, 1985, London, England.
80. Wright VA, Chamberlain MA. Behçet's syndrome. *Bull Rheum Dis* 1978–79; 29:972–977.
81. Yassin A, Girgis I. Behçet's disease. *J Laryngol Otol* 1966; 80:481–494.
82. Katzenellenbogen I. Recurrent aphthous ulceration of oral mucous membrane and genitals associated with recurrent hypopyon iritis (Behçet's syndrome). Report of three cases. *Br J Dermatol* 1946; 58:161–172.
83. McDonald GSA, Gad-Al-Rab J. Behçet's disease with endocarditis and the Budd-Chiari syndrome. *J Clin Pathol* 1980; 33:660–669.
84. Ramírez V, Peredo J, Cetina JA, Alarcón-Segovia D. Sjögren's syndrome in Behçet's disease (letter). *Lancet* 1973; 2:732.
85. Yashiro K, Nagasako K, Hasegawa K, et al. Esophageal lesions in intestinal Behçet's disease. *Endoscopy* 1986; 18:57–60.
86. Kansu E, Özer FL, Akalin E, et al. Behçet's syndrome with obstruction of the venae cavae A report of seven cases. *Q J Med* 1972; 41:151–168.
87. Shimizu T. Behçet's disease: A systemic inflammatory disease. In Shiokawa Y, ed: *Vascular Lesions of Collagen Diseases and Related Conditions. Proceedings of the International Workshop on Vascular Lesions of Collagen Diseases and Related Conditions, February 6–7, 1976, Tokyo.* Tokyo, University Park Press, 1977:201–211.
88. Johnson DA, Everhart CW. Colitis in Behçet's syndrome (letter). *Gastrointest Endosc* 1986; 32:58–59.
89. Hyman NM, Sagar HJ. Behçet's syndrome: Unusual multisystem involvement and immune complexes. *Postgrad Med J* 1980; 56:182–184.
90. Stringer DA, Cleghorn GJ, Durie PR, et al. Behçet's syndrome involving the gastrointestinal tract—A diagnostic dilemma in childhood. *Pediatr Radiol* 1986; 16:131–134.
91. Fukuda Y, Watanabe I. Pathological studies on intestinal Behçet's (entero-Behçet's) disease. In Dilşen N, Koniçe M, Övül C, eds: *Behçet's Disease. Proceedings of an International Symposium on*

Behçet's Disease, Istanbul, 29–30 September 1977. Amsterdam-Oxford, Excerpta Medica, 1979:90–95.

92. Katoh K, Matsunaga K, Ishigatsubo Y, et al. Pathologically defined neuro-, vasculo-, entero-Behçet's disease. *J Rheumatol* 1985; 12:1186–1190.
93. Little AG, Zarins CK. Abdominal aortic aneurysm and Behçet's disease. *Surgery* 1982; 91:359–362.
94. Park JH, Han MC, Bettmann MA. Arterial manifestations of Behçet disease. *AJR* 1984; 143:821–825.
95. Tsuchiya M, Hibi T, Mizuno Y, et al. Comparative, immunological studies on lymphangiectasia of the small intestine revealed in protein losing gastroenteropathy and Behçet's disease. *Gastroenterol Jpn* 1976; 11:88–99.
96. Yamana S, Jones SL, Shimamoto T, et al. Immunohistological analysis of lymphocytes infiltrating the terminal ileum in a patient with intestinal Behçet's disease (abstract 32). Royal Society of Medicine international conference on Behçet's disease, September 5 and 6, 1985, London, England.
97. Yim CW, White RH. Behçet's syndrome in a family with inflammatory bowel disease. *Arch Intern Med* 1985; 145:1047–1050.
98. Beroniade V. Amyloidosis and Behçet's disease (letter). *Ann Intern Med* 1975; 83:904–905.
99. Nestor G, Beroniade V, Cârnaru S, Badea I. Behçet's disease with renal involvement (with reference to three anatomico-clinical cases). *Rom Med Rev* 1970; 14:27–32.
100. Williams DG, Lehner T. Renal manifestations of Behçet's syndrome. In Lehner T, Barnes CG, eds: *Behçet's Syndrome. Clinical and Immunological Features. Proceedings of a Conference Sponsored by the Royal Society of Medicine, February, 1979.* London, Academic Press, 1979:259–264.
101. Yurdakul S, Tüzüner N, Yurdakul I, et al. Amyloidosis in Behçet's syndrome (abstract 75). Royal Society of Medicine international conference on Behçet's disease, September 5 and 6, 1985, London, England.
102. Firestein GS, Gruber HE, Weisman MH, et al. Mouth and genital ulcers with inflamed cartilage: MAGIC syndrome. Five patients with features of relapsing polychondritis and Behçet's disease. *Am J Med* 1985; 79:65–72.
103. Reimer G, Djawari D. Lymphocytotoxicity for oral epithelial cells in Behçet's disease. A case report. *Dermatologica* 1982; 164:82–89.
104. Dilşen N, Koniçe M. Gazioğlu K, et al. Pleuropulmonary manifestations in Behçet's disease. In Dilşen N, Koniçe M, Övül C, eds: *Behçet's Disease. Proceedings of an International Symposium on Behçet's Disease, Istanbul, 29–30 September 1977.* Amsterdam-Oxford, Excerpta Medica, 1979:163–170.
105. Ferraris R, Colzani G, Galatola G, Fiorentini MT. Ascites with suprahepatic portal hypertension in a case of Behçet's disease. *Panminerva Med* 1985; 27:43–44.

106. Müftüoglu AÜ, Yurdakul S, Yazici H, et al. Vascular involvement in Behçet's disease (abstract 63). Royal Society of Medicine international conference on Behçet's disease, September 5 and 6, 1985, London, England.
107. Nakayama S, Sakata J, Kusumoto S, et al. Ultrasonic appearance of the liver in hepatic venous outflow obstruction (Budd-Chiari syndrome): A case of pseudo hepatic infarct associated with Behçet's disease. *JCU* 1986; 14:300–303.
108. Wilkey D, Yocum DE, Oberley TD, et al. Budd-Chiari syndrome and renal failure in Behçet disease. Report of a case and review of the literature. *Am J Med* 1983; 75:541–550.
109. Mitchell MC, Boitnott JK, Kaufman S, et al. Budd-Chiari syndrome: Etiology, diagnosis and management. *Medicine* 1982; 61:199–218.
110. Parker RGF. Occlusion of the hepatic veins in man. *Medicine* 1959; 38:369–402.
111. Manna R, Ghirlanda G, Bochicchio GB. Chronic active hepatitis and Behçet's syndrome. *Clin Rheumatol* 1985; 4:93–96.
112. Aksungur P. The determination of hepatitis surface antigen and antibody in patients with Behçet's disease. In Dilşen N, Koniçe M, Övül C, eds: *Behçet's Disease. Proceedings of an International Symposium on Behçet's Disease, Istanbul, 29–30 September 1977*. Amsterdam-Oxford, Excerpta Medica, 1979:249–253.
113. Hamza H, Ayed HB. Clinical and histological study of 55 cases of Behçet's disease (abstract). In Dilşen N, Koniçe M, Övül C, eds: *Behçet's Disease. Proceedings of an International Symposium on Behçet's Disease, Istanbul, 29–30 September 1977*. Amsterdam-Oxford, Excerpta Medica, 1979:107.
114. Larsson H, Bengtsson-Stigmar E. Behçet's disease and close contact with pigs. *Acta Med Scand* 1984; 216:541–543.
115. Öneş Ü, Urgancioğlu M, Yakacikli S, Yalçin I. Behçet's disease and hepatitis B antigen. In Dilşen N, Koniçe M, Övül C, eds: *Behçet's Disease. Proceedings of an International Symposium on Behçet's Disease, Istanbul, 29–30 September 1977*. Amsterdam-Oxford, Excerpta Medica, 1979:245–248.
116. Cupps TR, Fauci AS. Behçet's disease. In: *The vasculitides*. Philadelphia, WB Saunders, 1981:142–146.
117. Duffy J, Lidsky MD, Sharp JT, et al. Polyarthritis, polyarteritis and hepatitis B. *Medicine* 1976; 55:19–37.
118. Fauci AS. Vasculitis. *J Allergy Clin Immunol* 1983; 72:211–223.
119. Gower RG, Sausker WF, Kohler PF, et al. Small vessel vasculitis caused by hepatitis virus immune complexes. *J Allergy Clin Immunol* 1978; 62:222–228.
120. Sergent JS, Lockshin MD, Christian CL, Gocke DJ. Vasculitis with hepatitis B antigenemia: Long-term observations in nine patients. *Medicine* 1976; 55:1–18.
121. Shusterman N, London WT. Hepatitis B and immune-complex disease. *N Engl J Med* 1984; 310:43–45.
122. Cadman EC, Lundberg WB, Mitchell MS. Pulmonary manifestations

in Behçet syndrome. Case report and review of the literature. *Arch Intern Med* 1976; 136:944–947.
123. Plotkin GR, Patel BR, Shah VN. Behçet's syndrome complicated by cutaneous leukocytoclastic vasculitis. Response to prednisone and chlorambucil. *Arch Intern Med* 1985; 145:1913–1915.
124. Schiff S, Moffatt R, Mandell WJ, Rubin SA. Acute myocardial infarction and recurrent ventricular arrhythmias in Behçet's syndrome. *Am Heart J* 1982; 103:438–440.
125. Davies JD. Behçet's syndrome with haemoptysis and pulmonary lesions. *J Pathol* 1973; 109:351–356.
126. James DG, Spiteri MA. Behçet's disease. *Ophthalmology* 1982; 89:1279–1284.
127. Kiernan TJ, Gillan J, Murray JP, McCarthy CF. Behçet's disease and splenomegaly. *Br Med J* 1978; 2:1340–1341.
128. Rosenthal T, Bank H, Aledjem M, et al. Systemic amyloidosis in Behçet's disease. *Ann Intern Med* 1975; 83:220–223.
129. Fishof FE. Behçet's syndrome. Report of two cases. *J Int Coll Surg* 1960; 34:213–229.
130. Dowling GB. Behçet's disease. *Proc R Soc Med* 1961; 54:101–104.
131. Katzenellenbogen I. Behçet's syndrome. *Arch Dermatol Syphilol* 1950; 61:481–484.
132. Price CA. Behçet's syndrome—A distressing, intriguing malady. *J R Coll Gen Pract* 1969; 18:38–45.
133. Vella MA, James DG. Vascular and neurological involvement in 25 patients with Behçet's disease (abstract 67). Royal Society of Medicine international conference on Behçet's disease, September 5 and 6, 1985, London, England.
134. Carswell GF. A case of Behçet's disease involving the bladder. *Br J Urol* 1976; 48:199–202.
135. Piers A. Behçet's disease with arterial and renal manifestations. *Proc R Soc Med* 1977; 70:540–544.
136. Dunlop EMC. Genital and other manifestations of Behçet's disease seen in venereological practice. In Lehner T, Barnes CG, eds: *Behçet's Syndrome. Clinical and Immunological Features. Proceedings of a Conference Sponsored by the Royal Society of Medicine, February 1979.* London, Academic Press, 1979:159–181.
137. Wong RC, Ellis CN, Diaz LA. Behçet's disease. *Int J Rheumatol* 1984; 23:25–32.
138. Nazzaro P. Cutaneous manifestations of Behçet's disease. Clinical and histopathological findings. In Monacelli M, Nazzaro P, eds: *Behçet's Disease. International Symposium on Behçet's disease, Rome 1964.* Basel, S Karger, 1966:15–41.
139. Tokoro Y, Seto T, Abe Y, et al. Skin lesions in Behçet's disease. *Int J Dermatol* 1977; 16:227–244.
140. Yamana S, Jones SL, Aoi K, et al. Lymphocyte subsets in erythema nodosum from patients with Behçet's disease (abstract 30). Royal Society of Medicine international conference on Behçet's disease, September 5 and 6, 1985, London, England.

141. Marufi M. et al. Histopathological study of normal skin in Behçet's disease (abstract 33). Royal Society of Medicine international conference on Behçet's disease, September 5 and 6, 1985, London, England.

142. Yazici H, Tüzün Y, Pazarli H, et al. Influence of age of onset and patient's sex on the prevalence and severity of manifestations of Behçet's syndrome. *Ann Rheum Dis* 1984; 43:783–789.

143. Carr GR. Cellulitis and thrombophlebitis in Behçet's syndrome. *Lancet* 1957; 2:358–359.

144. Marchionini A, Müller E. The dermatological view of Morbus Hulusi Behçet. In Monacelli M, Nazzaro P, eds: *Behçet's Disease. International Symposium on Behçet's Disease, Rome 1964.* Basel, S Karger, 1966:6–14.

145. Masheter HC. Behçet's syndrome complicated by intercranial thrombophlebitis. *Proc R Soc Med* 1959; 52:1039–1040.

146. Jorizzo JL, Schmalstieg FC, Solomon AR Jr, et al. Thalidomide effects in Behçet's syndrome and pustular vasculitis. *Arch Intern Med* 1986; 146:878–881.

147. Enoch BA. Gangrene in Behçet's syndrome (letter). *Br Med J* 1969; 3:54.

148. Mowat AG, Hothersall TE. Gangrene in Behçet's syndrome. *Br Med J* 1969; 2:636.

149. Lever WF, Schaumburg-Lever G. Systemic diseases with cutaneous manifestations. In: *Histopathology of the Skin.* Philadelphia, JB Lippincott, 1983:190–197.

150. White JW Jr. Hypersensitivity and miscellaneous inflammatory disorders. In Moschella SL, Hurley HJ, eds: *Dermatology.* Philadelphia, WB Saunders, 1985:464–498.

151. Haim S. The pathogenesis of lesions in Behçet's disease. *Dermatologica* 1979; 158:31–37.

152. Haim S, Sobel JD, Friedman-Birnbaum R, Lichtig C. Histological and direct immunofluorescence study of cutaneous hyperreactivity in Behçet's disease. *Br J Dermatol* 1976; 95:631–636.

153. Lichtig C, Haim S, Gilhar A, et al. Mast cells in Behçet's disease: Ultrastructural and histamine content studies. *Dermatologica* 1981; 162:167–174.

154. Lichtig C, Haim S, Hammel I, Friedman-Birnbaum R. The quantification and significance of mast cells in lesions of Behçet's disease. *Br J Dermatol* 1980; 102:255–259.

155. Hammar S, Bockus D, Remington F, Bartha M. The widespread distribution of Langerhans cells in pathologic tissues: An ultrastructural and immunohistochemical study. *Hum Pathol* 1986; 17:894–905.

156. Holbrook KA, Wolff K. The structure and development of skin. In Fitzpatrick TB, Eisen AZ, Wolff K, et al, eds: *Dermatology in General Medicine.* New York, McGraw-Hill, 1987:93–131.

157. Jakubovic HR, Ackerman AB. Structure and function of skin. Section I: development, morphology, and physiology. In Moschella SL, Hurley HJ, eds: *Dermatology.* Philadelphia, WB Saunders, 1985:1–74.

158. Stingl G, Wolff K. Langerhans cells and their relation to other dendritic cells and mononuclear phagocytes. In Fitzpatrick TB, Eisen AZ, Wolff K, et al, eds: *Dermatology in General Medicine.* New York, McGraw-Hill, 1987:410–426.
159. Dinarello CA. Interleukin-1. *Rev Infect Dis* 1984; 6:51–95.
160. Kohn S, Haim S, Gilhar A, et al. Epidermal Langerhans' cells in Behçet's disease. *J Clin Pathol* 1984; 37:616–619.
161. Blobner F. Zur rezidivierenden hypopyon-iritis. *Zeitschrift Augenheilkd* 1937; 91:129–139.
162. Jensen T. Sur les ulcérations aphtheuses de la muqueuse de la bouche et de la peau génitale combinées avec les symptômes oculaires (syndrome de Behçet). *Acta Dermato-Venereologica* 1941; 22:64–79.
163. Sobel JD, Haim S, Shafrir A, Gellei B. Cutaneous hyperreactivity in Behçet's disease. *Dermatologica* 1973; 146:350–356.
164. Tüzün Y, Altaç M, Yazici H, et al. Nonspecific skin hyperreactivity in Behçet's disease. Iperreattivita cutanea aspecifica nel Morbo di Behçet. *Haematologica* 1980; 65:395–398.
165. Cooper D, Penny R, Fiddes P. Autologous-plasma sensitization in Behçet's disease (letter). *Lancet* 1971; 1:910.
166. Shimizu T, Katsuta Y, Oshima Y. Immunological studies on Behçet's syndrome. *Ann Rheum Dis* 1965; 24:494–500.
167. Suzuki K, Mizuno N. Intracutaneous test with physiological saline in Behçet's disease. In Inaba G, ed: *Behçet's Disease. Pathogenetic Mechanism and Clinical Future. Proceedings of the International Conference on Behçet's Disease, October 23–24, 1981, Tokyo.* Tokyo, University of Tokyo Press, 1982:333–342.
168. Franceschetti A, Jadassohn W, Hunziker N. The cutaneous reaction to "Behçetin." *Bull Soc Franç Ophtal* 1960; 73:380–384.
169. Dilşen N, Koniçe M, Aral O, Aykat S. Standardization and evaluation of skin pathergy test (SPT) in Behçet's disease (BD) and controls (abstract 42). Royal Society of Medicine international conference on Behçet's disease, September 5 and 6, 1985, London, England.
170. Altaç M, Tüzün Y, Yurdakul S, et al. The validity of the pathergy test (non-specific skin hyperreactivity) in Behçet's disease: A double blind study by independent observers. *Acta Derm Venereol* (Stockh) 1982; 62:158–159.
171. Davies PG, Fordham JN, Kirwan JR, et al. The pathergy test and Behçet's syndrome in Britain. *Ann Rheum Dis* 1984; 43:70–73.
172. France R, Buchanan RN, Wilson MW, Sheldon MB Jr. Relapsing iritis with recurrent ulcers of the mouth and genitalia (Behçet's syndrome). Review: With report of additional case. *Medicine* 1951; 30:335–355.
173. Jorizzo JL, Hudson RD, Schmalstieg FC, et al. Behçet's syndrome: Immune regulation, circulating immune complexes, neutrophil migration, and colchicine therapy. *J Am Acad Dermatol* 1984; 10:205–214.
174. Jorizzo JL, Solomon AR, Cavallo T. Behçet's syndrome. Immunopathologic and histopathologic assessment of pathergy lesions

is useful in diagnosis and follow-up. *Arch Pathol Lab Med* 1985; 109:747–751.

175. Aksungur L, Çayhan A, Şentut L. A clinical and histopathological study of 35 patients with Behçet's disease. In Dilşen N, Koniçe M, Övül C, eds: *Behçet's Disease. Proceedings of an International Symposium on Behçet's Disease, Istanbul, 29–30 September 1977.* Amsterdam-Oxford, Excerpta Medica, 1979:114–119.

176. Yazici H, Tüzün T, Tanman AB, et al. Male patients with Behçet's syndrome have stronger pathergy reactions. *Clin Exp Rheumatol* 1985; 3:137–141.

177. Djawari D, Hornstein OP, Schötz J. Enhancement of granulocyte chemotaxis in Behçet's disease. *Arch Dermatol Res* 1981; 270:81–88.

178. Fellner MJ, Kantor I. Behçet's syndrome: Skin puncture test as guide in therapy. *NY State J Med* 1964; 64:1760–1761.

179. Aral O, Dilşen N, Koniçe M. Positive skin pathergy reactivity is a genetic marker of Behçet's disease (BD) (abstract 43). Royal Society of Medicine international conference on Behçet's disease, September 5 and 6, 1985, London, England. *J Roy Soc Med* 1984; 77:816–819.

180. Barnes CG. Behçet's syndrome. *J Roy Soc Med* 1984; 77:816–819.

181. Tüzün Y, Yazici H, Pazarli H, et al. The usefulness of the nonspecific skin hyperreactivity (the pathergy test) in Behçet's disease in Turkey. *Acta Derm Venereol* (Stockh) 1978; 59:77–79.

182. Yazici H, Akokan G, Yalçin B, Müftüoglu A. The high prevalence of HLA-B5 in Behçet's disease. *Clin Exp Immunol* 1977; 30:259–261.

183. Yazici H, Chamberlain MA, Schreuder I, et al. HLA antigens in Behçet's disease: A reappraisal by a comparative study of Turkish and British patients. *Ann Rheum Dis* 1980; 39:344–348.

184. Yazici H, Chamberlain MA, Tüzün Y, et al. A comparative study of the pathergy reaction among Turkish and British patients with Behçet's disease. *Ann Rheum Dis* 1984; 43:74–75.

185. Yazici H, Tüzün Y, Pazarli H, et al. The combined use of HLA-B5 and the pathergy test as diagnostic markers of Behçet's disease in Turkey. *J Rheumatol* 1980; 7:206–210.

186. Powell FC, Schroeter AL, Su WPD, Perry HO. Pyoderma gangrenosum: A review of 86 patients. *Q J Med* 1985; 217:173–186.

187. Domonkos AN, Arnold HL Jr, Odom RB. Cutaneous vascular diseases. In: *Andrews' Diseases of the Skin. Clinical Dermatology.* Philadelphia, WB Saunders, 1982:1003–1047.

188. James DG, Williams WJ. The skin. In: *Sarcoidosis and Other Granulomatous Disorders.* Philadelphia, WB Saunders, 1985:97–111.

189. Isobe T, Matsumoto J, Tomita M, et al. Intradermal tests in Behçet's disease. *Jpn J Med* 1982; 21:86–88.

190. Kaplinsky N, Movshovitis M, Frankel O. False-positive tuberculin test in Behçet's syndrome. *Cutis* 1980; 25:529–530.

191. Lee S, Kim DG, Band DS, et al: Immunological aspects in each type of Behçet's disease (abstract 11). Royal Society of Medicine international conference on Behçet's disease, September 5 and 6, 1985, London, England.

192. Haim S, Gilhar A. Clinical and laboratory criteria for the diagnosis of Behçet's disease. *Br J Dermatol* 1980; 102:361–363.
193. Sharquie KE. Suppression of Behçet's disease with dapsone. *Br J Dermatol* 1984; 110:493–494.
194. Reimer G, Luckner L, Hornstein OP. Direct immunofluorescence in recurrent aphthous ulcers and Behçet's disease. *Dermatologica* 1983; 167:293–298.
195. Yazaki K. Histopathologic studies on the non-specific skin sensitivity in Behçet's disease. *Jpn J Dermatol Ser B* 1970; 80:116–119.
196. Saito T, Honma T, Saigo K. Epidermal Langerhans' cells after the prick test for Behçet's disease. *Dermatologica* 1980; 161:152–156.
197. Djawari D, Hornstein OP, Luckner L. Skin window examination according to Rebuck and cutaneous pathergy tests in patients with Behçet's disease. *Dermatologica* 1985; 170:265–270.
198. Warabi H, Yamada E, Schiffman E, Shiokawa Y. Increased chemotactic activity of peripheral blood monocytes in Behçet's disease. In Inaba G, ed: *Behçet's Disease. Pathogenetic Mechanism and Clinical Future. Proceedings of the International Conference on Behçet's Disease, October 23–24, 1981, Tokyo.* Tokyo, University of Tokyo Press, 1982: 317–322.
199. O'Duffy JD, Lehner T, Barnes CG: Summary of the third international conference on Behçet's disease. Tokyo, Japan, October 23–24, 1981. *J Rheumatol* 1983; 10:154–158.

13

Miscellaneous Clinical Manifestations, Part III: Neuro-Behçet, Systemic Amyloidosis, Lymphoreticular System

Robert S. Lesser and Raphael J. DeHoratius

Neuro-Behçet's Syndrome

CENTRAL NERVOUS SYSTEM (CNS) INVOLVEMENT in Behçet's disease (BD) is one of the most serious complications of this illness. Much of the literature supports neuro-Behçet's syndrome (NBS) as having a variable and often poor prognosis with only the administration of immunosuppressive agents offering some clinical benefit. The diagnosis is frequently difficult to establish and is usually entertained after a thorough laboratory evaluation has excluded other more common infectious and noninfectious etiologies of nervous system pathology. Notwithstanding these qualifications and under the appropriate clinical setting, a thorough history and physical examination remain the sine qua non in arriving at the correct diagnosis of NBS.

From *Behçet's Disease: A Contemporary Synopsis*, edited by Gary R. Plotkin, M.D., John J. Calabro, M.D., and J. Desmond O'Duffy, M.B. © 1988, Futura Publishing Company, Inc., Mount Kisco, NY.

Clinical Presentation

Behçet in 1937 described a triple symptom complex of oral aphthous ulcers, genital ulcerations, and hypopyon iritis; and in 1944, Berlin[1] described the first necropsy results of a Behçet's disease patient with concurrent CNS involvement. Although Behçet's disease may affect all parts of the neuraxis with multiple lesions occurring simultaneously,[1-40] the following three patterns were proposed in 1956 to characterize the various forms of NBS[2]:

1. A brain-stem syndrome, which may be either episodic or progressive. Cranial nerve palsies, diplopia, nystagmus, dysarthria, ataxia, limb weakness, and pyramidal signs may be present.[2,5,13]

2. A meningomyelitic syndrome characterized by paraplegia or quadriplegia, headache, fever, nuchal rigidity, and cerebrospinal fluid (CSF) pleocytosis. In addition, recurrent episodes of culture negative meningitis, encephalitis, and transient or terminal brain stem signs may occur in this subset of patients.[2,5,13]

3. Organic confusional syndrome, which may be transient or progressive to dementia.[2,5] Other investigators have characterized a wide spectrum of psychological and mental symptoms and signs including memory impairment, character disorders, apathy, lethargy, altered consciousness, disorientation, insomnia, delirium, euphoria, psychomotor agitation, depression, emotional lability, hallucinosis, euphoria, paranoid attitudes, anxiety, suicidal ideation, delusions, and hypochondriasis.[11,13,30,38]

Complicating the clinical picture of NBS is the occurrence of these three patterns of neurological complications in various combinations.[5,13] Additional reports have expanded the original neurological observations to include the simultaneous occurrence of motor and sensory symptoms and signs; papilledema resulting either from active uveitis or benign intracranial hypertension (pseudotumor cerebri), the latter of which may be secondary to cerebral venous sinus thrombosis; Bell's palsy; palatal myoclonus; spinal cord and spinal and peripheral nerve lesions with manifestations including the Brown-Séquard syndrome, cauda equina syndrome, and peripheral neuropathy; cerebellar signs including nystagmus, tremor, and ataxia; pyramidal tract syndrome with Babinski sign, clonus, spastic paralysis, and altered speech; extrapyramidal signs; mixed pyramidal and extrapyramidal features; transient ischemic attacks; hemiparesis or quadriparesis; Weber's syndrome; bulbar paralysis; pseudobulbar palsy; paralysis of bladder and bowel; focal or generalized seizures; aphasia; dysphagia; hyperesthesia; coma; and subarachnoid and intracranial hemorrhages.[5-14,16-18,20,41] Signs of spinal cord involvement, besides including the Brown-Séquard syndrome, may consist of depressed sensations below a certain dermatome, hyperactive patellar reflexes, absent lower abdominal reflexes, and paralysis of the bladder with urinary retention.[30]

Hearing impairment and vertigo secondary to cochlear and vestibular abnormalities, respectively, have been reported in Behçet's disease. Although this inner-ear involvement is a late complication, it tends to progress during the ensuing years. Although the episodes of vertigo may become more frequent, they may decrease in duration and intensity.[28] The autonomic nervous system may also be affected in BD with reduction of the sympathetic excitability at the level of the hypothalamus and enhancement of peripheral parasympathetic reactivity including the presence of a cholinomimetic pupil.[36,39] Dilşen[40] has shown significant hyperactivity of the peripheral sympathetic system in BD.

The vascular lesions of Behçet's syndrome, which include aneurysms and arterial occlusions, may also affect the cerebral and vertebrobasilar circulations. Symptoms and signs are dependent upon the sites of arterial involvement, such as hemiplegia and syncope due to an aneurysm of the common carotid artery and occlusion of the subclavian artery, respectively.[13] In a series of 31 patients with NBS, the symptoms and signs in order of decreasing frequency were increased tendon reflexes, spastic paresis, headache, sensory impairment, extensor planter reflexes, ankle clonus, absent abdominal reflexes, dysarthria, difficulty in urination and defecation, nystagmus, diplopia, facial nerve palsy, coordination difficulties, dysphagia, focal convulsions, vertigo, and impaired visual acuity.[13] In another series, the most common clinical picture of NBS was transient or persistent episodes of brainstem dysfunction.[20]

Epidemiology, Clinical Correlates, and Histopathology

Central nervous system involvement affects approximately 4 to 42% of patients suffering from BD, and the onset of the neurological symptoms occurs from 1 to 11 years after the initial presentation of the triple symptom complex.[9,13,20] The mean age of the onset of CNS involvement is in the fourth decade, and the natural history of NBS is noteworthy for both spontaneous remissions and exacerbations.[9,31] However, three distinct clinical patterns of NBS have been recently described; these have consisted of exacerbations and remissions, transition into a chronic progressive stage after a phase of exacerbations and remissions, and a chronic progressive course from the onset.[37] The mortality associated with NBS has ranged from 47 to 66%[2]; however, more recently, Hughes[20] and Kalbian[7] have reported a more favorable outcome in their series of patients with various neurological deficits.

Pathologically, the CNS lesions may be distributed diffusely; a review of the autopsy literature has shown involvement of cerebral gray and white matter, hippocampus, basal ganglia, optic nerves, internal capsule, midbrain, pons, cerebellum, medulla, and spinal cord.[4,13,21,29,32–35,42] Histopathological examination has been remarkable for lymphocytic meningeal infiltration, scattered small necrotic or softened foci in the white matter, perivascular lymphocytic cuffing, especially around venules, and diffuse axonal demyelination and degeneration.[4,13] Swelling of the neuronal cells and the presence of pontine multinucleated nerve cells have been observed on tissue section.[13] Essentially, most authorities have viewed vasculitis as the main underlying pathogenic mechanism to explain the nervous system complications of BD, with thrombophlebitis contributing to certain manifestations, such as pseudotumor cerebri.[2,6,9,13,20]

Laboratory Evaluation

The laboratory evaluation of NBS involves investigation of the CNS as well as the peripheral blood, with examination of the cerebrospinal fluid (CSF) being one of the most widely applied modalities. Pleocytosis is generally observed in the CSF in NBS except in certain patients including those who present solely with benign intracranial hypertension.[2,6,10,16,26] In pseudotumor cerebri the fluid pressure is of course elevated.[16] In summary, the features of CSF analysis in NBS can be viewed as follows[6,8,10,20]:

1. Pleocytosis is found in 80% to 100% of patients,[6,10] except in one series[26] where only 20% had this feature.
2. Pleocytosis is predominantly monouclear or neutrophilic in character with cell counts averaging less than 100 and rarely greater than 500.[6,26]
3. Normal to moderately increased protein levels are present.
4. CSF is culture negative.
5. Glucose concentration is normal.

Cerebrospinal fluid immunoglobulin A (CSF-IgA), CSF-C3 and its conversion rate, and CSF-alpha II macroglobulin have been reported as useful parameters of severity of CNS involvement in BD.[13] A recent study[43] observed that the cerebrospinal immunoglobulin M (CSF IgM) index (CSF Ig × serum albumin) (serum Ig × CSF albumin), an indicator of intrathecal immunoglobulin synthesis, was not only significantly elevated in patients with active NBS, but also diminished with abatement of the neurological manifestations. Thus, this determination may assist in the evaluation of CNS activity. In addition, these investigators,[43] in contrast to earlier reports,[13] concluded that elevated levels of CSF-IgA resulted from a damaged blood-brain barrier and reflected raised serum IgA values rather than primary CNS endogenous IgA production.

The presence of myelin basic protein in the CSF has been assessed in patients with NBS, and in four of four patients with active nervous system disease, there were increased levels of this protein with the degree of elevation correlating with clinical activity at least in the one patient studied serially during a period of five months. Levels of the myelin basic protein did not attain significant elevation in 38 patients with BD who lacked CNS symptoms and signs.[44] Peripheral demyelinating antibodies have been detected in more than 70% of patients with NBS; however, these antibodies were similarly found in the sera of patients with multiple sclerosis, especially during the active phase of disease. The putative role of these antibodies may be myelin destruction and the inhibition of myelinization, and although both actions may occur in multiple sclerosis, inhibition of myelinization probably does not develop in NBS.[13] An antimyelin serum factor (AMSF) has been found in three of seven patients with NBS, but in neither 64 patients with BD who lacked active CNS disease nor in patients with multiple sclerosis. Affinity chromotography has also separated a cerebroside-binding serum factor (CBSF) from 71% (five patients) with NBS. However, this factor was less specific than AMSF, since it was present in 17% of patients with BD without neurological complications, 33% of those with multiple sclerosis, and 36% of patients who sustained a cerebrovascular accident.[13] Serum antiglycolipid antibodies including antibody with activity against the asialo GM_1 (GA_1) brain ganglioside have been determined in patients with various neurological disorders.[45,46] Although these antibodies may be elevated during the active phase of NBS, they are not specific for this disease,[45,46] and additional prospective studies are needed to assess their utility further in the diagnosis and management of NBS. More recently, Kansu et al.[47] have studied certain immunological markers including immunoglobulins, immune complexes, T and B lymphocytes, and T-helper and T-suppressor cells in BD. According to their preliminary data, pathognomonic abnormalities were not detected in patients with NBS.

Computerized tomography (CT) of the brain has been helpful in NBS in detecting focal lesions in the basal ganglia and cerebral gray matter, disclosing paraventricular edema, assisting in diagnosing benign intracranial hypertension, and delineating cerebral and brain-stem atrophy.[11,13,14,19] Ota et al.[48] have reported the radiographic abnormalities of computed tomography in nine patients with NBS, and these findings have consisted of atrophy of the brain stem and diencephalon, enlargement of the ventricles especially of the third, and minimal alteration of the cerebral cortex and cerebellum. Cerebral computerized tomography of another patient with NBS revealed contrast-enhancing lesions in the left basis pontis and at the level of the thalamus during acute exacerbations of the neurological deficits[49]; however, one must consider other infectious and noninfectious etiologies in the differential diagnosis of these radiographic abnormalities before ascribing the lesions to primary Behçet's syndrome. Nevertheless, the authors[49] postulated that the contrast-enhancing lesions were the sequelae of the BD vasculitis.

The electroencephalographic tracings of patients with NBS have ranged from normal results to those demonstrating diffuse alpha-wave patterns and mild to moderate increases of diffuse slow waves (slow alpha and theta). The EEG patterns have often correlated with the clinical signs and underlying brain pathology, and the presence of diffuse alpha waves may be dependent upon the preserved functioning of the brain-stem reticular-activating system.[50] Digital subtraction angiography (DSA) may eventually supplant cerebral arterial angiography in diagnosing cerebral sinus venous thrombosis of BD[16] since it is relatively noninvasive, may be performed as an outpatient procedure, and has been associated with favorable results.

Approach to Diagnosis of NBS

The first priority is to decide whether BD is the most probable working diagnosis, and since the CNS manifestations of NBS are so variable, definitive diagnosis is not possible unless the major and minor critreia are satisfied clinically. Assuming these criteria are present, then an examination of the CSF would be most propitious. As discussed above, results of the CSF opening pressure, cell count with differential, and protein and glucose determinations are mandatory in evaluating patients with NBS. Depending upon the differential diagnosis of the CNS disease, the fluid may be cultured for bacteria, fungi, mycobacteria, and viruses. Determination of the CSF-IgM index and myelin basic protein can also be helpful, although their absolute utility has not yet been defined. CNS imaging is important to localize the neuropathology and can include computed tomography, magnetic resonance imaging (MRI), and either standard arterial angiography or DSA. Since NBS is a disease of remissions and exacerbations, and in light of the limitations of many of the above serologic and immunological laboratory parameters, the clinician should be cautious in using these results to arrive at major therapeutic decisions.

Systemic Amyloidosis

Amyloidosis is a well-recognized complication of certain chronic inflammatory disorders, but has only recently been described in BD. Of the various organs that may be affected, renal amyloidosis has received much attention in the current literature; however, amyloid deposition within the spleen, intestine, breast, heart, adrenal glands, thyroid, and walls of blood vessels have been noted in tissue specimens from patients with BD.[51-61] Although amyloidosis has been amply reported in patients with BD, there remains debate as to the characterization of the amyloid deposit. Rosenthal et al.[51] argued in favor of the concept that amyloidosis was an inherent complication of the disease. This was supported, according to their observations, by the absence of other chronic conditions in the three reported autopsied cases. However, later investigators isolated amyloid AA protein, which is the secondary type, from renal biopsy material.[53,56]

The pathogenesis of the AA type of amyloidosis involves the action of an inflammatory stimulus on the macrophage to produce interleukin-1. This substance subsequently acts on hepatocytes to produce serum amyloid A protein (SAA), an acute-phase protein, which is the precursor molecule of secondary amyloid. SAA undergoes proteolytic cleavage to the smaller AA amyloid protein which is eventually deposited as an amyloid fibril.[53,62] This type of amyloid is associated with rheumatoid arthritis, seronegative spondyloathropathy, and familial Mediterranean fever as well as occurring uncommonly in systemic lupus erythematosus and other chronic inflammatory and neoplastic disorders.[63]

Those patients with BD complicated by renal amyloidosis characteristically have marked proteinuria, usually in the nephrotic range, and an occasional patient has required maintenance hemodialysis.[53] Although there is no ideal treatment modality for secondary amyloidosis, the main goal is to reverse the underlying inflammatory process. In addition, administration of colchicine has been associated with clinical improvement of amyloidosis secondary to various underlying disorders including BD and familial Mediterranean fever.[56,64]

Lymphoreticular System: Splenomegaly, Lymphadenopathy, and Thymus Gland

The involvement of the spleen and lymph nodes in BD has only been briefly mentioned in the literature. Two patients were reported in whom splenomegaly was detected clinically, and subsequent examinations of tissue specimens failed to reveal any histologic abnormality.[65] Two earlier cases of splenomegaly in BD were reported, but in one patient there was documented thrombosis of the superior vena cava[66] while the other one had congenital thalessemia.[9] Amyloidosis may also affect the spleen in BD.[51]

Lymphadenopathy has also been uncommon in BD, and in their series of 41 patients with BD, Chajek and Fainaru[9] described three with lymphadenopathy. The lymph node biopsies demonstrated nonspecific reactive changes. Lymphoid hyperplasia with germinal centers has been described in the thymus gland in BD, especially in those who had not received corticosteroids systemically. Also, hyperplasia of spindle-shaped epithelial cells with the disappearance of Hassall's corpuscles has been reported in the thymus glands of both corticosteroid-treated and untreated Behçet's disease patients. Investigators have hypothesized that the presence of thymic lymphoid follicles and spindle-shaped epithelial cells may contribute to certain immunological abnormalities characteristic of BD.[67-69]

References

1. Berlin C. Behçet's syndrome with involvement of the central nervous system. Report of a case, with necropsy, of lesions of the mouth, genitalia and eyes; Review of the literature. *Arch Dermatol Syphilol* 1944; 49:227-233.
2. Pallis CA, Fudge BJ. The neurological complications of Behçet's syndrome. *Arch Neurol Psychiat* 1956; 75:1-14.
3. Evans AD, Pallis CA, Spillane JD. Involvement of the nervous system in Behçet's syndrome. Report of three cases and isolation of virus. *Lancet* 1957; 2:349-353.
4. McMenemey WH, Lawrence BJ. Encephalomyelopathy in Behçet's disease. Report of necropsy findings in two cases. *Lancet* 1957; 2:353-358.
5. Strachan RW, Wigzell FW. Polyarthritis in Behçet's multiple symptom complex. *Ann Rheum Dis* 1963; 22:26-35.
6. Wolf SM, Schotland DL, Phillips LL. Involvement of nervous system in Behçet's syndrome. *Arch Neurol* 1965; 12:315-325.
7. Kalbian VV, Challis MT. Behçet's disease. Report of twelve cases with three manifesting as papilledema. *Am J Med* 1970; 49:823-829.
8. O'Duffy JD, Carney JA, Deodhar S. Behçet's disease. Report of 10 cases, 3 with new manifestations. *Ann Intern Med* 1971; 75:561-570.

9. Chajek T, Fainaru M. Behçet's disease. Report of 41 cases and a review of the literature. *Medicine* 1975; 54:179–196.
10. O'Duffy JD, Goldstein NP. Neurological involvement in seven patients with Behçet's disease. *Am J Med* 1976; 61:170–178.
11. Kozin F, Haughton V, Bernhard GC. Neuro-Behçet disease: Two cases and neuroradiologic findings. *Neurology* 1977; 27:1148–1152.
12. Wright VA, Chamberlain MA. Behçet's syndrome. *Bull Rheum Dis* 1978–79; 29:972–977.
13. Shimizu T, Ehrlich GE, Inaba G, Hayashi K. Behçet disease (Behçet syndrome). *Semin Arthritis Rheum* 1979; 8:223–260.
14. Pamir MN, Kansu T, Erbengi A, Zileli T. Papilledema in Behçet's syndrome. *Arch Neurol* 1981; 38:643–645.
15. O'Duffy JD, Robertson DM, Goldstein NP. Chlorambucil in the treatment of uveitis and meningoencephalitis of Behçet's disease. *Am J Med* 1984; 76:75–84.
16. Harper CM, O'Neill BP, O'Duffy JD, Forbes GS. Intracranial hypertension in Behçet's disease: Demonstration of sinus occlusion with the use of digital subtraction angiography. *Mayo Clin Proc* 1985; 60:419–422.
17. Wechsler B, Bousser MG, Huong Du LT, et al. Central venous sinus thrombosis in Behçet's disease (letter). *Mayo Clin Proc* 1985; 60:891.
18. Shuttleworth EC, Voto S, Sahar D. Palatal myoclonus in Behçet's disease. *Arch Intern Med* 1985; 145:949–950.
19. O'Duffy JD, Lehner T, Barnes CG. Summary of the third international conference on Behçet's disease, Tokyo, Japan, October 23–24, 1981. *J Rheumatol* 1983; 10:154–158.
20. Hughes RAC, Lehner T. Neurological aspects of Behçet's syndrome. In Lehner T, Barnes CG, eds: *Behçet's Syndrome. Clinical and Immunological Features. Proceedings of a Conference Sponsored by the Royal Society of Medicine, February 1979.* London, Academic Press, 1979:241–258.
21. Rubinstein LJ, Urich H. Meningo-encephalitis of Behçet's disease: Case report with pathological findings. *Brain* 1963; 86:151–160.
22. Salvarani C, Iori I, Rossi F, et al. Neurologic involvement as first sign of Behçet's syndrome (letter). *Clin Exp Rheumatol* 1984; 2:353–354.
23. Mamo JG, Baghdassarian A. Behçet's disease. A report of 28 cases. *Arch Ophthalmol* 1964; 71:4–14.
24. Emura A, Takeuchi A, Hashimoto T, et al. A case of Behçet's disease with Weber's syndrome. *J Rheumatol* 1986; 13:459–461.
25. Strouth JC, Dyken M. Encephalopathy of Behçet's disease. Report of a case. *Neurology* 1964; 13:794–805.
26. Schotland DL, Wolf SM, White HH, Dubin HV. Neurologic aspects of Behçet's disease. Case report and review of the literature. *Am J Med* 1963; 34:544–553.
27. Bienenstock H, Margulies ME. Behçet's syndrome. Report of a case with extensive neurologic manifestations. *N Engl J Med* 1961; 264:1342–1345.
28. Brauma I, Fainaru M. Inner ear involvement in Behçet's disease. *Arch Otolaryngol* 1980; 106:215–217.

29. Katoh K, Matsunaga K, Ishigatsubo Y, et al. Pathologically defined neuro-, vasculo-, entero-Behçet's disease. *J Rheumatol* 1985; 12:1186–1190.
30. Mavioğlu H. Behçet's recurrent disease. Analytical review of the literature. *Mo Med* 1958; 55:1209–1222.
31. Alemà G, Bignami A. Involvement of the nervous system in Behçet's disease. In Monacelli M, Nazzaro P, eds: *Behçet's Disease. International Symposium on Behçet's Disease, Rome, 1964.* Basel, S Karger, 1966:52–66.
32. Normal RM, Campbell AMG. The neuropathology of Behçet's disease. In Monacelli M, Nazzaro P, eds: *Behçet's Disease. International Symposium on Behçet's Disease, Rome, 1964.* Basel, S Karger, 1966:67–78.
33. Fukuda Y, Hayashi H, Kuwabara N. Pathological studies on neuro-Behçet's disease. In Inaba G, ed: *Behçet's Disease. Pathogenetic Mechanism and Clinical Future. Proceedings of the International Conference on Behçet's Disease, October 23–24, 1981, Tokyo.* Tokyo, University of Tokyo Press, 1982:127–143.
34. Totsuka S, Hattori T, Yazaki M, Nagao K. Clinicopathology of neuro-Behçet's disease. In Inaba G, ed: *Behçet's Disease. Pathogenetic Mechanism and Clinical Future. Proceedings of the International Conference on Behçet's Disease, October 23–24, 1981, Tokyo.* Tokyo, University of Tokyo Press, 1982:183–196.
35. Hayashi H, Fukuda Y, Kuwabara N. Pathological studies on neuro-Behçet's disease: With special reference to leukocytic reaction. In Inaba G, ed: *Behçet's Disease. Pathogenetic Mechanism and Clinical Future. Proceedings of the International Conference on Behçet's Disease, October 23–24, 1981, Tokyo.* Tokyo, University of Tokyo Press, 1982:197–211.
36. Sugiura S, Ohno S, Ohguchi M, et al. Autonomic nervous system in Behçet's disease. In Inaba G, ed: *Behçet's Disease. Pathogenetic Mechanism and Clinical Future. Proceedings of the International Conference on Behçet's Disease, October 23–24, 1981, Tokyo.* Tokyo, University of Tokyo Press, 1982:81–88.
37. Inaba G. Clinical investigation in neuro-Behçet's syndrome (abstract 60). Royal Society of Medicine international conference on Behçet's disease, September 5 and 6, 1985, London, England.
38. Siva A, Özdogan H, Yacici H, et al. The neurological and psychiatric complications of Behçet's disease and neuro-CT findings (abstract 61). Royal Society of Medicine international conference on Behçet's disease, September 5 and 6, 1985, London, England.
39. Tabuchi S, Ishikawa S. Pupillary study of Behçet's disease (abstract 65). Royal Society of Medicine international conference on Behçet's disease, September 5 and 6, 1985, London, England.
40. Dilşen G. Autonomic nervous system in Behçet's disease (abstract 66). Royal Society of Medicine international conference on Behçet's disease, September 5 and 6, 1985, London, England.
41. Nagata K. Recurrent intracranial hemorrhage in Behçet disease (letter). *J Neurol Neurosurg Psychiatry* 1985; 48:190–191.
42. Lakhanpal S, Tani K, Lie JT, et al. Pathologic features of Behçet's

syndrome: A review of Japanese autopsy registry data. *Hum Pathol* 1985; 16:790–795.

43. Hirohata S, Takeuchi A. Miyamoto T. Association of cerebrospinal fluid IgM index with central nervous system involvement in Behçet's disease. *Arthritis Rheum* 1986: 29:793–796.

44. Ohta M, Nishitani H, Matsubara F, Inaba G. Myelin basic protein in spinal fluid from patients with neuro-Behçet's disease (letter). N Engl J Med 1980; 302:1093.

45. Inaba G, Aoyama J. Anti-glycolipid antibodies in neuro-Behçet's syndrome. In Inaba G, ed: *Behçet's Disease. Pathogenetic Mechanism and Clinical Future. Proceedings of the International Conference on Behçet's Disease, October 23–24, 1981, Tokyo.* Tokyo, University of Tokyo Press, 1982:145–152.

46. Yasuda T, Ueno J, Matuhasi T. Antiglycolipid antibodies in Behçet's disease. In Inaba G, ed: *Behçet's Disease. Pathogenetic Mechanism and Clinical Future. Proceedings of the International Conference on Behçet's Disease, October 23–24, 1981, Tokyo.* Tokyo, University of Tokyo Press, 1982:413–420.

47. Kansu E, Kayserili B, Aktan S, et al. Immunological features of neuro-Behçet's syndrome (abstract 14). Royal Society of Medicine international conference on Behçet's disease, September 5 and 6, 1985, London, England.

48. Ota T, Kashiwamura K, Nakamura Y, et al. Computed tomography in neuro-Behçet's syndrome. In Inaba G, ed: *Behçet's Disease. Pathogenetic Mechanism and Clinical Future. Proceedings of the International Conference on Behçet's Disease, October 23–24, 1981, Tokyo.* Tokyo, University of Tokyo Press, 1982:213–218.

49. Dobkin BH. Computerized tomographic findings in neuro-Behçet's disease. *Arch Neurol* 1980; 37:58–59.

50. Matsumoto K, Matsumoto H, Morofushi K. The clinicoelectroencephalographical correlation to the underlying neuropathology in neuro-Behçet's syndrome. In Inaba G, ed: *Behçet's Disease. Pathogenetic Mechanism and Clinical Future. Proceedings of the International Conference on Behçet's Disease, October 23–24, 1981, Tokyo.* Tokyo, University of Tokyo Press, 1982:219–231.

51. Rosenthal T, Bank H, Aladjem M, et al. Systemic amyloidosis in Behçet's disease. *Ann Intern Med* 1975; 83:220–223.

52. Beroniade V. Amyloidosis and Behçet's disease (letter). *Ann Intern Med* 1975; 83:904–905.

53. Peces R, Riesgo I, Ortega F, et al. Amyloidosis in Behçet's disease. *Nephron* 1984; 36:114–117.

54. Sözen T, Dündar S, Oto MA, et al. Amyloidosis in Behçet's disease (letter). *Nephron* 1985; 39:402.

55. Sözen T, Dündar S, Oto A, et al. Behçet's disease associated with amyloidosis. *Is J Med Sci* 1984; 20:1071–1072.

56. Case records of the Massachusetts General Hospital. Weekly clinicopathological exercises. Case 19-1982. Recent onset of proteinuria in a young woman with a chronic, multisystemic disease. *N Engl J Med* 1982; 306:1162–1167.

57. Williams DG, Lehner T. Renal manifestations of Behçet's syndrome. In Lehner T, Barnes CG, eds: *Behçet's syndrome. Clinical and Immunological Features. Proceedings of a Conference Sponsored by the Royal Society of Medicine, February 1979.* London, Academic Press, 1979:260–264.

58. Nestor G, Beroniade V, Cârnaru S, Badea I. Behçet's disease with renal involvement (with reference to three anatomico-clinical cases). *Rom Med Rev* 1970; 14:27–32.

59. Dilşen N, Koniçe M, Erbengi T, et al. Amyloidosis in two cases of Behçet's disease. In Dilşen N, Koniçe M, Övül C, eds: *Behçet's Disease. Proceedings of an International Symposium on Behçet's Disease, Istanbul, 29–30 September 1977.* Amsterdam-Oxford, Excerpta Medica, 1979:171–177.

60. Dilşen N, Koniçe M, Övül C, et al. Three cases of Behçet's disease with amyloidosis. In Inaba G, ed: *Behçet's Disease. Pathogenetic Mechanism and Clinical Future. Proceedings of the International Conference on Behçet's disease, October 23–24, 1981, Tokyo.* Tokyo, University of Tokyo Press, 1982:449–457.

61. Yurdakul S, Tüzüner N, Yurdakul I, et al. Amyloidosis in Behçet's syndrome (abstract 75). Royal Society of Medicine International conference on Behçet's disease, September 5 and 6, 1985, London, England.

62. Dinarello CA. Interleukin-1. *Rev Infect Dis* 1984; 6:51–95.

63. Wright JR, Calkins E. Clinical-pathologic differentiation of common amyloid syndromes. *Medicine* 1981; 60:429–448.

64. Zemer D, Pras M, Sohar E, et al. Colchicine in the prevention and treatment of the amyloidosis of familial Mediterranean fever. *N Engl J Med* 1986; 314:1001–1005.

65. Kiernan TJ, Gillan J, Murray JP, McCarthy CF. Behçet's disease and splenomegaly. *Br Med J* 1978; 2:1340–1341.

66. Kansu E, Özer FL, Akalin E, et al. Behçet's syndrome with obstruction of the venae cavae. A report of seven cases. *Q J Med* 1972; 41:151–168.

67. Tamaoki N, Habu S, Yoshimatsu H, et al. Thymic change in Behçet's disease. *Keio J Med* 1972; 21:201–213.

68. Morgenstern NL, Shearn MA. Thymic hyperplasia in Behçet's syndrome (letter). *Lancet* 1973; 1:482.

69. Kaneko H, Nakajima H, Okamura A, et al. Histopathology of Behçet's disease. Review of the literature with a case report. *Acta Pathol Jpn* 1976; 26:765–779.

14

TREATMENT AND PROGNOSIS

J. Desmond O'Duffy

THE DECISION TO TREAT BEHÇET'S disease must be based on a secure clinical diagnosis. Typically, the diagnosis depends on the documentation of recurrent oral aphthous ulcerations with at least two of the following: genital ulcerations, uveitis, synovitis, cutaneous vasculitis, meningitis or meningoencephalitis, and large-vessel inflammation, i.e., phlebitis or arteritis. The most appropriate management of Behçet's disease uses a multidisciplinary approach. The team may, at various stages, consist of an ophthalmologist, dermatologist, neurologist, vascular radiologist, rheumatologist, or a surgeon. Errors in diagnosis are minimized by this team approach. It is estimated that among 100 patients referred to a major medical center in this country with a possible diagnosis of Behçet's disease, at most 50 will have this illness. Patients with Crohn's disease of the colon, viral diseases, pustular dermatoses, and "nondisease" comprise most of the remainder.

Based on the principle "primum non nocere," the treatment of Behçet's disease is tailored to the severity of the illness. Mucosal ulceration, cutaneous vasculitis, and synovitis require less drastic treatment than uveitis, meningoencephalitis, and arteritis. The most effective treatment, alkylation therapy, is almost always reserved for those patients with the most serious pathological complications, i.e., uveitis and meningoencephalitis. These two

From *Behcet's Disease: A Contemporary Synopsis*, edited by Gary R. Plotkin, M.D., John J. Calabro, M.D., and J. Desmond O'Duffy, M.B. © 1988 , Futura Publishing Company, Inc., Mount Kisco, NY.

manifestations are confirmed by techniques available for detecting antemortem pathology; the former by slit lamp biomicroscopy and fundoscopy, and the latter by examining the cerebrospinal fluid for pleocytosis. Although treatment does not produce a cure, the disease may also enter a spontaneous remission after many years of recurrent attacks.

Antiinflammatory Drugs

Moderate doses of prednisone (i.e., 10 to 30 mg daily) usually suppress synovitis and cutaneous vasculitis. For the aphthous oral ulcers, topical corticosteroids are disappointing; however, early and frequent application (up to four times daily) of a dental paste of 0.1% triamcinolone acetonide to the emerging oral ulcers is palliative. Oral prednisone can suppress aphthae in the mouth or genitalia, but the dosage required may exceed 30 mg daily and thus may result in hypercortisolism. A few patients with discrete ulcerative episodes can use brief tapering schedules such as 40-30-20-10-5-0 mg daily for their attacks.

Anterior uveitis, documented by cells in the anterior chamber of the eye, is successfully treated with topical corticosteroid drops, especially 1% prednisolone acetate ophthalmic suspension. However, posterior uveitis, with associated retinal vasculitis, is the main cause of blindness and is only ameliorated by large doses of oral prednisone since corticosteroids do not prevent eventual loss of vision.[1] Nonsteroidal antiinflammatory drugs such as aspirin and indomethacin have a minimal effect on the benign lesions, but may be beneficial as the dosage of prednisone is being reduced. If the patients are premenopausal women, the risk of symptomatic osteoporosis from chronic low-dose prednisone is not significant. Nevertheless, since corticosteroids inhibit calcium absorption through the gastrointestinal tract, the physician is advised to prescribe supplemental calcium carbonate.

Colchicine has been used, chiefly by Japanese physicians, because polymorphonuclear chemotactic function is increased in Behçet's disease.[2,3] Modest clinical improvement using a dosage of 0.5 mg twice daily was claimed in these uncontrolled studies,[2,3] and a reduction in the number of attacks of uveitis was reported by other Japanese workers in an uncontrolled trial.[4] In other studies[5,6] colchicine has been moderately efficacious in ameliorating oral aphthosis, erythema nodosum-like lesions and the genital erosions. Most patients in the United States are prescribed colchicine at some time during their illness, but there is no convincing evidence of its efficacy.

The use of levamisole, an antihelminthic that can cause severe granulocytopenia, was based on its effect of normalizing impaired immune responses. In an uncontrolled trial using various dosing regimens, there was some improvement, especially in the mucosal ulcerations, but it has not been shown to prevent blindness or death from meningoencephalitis.[7]

Dapsone, 100 mg daily for 4 to 7 months, was used in seven men with Behçet's disease in an uncontrolled study.[8] It had a beneficial effect, especially on the mucocutaneous lesions. However, its effect on major organ involvement in Behçet's disease awaits controlled studies.

Thalidomide, the ill-fated sedative that caused teratogenesis, has at times a remarkable benefit on the mucosal and cutaneous lesions of Behçet's disease at dosages of 100 to 300 mg daily.[9-11] Pustular vasculitis[12] and also the arthritis of Behçet's disease[11] have improved with thalidomide therapy; however, this drug is not effective in suppressing uveitis.[13] The mechanism of action is unknown, but it has been proposed to inhibit neutrophil chemotaxis[14] or, alternatively, to block the action of activated T lymphocytes.[15] Thalidomide survived the phocomelia epidemic because it can suppress the erythema nodosum leprosum reaction that may occur in leprosy patients treated with sulfones. Besides phocomelia, its main toxicity is an irreversible neuropathy. The drug is not generally available as the limited supplies are rigidly controlled by the World Health Organization which strictly provides it to leprosariums.

Immunosuppressive Therapy

Although prednisone can suppress inflammation in most phases of the disease, especially the acute ones, it is not dependable for long-term suppression of posterior uveitis or meningoencephalitis. Since these serious complications are incompletely maintained in remission, other immunosuppressive therapies have been extensively studied.[16,17] Therapy with azathioprine, 2 to 2.5 mg/kg/day, gave encouraging results in the management of uveitis in a small open trial.[18] Intravenous methotrexate, 2.5 mg/m² every four days for six weeks, temporarily reduced uveitis activity.[19] In the same study, Wong[19] reported that cyclophosphamide, 0.1 g/m² body surface area weekly for six weeks, resulted in a response in five of six patients. Hijikata and Matsuda[4] reported that oral cyclophosphamide, 50 to 100 mg/day, also improved the visual prognosis. However, the results were not superior to those of patients treated with oral colchicine. Penicillamine, 300–600 mg daily, has not demonstrated adequate activity in controlling the chronic arthritis of Behçet's disease.[20]

Mamo and Azzam[16] from Lebanon first reported the results of chlorambucil therapy in Behçet's disease. In a dosage of 0.1 to 0.2 mg/kg/day uveitis was controlled, and after several months corticosteroids were discontinued. Bonnet[21] from France confirmed these results in a study of 18 patients followed for a mean of 4.5 years after the onset of treatment. An impressive feature of Bonnet's series was that eight of her patients were already blind in one eye at the beginning of treatment.

The Mayo Clinic group[22] confirmed the efficacy of chlorambucil, 0.1 mg/kg/day, in 21 patients. Both uveitis and meningoencephalitis activity were abolished during treatments lasting a mean of 20 to 21 months. These results have been reinforced by most other workers.[23,24] Bonnet[21] believed that chlorambucil was more effective for uveitis when given alone than when administered with corticosteroids. Patients with meningoencephalitis are usually begun on both prednisone and chlorambucil therapy. However, if patients being treated with prednisone alone are evaluated during a period of temporary suppression of their central nervous system symptoms, it should be possible, by adding chlorambucil, to taper the dosage of corticosteroid. Most, but not all, chlorambucil-treated patients can be weaned off prednisone.[22]

Nevertheless, Tabbara[25] raised a question regarding the efficacy of chlorambucil therapy. He saw 10 patients who had taken this agent for uveitis before his intervention and was impressed by chlorambucil's toxicity and apparent failure to prevent blindness.

However, specific details of the prior treatment were not provided by the author.[25]

Chlorambucil therapy begun at 0.1 mg/kg/day will, if tolerated, usually suppress uveitis and episodes of meningoencephalitis after three months. When the ophthalmologist reports a quiet fundus with declining cells in the vitreous and improving visual acuity at three to six months, the dose of chlorambucil can be reduced by 25 to 33%. Subsequent reductions usually cease at 2 mg/day which is continued for one to two years. Most patients have inactive disease with few or no aphthous ulcers at 2 to 2½ years, and at that time chlorambucil may be discontinued. Uveitis flare-ups can recur and generally commence after a period of reactivation in aphthosis. Some patients require two or more courses of chlorambucil for proper control of their symptoms.[22]

About 20 to 25% of patients experience toxicity during chlorambucil treatment. Cytopenias, especially leukopenia and thrombocytopenia, with infections require at least temporary stoppage of treatment. The dropout rate from chlorambucil is much higher, perhaps 50%, if each episode of cytopenia is considered the end of treatment. Thus, the mainstay of successful three-year treatment is frequent careful monitoring of blood counts with decisive action consisting of temporary drug withdrawals for leukocyte counts below 3,500 and platelets below 100,000/mm^3. Then, with return of counts to normal, chlorambucil may be restarted at a lesser dosage.

The major long-term hazards of chronic chlorambucil treatment are sterility in both sexes and the occurrence of leukemia. Although the latter dire outcome was frequently seen from chlorambucil treatment of polycythemia vera,[26] it has also been reported in at least three treated patients with Behçet's disease.[27] It appears that acute leukemia is more likely to occur in patients who initially receive 0.2 mg/kg/day.[27]

Twenty-eight of the Mayo Clinic's Behçet's disease patients, begun at 0.1 mg/kg/day of chlorambucil, were treated an average of 2.5 years. Computing an "at-risk" period of 150 years, one malignancy occurred, with the patient developing a uterine adenocarcinoma but surviving its treatment. Although there was no significant increased association of malignancy with chlorambucil therapy as compared to an appropriate control population, further follow-up is necessary. Since both the myelodysplastic syndrome and acute myeloid leukemia from alkylation therapy have grave prognoses,[28] alternative therapeutic modalities must be developed in the therapy of Behçet's disease.[29]

Since lymphocytes are the predominant cells in the chronic uveal and neural lesions of Behçet's disease, and since there are numerical and functional T-cell aberrations, it was logical to use cyclosporine A in the treatment of Behçet's disease. Experimental autoimmune uveitis induced in animals by injections of retinal S antigen was prevented by cyclosporine A. Nussenblatt and colleagues[30] used 10 mg/kg/day, achieving plasma levels of 50 to 200 ng/ml in seven Behçet's disease patients with posterior uveitis. Attacks of uveitis were controlled, but relapses occurred in patients in whom the medication was discontinued.[30] As a result of the initial enthusiasm for cyclosporin A therapy in controlling the acute episodes of ocular inflammation and decreasing the recurrence rate of these attacks, other investigators have reported similar and favorable experience at the 1985 International Conference on Behçet's Disease held in London.[31] The disadvantages of cyclosporine A therapy are its expense and renal toxicity.[30–32] Thus, whether the cost-effectiveness of this treatment will merit its preference over other cytotoxic components awaits further studies. Systemic acyclovir,[32–35] recombinant leukocyte alpha-interferon,[36] plasmapheresis,[37] total lymphoid irradiation,[38] and transfer factor,[39] are other modaldities that have been used in controlling the acute attacks of Behçet's disease; however, the study samples have been limited and the results variable.

Prognosis

Evaluating the prognosis of Behçet's disease is hindered by differences existing among patients reported from various areas of the world. These important geographic peculiarities may be summarized as follows:

1. A greater prevalence among males in countries where the disease is most common; e.g., Japan[40] (1.2–2 to 1) and Turkey[41] (over 2 to 1). Among North American patients the ratio

is reversed; females with the disease outnumber males 2 to 1.[42]

2. The prognosis for visual retention appears much worse in the countries of highest prevalence. Thus, among Japanese patients reported in 1979 by Shimizu and colleagues,[40] blindness resulted in 50 to 80% of uveitis patients. Somewhat similar results were reported from a recent Turkish series,[41] as well as series from Tunisia[43] and Italy.[44] Although in North America, as elsewhere, uveitis is more common among male than among female patients, the prognosis for vision is much better than in the other aforementioned foreign countries. Colvard,[45] reporting from the Mayo Clinic in 1977 on 21 uveitis patients who had been followed for 4.5 years from onset, found that only three patients had become legally blind. Legal blindness is defined as a visual acuity score of 20/200 or worse in both eyes. Since most patients then had not received cytotoxic drugs, it appears that even before the liberal use of chlorambucil, North American patients were faring better than those from "endemic" areas. Since the manifestations of the disease are quite similar regardless of geography, there is no reason to believe that the disease comprises different patient subsets from around the world, nor is there likely to be an "ascertainment bias" toward milder cases in our tertiary care centers. Instead, it is more likely that genetic predisposition to the disease determines both incidence and severity. At present the only biological clue that parallels both incidence and severity is the association with HLA-B5 or Bw51. In certain regions where the disease is both prevalent and severe, HLA-B5 is more common, in both the patients and the population at large. Moreover, there is no increased association of specific HLA-A, B, C, and D-locus antigens in North American patients with Behçet's disease.[46]

Irrespective of the geographic differences in uveitis severity, the prognosis now appears considerably better than that reported by Mamo[16] in 1970. His study included the era of corticosteroid therapy and vision was lost an average of 3.4 years after the onset of eye symptoms. A life-table analysis of prognosis for life compared patients with Behçet's disease from the Mayo Clinic (N = 37) with geographic controls.[42] The prognosis for life was worse in Behçet's disease patients but the difference was of borderline significance. Among six patients who died, four had central nervous system involvement. It is reasonable to postulate that patients with early-diagnosed Behçet's uveitis or meningoencephalitis, if treated promptly and followed meticulously, should expect to retain both vision and neurological function.

References

1. Mamo JG. The rate of visual loss in Behçet's disease. *Arch Ophthalmol* 1970; 84:451–452.
2. Matsumura N, Mizushima Y. Leukocyte movement and colchicine treatment in Behçet's disease (letter). *Lancet* 1975; 2:813.
3. Mizushima Y, Matsumura N, Mori M, et al. Colchicine in Behçet's disease (letter). *Lancet* 1977; 2:1037.
4. Hijikata K, Masuda K. Visual prognosis in Behçet's disease. Effects of cyclophosphamide and colchicine. *Jpn J Ophthalmol* 1978; 22:506–519.
5. Miyachi Y, Taniguchi S, Ozaki M, Horio T. Colchicine in the treatment of the cutaneous manifestations of Behçet's disease. *Br J Dermatol* 1981; 104:67–69.
6. Sander HM, Randle HW. Use of colchicine in Behçet's syndrome. *Curtis* 1986; 37:344–348.
7. de Merieux P, Spitler LE, Paulus HE. Treatment of Behçet's syndrome with levamisole. *Arthritis Rheum* 1981; 24:64–70.
8. Sharquie KE. Suppression of Behçet's disease with dapsone. *Br J Dermatol* 1984; 110:493–494.
9. Mascaro JM, Lecha M, Torras H. Thalidomide in the treatment of recurrent, necrotic, and giant mucocutaneous aphthae and aphthosis (letter). *Arch Dermatol* 1979; 115:636–637.
10. Allen BR. Thalidomide in orogenital ulceration (abstract 96). Royal Society of Medicine international conference on Behçet's disease, September 5 and 6, 1985, London, England.
11. Hamza M. Treatment of Behçet's disease with thalidomide (abstract 97). Royal Society of Medicine international conference on Behçet's disease, September 5 and 6, 1985, London, England.
12. Jorizzo JL, Schmalstieg FC, Solomon AR Jr, et al. Thalidomide effects in Behçet's syndrome and pustular vasculitis. *Arch Intern Med* 1986; 146:878–881.
13. Saylan T, Saltik I. Thalidomide in the treatment of Behçet's syndrome (letter). *Arch Dermatol* 1982; 118:536.
14. Hendler SS, McCarty MF. Thalidomide for autoimmune disease. *Med Hypotheses* 1983; 10:437–443.
15. Moncada B, Baranda ML, González-Amaro R, et al. Thalidomide-

effect on T cells subsets as a possible mechanism of action. *Int J Lepr* 1985; 53:201–205.

16. Mamo JG, Azzam SA. Treatment of Behçet's disease with chlorambucil. *Arch Ophthalmol* 1970; 84:446–450.
17. O'Duffy JD, Goldstein NP. Neurologic involvement in seven patients with Behçet's disease. *Am J Med* 1976; 61:170–178.
18. Rosselet E, Saudan Y, Zenklusen G. Les effets de l'azathioprine ("Imuran") dans la maladie de Behçet. Premiers résultats thérapeutiques. *Ophthalmologica* 1968; 156:218–226.
19. Wong VG. Immunosuppressive therapy of ocular inflammatory diseases. *Arch Ophthalmol* 1969; 81:628–637.
20. Yurdakul S, Özdoğan H, Yazici H. d-Penicillamine in the arthritis of Behçet's syndrome (abstract 82). Royal Society of Medicine international conference on Behçet's disease. September 5 and 6, 1985, London, England.
21. Bonnet M. Immunosuppressive therapy of Behçet's disease: long-term follow-up evaluation. In Inaba G, ed: *Behçet's Disease. Pathogenetic Mechanism and Clinical Future. Proceedings of the International Conference on Behçet's Disease, October 23–24, 1981, Tokyo*. Tokyo, University of Tokyo Press, 1982:487–498.
22. O'Duffy JD, Robertson DM, Goldstein NP. Chlorambucil in the treatment of uveitis and meningoencephalitis of Behçet's disease. *Am J Med* 1984; 76:75–84.
23. Abdalla MI, Bahgat NE. Long-lasting remission of Behçet's disease after chlorambucil therapy. *Br J Ophthalmol* 1973; 57:706–711.
24. Tricoulis D. Treatment of Behçet's disease with chlorambucil. *Br J Ophthalmol* 1976; 60:55–57.
25. Tabbara KF. Chlorambucil in Behçet's disease. A reappraisal. *Ophthalmology* 1983; 90:906–908.
26. Berk PD, Goldberg JD, Silverstein MN, et al. Increased incidence of acute leukemia in polycythemia vera associated with chlorambucil therapy. *N Engl J Med* 1981; 304:441–447.
27. O'Duffy JD, Bowles CA, O'Fallon WM. The immunosuppressive treatment of Behçet's disease with emphasis on chlorambucil. In Lehner T, Barnes CG, eds: *Recent Advances in Behçet's Disease. Proceedings of an International Conference held at the Royal College of Physicians, London, 5–6 September 1985*. Royal Society of Medicine services international congress and symposium series No. 103. London, Royal Society of Medicine Services, 1986:301–306.
28. Michels SD, McKenna RW, Arthur DC, Brunning RD. Therapy-related acute myeloid leukemia and myelodysplastic syndrome: A clinical and morphological study of 65 cases. *Blood* 1985; 65:1364–1372.
29. Palmer RG, Doré CJ, Denman AM. Chlorambucil-induced chromosome damage to human lymphocytes is dose-dependent and cumulative. *Lancet* 1984; 1:246–249.
30. Nussenblatt RB, Palestine AG, Chan C-C, et al. Effectiveness of cyclosporine therapy for Behçet's disease. *Arthritis Rheum* 1985; 28:671–679.

31. Royal Society of Medicine. Abstracts of international conference on Behçet's disease, September 5 and 6, 1985, London, England.
32. Wechsler B, Mertani EB, le Hoang P, et al. Cyclosporine A is effective, but not safe, in the management of Behçet's disease (letter). *Arthritis Rheum* 1986; 29:574.
33. Resegotti L, Pistone M. Acyclovir and Behçet's syndrome (letter). *Ann Intern Med* 1984; 100:319.
34. Prieto J, Suárez J, Civeira P. Acyclovir and Behçet's disease (letter). *Ann Intern Med* 1984; 101:565–566.
35. Dürhrsen U, Kirch W, Brittinger G, Ohnhaus EE. Acyclovir in Behçet's syndrome (BS). Abstract 84. Royal Society of Medicine international conference on Behçet's disease, September 5 and 6, 1985, London, England.
36. Tsambaos, Eichelberg D, Goos M. Behçet's syndrome: Treatment with recombinant leukocyte alpha-interferon. *Arch Dermatol Res* 1986; 278:335–336.
37. Wizemann AJS, Wizemann V. Therapeutic effects of short-term plasma exchange in endogenous uveitis. *Am J Ophthalmol* 1984; 97:565–572.
38. Yurdakul S, Yazici H, Müftüoğlu A, et al. Total lymphoid irradiation for the treatment of intractable Behçet's syndrome (abstract 77). Royal Society of Medicine international conference on Behçet's disease, September 5 and 6, 1985, London, England.
39. Wolfe RE, Fudenberg HH, Welch TM, et al. Treatment of Behçet's syndrome with transfer factor. *JAMA* 1977; 238:869–871.
40. Shimizu T, Ehrlich GE, Inaba G, Hayashi K. Behçet's disease (Behçet's syndrome). *Semin Arthritis Rheum* 1979; 8:223–260.
41. Yazici H, Tüzün Y, Pazarli H, et al. Influence of age of onset and patient's sex on the prevalence and severity of manifestations of Behçet's syndrome. *Ann Rheum Dis* 1984; 43:783–789.
42. O'Duffy JD. Behçet's syndrome, comments (on V. Wright's summary). *Bull Rheum Dis* 1978–79; 29:972–979.
43. Daghfous MT, Ammar M, Kamoun M, Triki F. Aspects cliniques et évolution de la maladie d'Amantiades Behçet en Tunisia. A propos de 41 cas. *J Fr Ophthalmol* 1980; 3:463–468.
44. Pivetti Pezzi P, Gasparri V, De Liso P, Catarinelli G. Prognosis in Behçet's disease. *Ann Ophthalmol* 1985; 17:20–25.
45. Colvard DM, Robertson DM, O'Duffy JD. The ocular manifestations of Behçet's disease. *Arch Ophthalmol* 1977; 95:1813–1817.
46. Moore SB, O'Duffy JD. Lack of association between Behçet's disease and major histocompatibility complex class II antigens in an ethnically diverse North American Caucasoid patient group. *J Rheumatol* 1986; 13:771–773.